Regeneration and Plasticity in the Mammalian Visual System

Proceedings of the Retina Research Foundation Symposia

Volume Four

Regeneration and Plasticity in the Mammalian Visual System

Proceedings of the Retina Research Foundation Symposia

Volume Four

edited by
Dominic Man-Kit Lam and Garth M. Bray

A Bradford Book
The MIT Press
Cambridge, Massachusetts
London, England

Contents

Participants

Albert J. Aguayo
McGill University Centre for
Research in Neuroscience
Montreal General Hospital
Montreal, Canada

Garth M. Bray
McGill University Centre for
Research in Neuroscience
Montreal General Hospital
Montreal, Canada

Manuel P. del Cerro
Department of Neurobiology
University of Rochester Medical
School
Rochester, New York

Douglas O. Frost
Department of Neurology
Kennedy Laboratory
Massachusetts General Hospital East
Charlestown, Massachusetts

Edward G. Jones
Department of Anatomy
University of California College of
Medicine
Irvine, California

Greg E. Lemke
Molecular Neurobiology Laboratory
Salk Institute
La Jolla, California

Raymond D. Lund
Department of Anatomy
University of Cambridge
Cambridge, England

Lamberto Maffei
Instituto di Neurofisiologia del
C.N.R.
Pisa, Italy

Randall N. Pittman
Department of Pharmacology
University of Pennsylvania School
of Medicine
Philadelphia, Pennsylvania

Louis F. Reichardt
Howard Hughes Medical Center
Neuroscience Unit
University of California
San Francisco, California

Eric M. Shooter
Department of Neurobiology
Stanford University School of
Medicine
Stanford, California

Kwok-Fai So
Department of Anatomy
University of Hong Kong
Hong Kong

James E. Turner
Department of Anatomy
Bowman Gray School of Medicine
Winston-Salem, North Carolina

Torsten Wiesel
Neurobiology Laboratories
Rockefeller University
New York, New York

Mark B. Willard
Department of Anatomy and
Neurobiology
Washington University School of
Medicine
St. Louis, Missouri

Preface

Studies of regeneration and plasticity in the mammalian visual system are relevant both as potential approaches to the diverse disorders that lead to visual loss and as models for the reconstitution of other parts of the nervous system. In contrast to certain amphibians and fish, loss of neurons in the visual system of adult mammals or the interruption of their connecting pathways leads to permanent loss of vision. This is primarily because postmitotic neurons, which are lost due to injury or disease, are not replaced, and interrupted central nervous system (CNS) fiber pathways do not regrow the distances necessary to reconnect, for example, the eye and the brain. This book highlights several of the strategies and experimental paradigms that are currently used to exploit and amplify the regenerative capacity of the adult mammalian visual system and reviews some of the exciting advances being made in understanding the molecular basis of CNS regeneration in general.

Several consequences of interrupting the optic nerve in adult rodents and other laboratory mammals contribute to the failure of structural or functional recovery. These include the retrograde degeneration and death of the axotomized ganglion cells in the retina, the failure of the interrupted axons to regrow in the milieu of the injured CNS, and the consequent disconnection between the retinal ganglion cells and their targets in the brain. Beginning in the early 1980s, Albert Aguayo and his colleagues applied anatomical tracing and electrophysiological techniques to show that CNS axons could elongate in peripheral nerve grafts. Furthermore, when guided to specific targets, these axons formed functional synapses, and retrograde loss of neurons could be ameliorated. The results of these experiments, together with the explosion of knowledge in cell and molecular biology over the past decade, have created the intellectual environment for studies of neural regeneration and plasticity such as those presented in this volume.

The chapters in the second section of this book address the problem of postinjury neuronal survival from several perspectives—the expanding number of target-derived trophic molecules, the neurotrophins, which interact with neuronal signaling systems to influence cell survival and differentiation; the exploration of novel trophic substances within the retina; and the effects of time and lesion site on the survival of axotomized retinal ganglion cells. The third section of the book deals with some of the recently defined molecules that are relevant to CNS regeneration in general—the growth-associated protein GAP-43; transcriptional controls of glial cells; the role of proteases in axonal growth; and the various cellular adhesion molecules. In the fourth section, the plasticity of retinal neurons is explored from the perspectives of their responses to axotomy, the capacity of transplanted retinas to integrate into the circuitry of the visual system and to replace lost retinal neurons. The fifth section deals with plasticity of visual cortex and other cortical areas that can be induced to form connections with the visual system.

In the Retina Research Foundation/Helmerich Lecture (chapter 16), Albert Aguayo summarizes the experimental studies of reformed connections between the eye and the superior colliculus, emphasizing the observations in this experimental system that may be relevant to the understanding of connectivity and neuron survival in general.

I Introduction

1 Historical Perspective on Regeneration and Plasticity in the Visual System

Harold J. Sheedlo and James E. Turner

This introductory chapter is an attempt to bring into perspective, from a historical point of view, some of the basic themes of this book in the field of regeneration and plasticity of the visual system. It is by no means an attempt to be all-inclusive, but only to give enough background to be helpful to those who may not be intimately involved in this area of neuroscience.

CENTRAL NERVOUS SYSTEM RESPONSE TO INJURY

Damage to the central nervous system (CNS) induces both physiological and pathological anomalies. Lower vertebrate species, such as some fish and amphibians, have been shown to readily regenerate damaged areas of the CNS, while the CNS of higher vertebrates, particularly in mammals, fails to respond adequately to such insults (Goss, 1969). On the other hand, all vertebrate species demonstrate some form of successful peripheral nervous system (PNS) regeneration. In response to injury to a CNS neuron, which may result from crushing or severing of its axon, disorganization of organelles, in particular the ribosomes, which become dislodged from endoplasmic reticulum, is initially observed. This process is referred to as chromatolysis (for reviews, see Liu, 1981; Barron, 1983). However, within a few days, RNA synthesis increases and ultimately protein production is enhanced within these neurons. In successfully regenerating neurons, these proteins are then conveyed along the axon by axoplasmic transport to be inserted as new membrane material.

As shown by microscopy, injury induced by a lesion, toxic substance, or an immunological insult to the CNS directly results in astrocytic hypertrophy or gliosis. The major role of the reactive astrocyte in response to the injury is thought to promote the restoration of the structural integrity of the damaged nervous system region (Lindsay, 1986; Reier, 1986). However, evidence remains inconclusive as to the biological function of the astrocytic scar. In some studies, axons have been shown to completely avoid the gliotic scar, while other investigations have documented axonal growth through this region and even into the contiguous PNS. Although the formation of an astrocytic scar may only be a secondary response to the injury, it is also possible that these astrocytes may play some role in the subsequent regenerative events, particularly in younger animals. In this regard, astrocytes have been shown to produce trophic agents which promote hippocampal neuron survival and neurite outgrowth in vitro (e.g. Banker, 1980).

In both the CNS and PNS, the proximal segment of severed nerves often survives and even regenerates to some extent. The axonal regenerative capacity in the PNS is much greater than that seen in the CNS. The distal segment of severed nerves undergoes wallerian degeneration, in which both the myelin and axons rapidly degenerate. In the CNS, wallerian degeneration has been demonstrated by enucleation of the eye in rats, with ultimate microscopic analysis of the optic nerve. In these optic nerves, the accumulated debris material was removed by either macrophages or other glial cells with phagocytic capacity (Barron, 1983).

After injury, axon regrowth is limited by the levels of actin and tubulin located at the growth cone. Therefore, these cytoskeletal proteins may play a significant role in axonal regeneration. In addition to astrocytes, several other cell types respond to CNS injury, including microglia, fibroblasts, and oligodendrocytes. All these cells appear to affect polymerization of cytoskeletal proteins (McQuarrie, 1983). However, axonal regeneration is the major event following axotomy, a phenomenon that is dependent on cytoskeletal protein synthesis. The area of CNS injury usually becomes surrounded by astrocytic processes; these processes contain an extensive array of glial fibrillary acidic protein (GFAP), which is an intermediate filament protein (Bignami et al., 1974). However, after resection of the spinal cord, a fibrous gliosis is rarely observed in those areas which exhibit axonal regeneration (McQuarrie, 1983).

Axonal regeneration occurs in three phases. First, axonal sprouting is characterized by growth cone movement, which is dependent on the length of microfilaments. Second, elongation of the axon occurs immediately behind the advancing growth cone. This region consists primarily of microtubules surrounded by axolemma with a few mitochondria. The final phase is axonal elongation, which involves an axonal thickening or radial growth. This phase is dependent on the accumulation of neurofilaments, which are exclusive to neurons and axons (Liu, 1981).

RETINAL REGENERATION IN LOWER VERTEBRATES

During the development of the vertebrate retina, the optic cup is formed by the invagination of a single layer of neuroepithelial cells. This region consists of two closely apposed layers of epithelial cells that will subsequently differentiate into morphologically distinct cell types. The multilayered neural retina develops from the proliferation of the innermost layer. While the outermost layer proliferates, it continues as a monolayer structure, and ultimately results in the formation of the retinal pigment epithelium (RPE) (Stroeva and Mitashova, 1983). Interest in the RPE cells has arisen because these cells can transdifferentiate into a new neural retina, which has been observed in newts and salamanders (Stone, 1957). This regenerative phenomenon has been demonstrated both in vitro (Okata, 1980) and in vivo (Stone, 1957). The factor(s) responsible for this regenerative effect and its mode of action have yet to be discerned. The capacity of RPE cells to transdifferentiate into a neural retina after retinectomy has been reported in fish and embryonic birds, as well as in some mammals. Prior to this phenomenon, the RPE cells undergo depigmentation, which is immediately followed by increased DNA synthesis and elevated mitotic activity. Thus, loss of the original differentiated traits and several mitotic divisions must precede this RPE cell transdifferentiation event. In some species, a stimulus from a donor neural retina is required for transdifferentiation of RPE cells when the whole host retina is removed. However, for this event to occur in vitro, a stimulus from a neural retina is not necessary. In newts, two ocular areas are capable of regenerating into neural retina. These regenerative areas consist of cells at the ora serrata and ciliary body and cells of the pigment epithelium (Stroeva and Mitashova, 1983).

Fish also have the potential to regenerate their retinas. The fish retina, in particular that of the goldfish, has been extensively studied, including pharmacological and microscopic analyses. In these retinas, cell division ceases at hatching and cell differentiation begins. The fish retina at this stage consists of an inner and outer nuclear layer and a ganglion cell layer (Raymond, 1991). To study the regenerative capacity of the fish retina, neurons have been destroyed by a surgical lesion or chemical injections. The degenerated goldfish retina, damaged by the cardiac glycoside ouabain, retains its capacity to regenerate. In these studies, high doses of ouabain cause destruction of photoreceptor cells, which are subsequently phagocytized by RPE cells. Regeneration of the damaged retina originates from the marginal growth zone, at the ora serrata, not the RPE cells. In this peripheral retinal region, the cells remain in a neuroblastic state. With retinal degeneration, cell mitosis increases resulting in a spreading out of cells over the fundus of the eye. In this regeneration process, mitotic division continues radially, resulting in thickening and normal layering, to form a new retina (Maier and Wolburg, 1979).

RPE cells of the chick also have the capacity to form a neural retina. For example, RPE cells of 4-day-old chick embryo differentiate into retinas after removal of the retina and subsequent transplantation of retina from either mice or chicks. Also, RPE cells removed from embryonic chicks have the capacity to transdifferentiate into neural retina and lens in vitro. Results of these studies suggest that RPE cells in embryonic chicks are of two classes, one that can transdifferentiate and another which is stable or fully differentiated (Tsunematsu and Coulombre, 1981). More recent studies have indicated that fibroblast growth factor, administered intraocularly to the chick embryo when the retina had been removed stimulates retinal regeneration from the host RPE cells (Park and Hollenberg, 1989).

In addition to their ability to transdifferentiate, RPE cells perform several essential activities which preserve ocular function, such as microvillar interdigitation with photoreceptor cell outer segments, phagocytosis of shed outer segments, and serving as a barrier between the choroid and neural retina. RPE cell biochemical functions include vitamin A metabolism, transportation of metabolites, and enzyme synthesis (Stroeva and Mitashova, 1983).

OPTIC NERVE REGENERATION

Optic nerve regeneration is a robust and successful event in many lower vertebrate species (Gaze 1959; Goss, 1969; Mattley, 1925; Sperry, 1943a,b, 1945; Stone, 1948, 1953, 1957). In some mammals, axons of ganglion cells have been shown to possess a limited regenerative capacity after damage to the optic nerve. In these studies, crushing the adult rat optic nerve causes axons of ganglion cells to undergo a slow degenerative process away from the site of the damage, toward the cell body, while the distal axonal region undergoes a much more rapid degenerative phase. In contrast, severing the optic nerve causes a more rapid degeneration of the proximal ganglion cells. Interestingly, ganglion cell axons have the capacity to regenerate short fibers for at least 3 months after lesion of the optic nerve (McConnell and Berry, 1982). It has been shown that ganglion cells regenerate their axons more dramatically when axotomy is performed in close proximity to the cell body than when the axons are severed distant from the cell body (Richardson et al., 1982).

The regenerative potential of severed CNS axons has been studied with the utilization of nerves of the PNS serving as a bridge between the two axonal ends (So and Aguayo, 1985; see chapter 16). In these experiments, a sciatic nerve from an adult rat was inserted into a lesioned retina of the same rat in which the optic nerve was severed near the optic disc. It was found that axons of ganglion cells of the surgically manipulated retina regrew to an approximate normal length by extending their axons into the sciatic nerve graft, as was shown by retrograde labeling with horseradish peroxidase. These regrowing axons were observed to survive for considerable time periods after optic nerve severing and peripheral nerve graft placement.

Embryonic rat retina transplanted into adult cerebral cortex survived for several weeks and developed a normal-appearing laminated pattern. Axons from the retinal ganglion cells of these transplants grew over the superior colliculus, and into the stratum opticum and lateral geniculate nucleus. It is of interest that neonatal retinal transplants in neonatal hosts undergo reduced differentiation, with few axonal projections into the host brain (McLoon and Lund, 1980).

REPLACEMENT AND RESCUE WITHIN THE DAMAGED VISUAL SYSTEM

Transplantation studies within damaged mammalian retinas, either artificially or genetically induced, have varied as to the source and intact nature of the donor tissue. For example, partially intact retina or single- or multiple-cell suspensions have been grafted into these retinas. Also, different methods of delivering the donor tissue into these retinas have been employed (del Cerro et al., 1985; Li and Turner, 1988; Silverman and Hughes, 1990).

The first to investigate the survivability of fetal retinas transplanted into the anterior chamber were Royo and Quay (1959). This transplantation work was subsequently extended by del Cerro and co-workers (1985). In addition, whole embryonic or neonatal retina grafted into a retinal lesion, at the interface with the vitreous, survived and even integrated with the adjoining host retina (for review, see Turner et al., 1988). Host animals in these studies were usually adult rats. However, ganglion cells of the transplanted retina did not survive. Furthermore, neonatal rat neural retina, devoid of the overlying RPE cells, survived for up to 3 months when transplanted in retinas of adult rats damaged by high intensity light. It has been shown that the photoreceptor cells are eliminated by exposing rats to extreme lighting conditions for even short periods of time (O'Steen, 1970). However, the extent of integration with the host retina has not yet been reported (Gouras et al., 1990).

Results of the above studies have provided extensive knowledge of retinal development and retinal cell interactions. However, for practical application to mammalian eyes, especially in humans, studies need to be directed toward replacing those specific cell types which are deficient or lost in a large number of diseased retinas. More specifically, research has to be directed toward diminishing the time of onset or replacing lost or degenerating photoreceptor cells, or at least those cells which are important in photoreceptor cell survival and function, in particular, the RPE cell. In this regard, an intact layer of photoreceptor cells transplanted into the subretinal space of adult light-damaged and Royal College of Surgeons (RCS) dystrophic rats has been shown to survive for up to 2 months (Silverman and Hughes, 1990). This procedure, if developed in a consistent manner, relating to time of survival, limiting ocular damage resulting from the transplantation method, and integration with the host retina, will be especially applicable in those retinas which lack photoreceptor cells or wherein photoreceptor cell degeneration is far too extensive for transplantation-induced rescue. A second laboratory has reported survival of photoreceptor cells in a single-cell suspension when transplanted into retinas of adult RCS dystrophic rats (Gouras et al., 1990). To date, however, no studies have been performed documenting long-term survival of these transplanted photoreceptor cells or that they make appropriate synaptic connections. Of course, these studies are necessary and essential before transplantation techniques of this nature can be attempted in humans.

The major focus of cell transplantation studies in diseased retinas over the past 5 years has been concerned with RPE cells. These studies have been primarily performed in retinas of Royal College of Surgeons (RCS) rats in which photoreceptor cell loss begins in the third postnatal week (LaVail, 1981). RPE cells are defective in this inherited disease model, in that these cells do not phagocytize shed photoreceptor cell outer segments (Bok and Hall, 1971). Li and Turner (1988) were the first to show that replacement of defective RPE cells with their normal counterparts in retinas of young RCS dystrophic rats caused rescue of photoreceptor cells. Subsequent studies showed that transplanted RPE cells interacted structurally and possibly in a trophic manner with the surviving photoreceptor cells, as cell rescue was observed lateral to, as well as directly beneath the donor normal RPE cell (Sheedlo et al., 1989). Also, surviving photoreceptor cells were detected for one year after transplantation in these dystrophic retinas (Li and Turner, 1991), a finding which should provide a stimulus for similar experimentation in other retinal disease models and possible application to human patients. In this regard, Peyman and associates (1991) performed the first RPE-cell transplantation in five human patients suffering with age-related macular degeneration (ARMD). a disease in which photoreceptor cell loss is thought to arise as a result of defective RPE cells. Interestingly, vision was reported to be improved in three of these ARMD transplant patients.

Retinal disease models in mice (Sanyal, 1987), cats (Narfstrom, 1983), and dogs (Buyukmihci et al., 1980) have been well characterized microscopically. However, even though some of these retinal models may involve an RPE cell deficiency directly or indirectly leading to photoreceptor cell loss, transplantation of photoreceptor or RPE cells has not yet been performed in these diseased retinas.

PLASTICITY WITHIN THE VISUAL SYSTEM

Neuroplasticity, broadly defined, involves the ability of the nervous system to adapt its structural organization to altered circumstances arising from either developmental, environmental, or traumatic phenomena. Plasticity changes within the nervous system are exhibited in the form of (1) collateral axon sprouting; (2) regeneration; (3) continued axon growth or turnover, or both; and (4) synaptic displacement. The visual system has been an area that has contributed much to the understanding of neuroplasticity. Some of the classic studies in this area have shown that during brain development a number of environmental factors have been found to influence the visual centers. Specifically, data obtained from work in which one eye was removed or sutured during development suggest that binocular competition between the afferent inputs to the lateral geniculate body and visual cortex profoundly affect the morphological and physiological development of the neurons in these visual centers (Friedlander et al., 1982; Guillery and Stelzner, 1970; Kalil, 1980; Shatz and Stryker, 1978; Wiesel and Hubel, 1963a,b, 1965). In addition, visual or light deprivation also affects the morphology and physiological properties of these cells (Borges and Berry, 1976, 1978; Gabbott and Stewart, 1987; Hickey et al., 1977; Leventhal and Hirsch, 1977; Valverde, 1967).

The degree of neuronal activity has also been found to influence the level of development and maturation within the visual system. Specifically, the use of tetrodotoxin, a compound used to abolish sodium-mediated action potentials, was found in experimental animals to prevent (1) the formation of eye-specific layers in the lateral geniculate body (Shatz and Stryker, 1988); (2) the formation of ocular dominance columns in the visual cortex (Stryker and Harris, 1986); (3) the formation of restricted axon arbors of retinal ganglion cells in the lateral geniculate nucleus (Sretavan et al., 1988); and (4) the formation of mature retinogeniculate synaptic structures in the lateral geniculate nucleus (Kalil et al., 1986).

In addition, the *N*-methyl-D-aspartate (NMDA) receptors on neurons of the visual system have been found to influence its plasticity during development. For example, by applying an NMDA antagonist to the tecta of three-eye tadpoles, desegregation of the retinal ganglion cell terminals was found which was reversible after the removal of the antagonist (Cline et al., 1987). Also, an NMDA antagonist prevented the matching of the ipsilateral map to the contralateral map in the tecta of *Xenopus* during development (Scherer and Udin, 1989). Furthermore, in adult *Xenopus*, plasticity for the matching of the binocular maps can even be restored after the rotation of the contralateral eye by the application of NMDA to the tecta (Udin and Scherer, 1990).

The age of the animal may determine to what degree the visual system retains its plasticity. For example, if the afferents from one eye to the superior colliculus are restricted early in development, the remaining optic afferents undergo considerable reorganization, which does not occur in older animals (Goodman et al., 1973). However, despite the absence of extensive plasticity in the termination of retinal afferents, there is an indication of considerable mobility of synaptic connections after optic deafferentation in the adult (Lund and Lund, 1971a,b). These results show that a bare postsynaptic site can be reoccupied by a wide variety of other profiles in the area, including other axon terminals. It is possible that the main function of the plasticity shown in the colliculus is to silence hyperactive postsynaptic sites (Lund, 1978).

Perhaps one of the most remarkable examples of visual system plasticity is the response of the lower vertebrate optic nerve to trauma. More specifically, the plasticity response in this situation was in the form of vigorous optic nerve regeneration. This response was first reported by Mattley (1925), who observed that if an optic nerve in adult newts is cut, it regenerates and vision is restored. Sperry (1944) noted that the axons appear to grow across the severed optic nerve in a disorganized manner and yet the final connections to the visual centers are sufficient for the animal to regain its normal visuomotor orienting responses. Subsequent neurophysiological studies (Gaze, 1959) showed that this order was reestablished by the optic axons themselves, since the regenerating optic terminals distribute over the tectum, presenting a normal visuotopic map. However, in subsequent experiments dealing with the experimental modification of central-peripheral relations, such as rotating the retina (Sperry, 1943a,b; 1944, 1945; Stone, 1948, 1953), the animal's behavior was misdirected and not corrected by training. Under these postregeneration conditions the specification of the neurons from the retinal ganglion cells was essentially irreversible and thus demonstrates a lack of plasticity.

The above examples serve to demonstrate the extent to which the developing and maturing visual system possesses the vigor of plasticity through altered circumstances arising from either developmental, environmental, or traumatic phenomena. It appears probable that function before and after birth is important in maintaining visual pathways during early development and continuing neuronal specification. Function (behavior) might even play a role in selecting pathways. Behavior and learning appear to play important roles in the emergence of order within the visual system, which continues to develop postnatally. What we have learned about the plasticity of the visual system now allows for the formation of a working hypothesis which states that the final order attained in the brain, as reflected in normal adult behavior, results from interaction between the inherited nervous system and the external environment. Continuing plasticity studies in the visual system will undoubtedly reveal many more themes central to brain function and behavior. The extent to which the "plastic quality" of the human visual system can be manipulated to correct defects caused by trauma or disease is an intriguing and challenging question which is yet to be fully answered.

CURRENT AND FUTURE PERSPECTIVES AND APPROACHES

The chapters that follow are organized in a way to give the reader a feeling for the cutting edge of science as it relates to regeneration and plasticity in the visual system. Each of the four sections: Cells and Molecules That Influence Neuronal Survival; Molecular Mechanisms of Axonal Regeneration; Retinal Responses to Injury and Transplantation; and Plasticity of Connectivity in the Visual System are current approaches that are essential to our understanding of regeneration and plasticity. In turn, they provide insight into future perspectives for carrying this field into new and exciting arenas of science.

REFERENCES

Banker, G.A. (1980). Trophic interactions between astroglial cells and hippocampal neurons in culture. *Science* 209:809–810.

Barde, Y.-A. (1989). Trophic factors and neuronal survival. *Neuron* 2:1525–1534.

Barron, K.D. (1983). Axon reaction and central nervous system regeneration. In *Nerve, Organ, and Tissue Regeneration: Research Perspective*, ed. F.J. Seil, 3–50. New York: Academic Press.

Bignami, A., Forno, L., and Dahl, D. (1974). The neuroglial response to injury following spinal cord transection in the goldfish. *Exp. Neurol.* 44:60–70.

Bok, D., and Hall, M. (1971). The role of the pigment epithelium in the etiology of inherited retinal dystrophy in the rat. *J. Cell Biol.* 49:664–682.

Borges, S., and Berry, M. (1976). Preferential orientation of stellate cell dendrites in the visual cortex of the dark-reared rat. Brain Res. 112:141–147.

Borges, S. and Berry, M. (1978). The effects of dark rearing on the development of the visual cortex of the rat. *J. Comp. Neurol.* 180:277–300.

Buyukmihci, N., Aguirre, G., and Marshall, J. (1980). Retinal degenerations in the dog. II. Development of the retina in rod-cone dysplasia. *Exp. Eye Res.* 30:575–586.

Carmignoto, G., Maffei, L., Candeo, C., Canella, R., and Comelli, C. (1989). Effect of NGF on the survival of retinal ganglion cells following optic nerve section. *J. Neurosci.* 9:1263–1273.

Cline, H.T., Debski, E.A., and Constantine-Paton, M. (1987). N-Methyl-D-aspartate receptor antagonist desegregates eye-specific stripes. *Proc. Natl. Acad. Sci. U.S.A.* 84:4342–4345.

del Cerro, M., Gash, D.M., Rao, G.N., Notter, M.F., Wiegand, S.J., and del Cerro, C. (1985). Intraocular retinal transplants. *Invest. Ophthalmol. Vis. Sci.* 26:1182–1185.

Friedlander, M.J., Stanford, L.R., and Sherman, S.M. (1982). Effects of monocular deprivation on the structure-function relationship of individual neurons in the cat's lateral geniculate nucleus. *J. Neurosci.* 2:321–331.

Gabbott, P.L.A., and Stewart, M.G. (1987). Quantitative morphological effects of dark-rearing and light exposure on the synaptic connectivity of layer 4 in the rat visual cortex (area 17). *Exp. Brain Res.* 68:103–114.

Gaze, R.M. (1959). Regeneration of the optic nerve in *Xenopus laevis. Q. J. Exp. Physiol.* 44:290–308.

Goodman, D.C., Bogdasarian, R.S., and Horel, J.A. (1973). Axonal sprouting of ipsilateral optic tract following opposite eye removal. *Brain Behav. Evol.* 8:27–50.

Goss, R.J. (1969). *Principles of Regeneration.* New York: Academic Press.

Gouras, P., Lopez, R., Du, J., Gelanze, M., Kwun, R., Brittis, M., and Kjeldbye, H. (1990). Transplantation of retinal cells. *Neuro Ophthalmol.* 10:165–176.

Guillery, R.W., and Stelzner, D.J. (1970). The differential effects of unilateral lid closure upon the monocular and binocular segments of the dorsal lateral geniculate nucleus in the cat. *J. Comp. Neurol.* 139:413–422.

Hallbook, F., Ibanez, C.F., and Persson, H. (1991). Evolutionary studies of the nerve growth factor family reveal a novel member abundantly expressed in *Xenopus* ovary. *Neuron* 6:845–858.

Hickey, T.L., Spear, P.D., and Kratz, K.E. (1977). Quantitative studies of cell size in the cat's dorsal lateral geniculate nucleus following visual deprivation. *J. Comp. Neurol.* 172:265–282.

Johnson, J.E., Barde, Y.-A., Schwab, M., and Thoenen, H. (1986). Brain derived neurotrophic factor supports the survival of cultured rat retinal ganglion cells. *J. Neurosci.* 6:3031–3038.

Kalil, R. (1980). A quantitative study of the effects of monocular enucleation and deprivation on cell growth in the dorsal lateral geniculate nucleus of the cat. *J. Comp. Neurol.* 189:483–524.

Kalil, R., Dubin, M.W., Scott, G., and Stark, L.A. (1986). Elimination of action potentials blocks the structural development of retinogeniculate synapses. *Nature* 323:156–158.

LaVail, M.M. (1981). Analysis of neurological mutants with inherited retinal degeneration. *Invest. Ophthalmol. Vis. Sci.* 21:638–657.

Leventhal, A.G., and Hirsch, H.V.B. (1977). Effects of early experience upon orientation sensitivity and binocularity of neurons in visual cortex of cats. *Proc. Natl. Acad. Sci. U.S.A.* 74:1272–1276.

Levi-Montalcini, R., and Booker, B. (1960). Destruction of the sympathetic ganglia in mammals by an anti-serum to a nerve-growth protein. *Proc. Natl. Acad. Sci. U.S.A.* 46:384–391.

Li, L., and Turner, J.E. (1988). Inherited retinal dystrophy in the RCS rat: Prevention of photoreceptor degeneration by pigment epithelial cell transplantation. *Exp. Eye Res.* 47:771–785.

Li, L., and Turner, J.E. (1991). Optimal conditions for long-term photoreceptor cell rescue in RCS rats: The necessity for healthy RPE transplants. *Exp. Eye Res.* 52:669–679.

Lindsay, R.M. (1986). Reactive gliosis. In *Astrocytes. Cell Biology and Pathology of Astrocytes,* ed. S. Fedoroff, and A. Vernadakis, 231–262. New York: Academic Press.

Liu, H.M. (1981). *Biology and Pathology of Nerve Growth.* New York: Academic Press.

Lund, R.D. (1978). *Development and Plasticity of the Brain. An Introduction.* New York: Oxford University Press.

Lund, R.D., and Lund, J.S. (1971a). Synaptic adjustment after deafferentiation of the superior colliculus of the rat. *Science* 171:804–807.

Lund, R.D., and Lund, J.S. (1971b). Modification of synaptic patterns in the superior colliculus of the rat during development and following deafferentiation. *Vision Res.* 11:281–298.

Maier, W., and Wolburg, H. (1979). Regeneration of the goldfish retina after exposure to different doses of ouabain. *Cell Tissue Res.* 202:99–118.

Mattley, R. (1925). Récupération de la vue après résection de nerfs optique chez le triton. *C.R. Soc. Biol. (Paris)* 93:904–906.

McConnell, P., and Berry, M. (1982). Regeneration of ganglion cell axons in the adult mouse retina. *Brain Res.* 241:362–365.

McLoon, S.L., and Lund, R.D. (1980). Specific projections of retinas transplanted to rat brain. *Exp. Brain Res.* 40:273–282.

McQuarrie, I.G. (1983). Role of the axonal cytoskeletal in the regenerating nervous system. In *Nerve, Organ, and Tissue Regeneration: Research Perspectives*, ed. F.J. Seil, 51–88. New York: Academic Press.

Narfstrom, K. (1983). Hereditary progressive retinal atrophy in the Abyssinian cat. *J. Hered.* 74:273–276.

Okata, T.S. (1980). Cellular metaplasia or transdifferentiation as a model for retinal cell differentiation. *Curr. Top. Dev. Biol.* 16:349–380.

O'Steen, W.K. (1970). Retinal and optic nerve serotonin and retinal degeneration as influenced by photoperiod. *Exp. Neurol.* 27:194–205.

Park, C.M., and Hollenberg, M.J. (1989). Basic fibroblast growth factor induces retinal regeneration *in vivo*. *Dev. Biol.* 134:201–205.

Peyman, G.A., Blinder, K.J., Paris, C.L., Alturki, W., and Nelson, N.C. (1991). A technique for retinal pigment epithelium transplantation for age-related macular degeneration secondary to extensive subfoveal scarring. *Ophthalmic Surg.* 22:102–108.

Raymond, P.A. (1991). Cell determination and positional cues in the teleost retina: Development of photoreceptors and horizontal cells. In *Development of the Visual System*, ed. D.-M.K. Lam, and C.J. Shatz, 59–78. Cambridge, Mass.: MIT Press.

Reichardt, L.F., Bossy, B., Cabonetto, S., deCurtis, I., Emmett, C., Hall, D.E., Ignatius, M.J., Large, T., Lefcort, F., Napolitano, E., Neugebauer, F.M., and Tomaselli, K.J. (1990). Neuronal receptors that regulate axon growth. *Cold Spring Harb. Symp. Quant. Biol.* 55:342–350.

Reier, P.J. (1986). Gliosis following CNS injury: The anatomy of astrocytic scars and their influences on axonal elongation . In *Astrocytes . Cell Biology and Pathology of Astrocytes*, ed. S. Federoff, and A. Vernadakis, 263–324. New York: Academic Press.

Richardson, P.M., Issa, V.M.K., and Shemie, S. (1982). Regeneration and retrograde degeneration of axons in the rat optic nerve. *J. Neurocytol.* 11:949–966.

Royo, P.E., and Quay, W.B. (1959). Retinal transplantation from fetal to maternal mammalian eye. *Growth* 23:313–336.

Sanyal, S. (1987). Cellular site of expression and genetic interaction of the rd and the rds loci in the retina of the mouse. In *Degenerative Retinal Disorders: Clinical and Laboratory Investigations*, ed. J.G. Hollyfield et al., 175–194. New York: Alan R. Liss.

Scherer, W.J., and Udin, S.B. (1989). N-Methyl-D-aspartate antagonists prevent interaction of binocular maps in *Xenopus* tectum. *J. Neurosci.* 9:3837–3843.

Shatz, C.J., and Stryker, M.P. (1978). Ocular dominance in layer IV of the cat's visual cortex and the effects of monocular deprivation. *J. Physiol.* 281:267–283.

Shatz, C.J., and Stryker, M.P. (1988). Prenatal tetrodotoxin infusion blocks segregation of retinogeniculate afferents. *Science* 242:87−89.

Sheedlo, H.J., Li, L., and Turner, J.E. (1989). Functional and structural characteristics of photoreceptor cells rescued in RPE-cell grafted retinas of RCS dystrophic rats. *Exp. Eye Res.* 48:841−854.

Silverman, M.S., and Hughes, S.E. (1990). Transplantation of retinal photoreceptors to light-damaged retina. *Invest. Ophthalmol. Vis. Sci.* 30:1684−1690.

Snider, W.D., and Johnson, E.M. (1989). Neurotrophic molecules. *Ann. Neurol.* 26:489−506.

So, K.F., and Aguayo, A.J. (1985). Lengthy regrowth of cut axons from ganglion cells after peripheral nerve transplantation into the retina of adults rats. *Brain Res.* 328:349−354.

Sperry, R.W. (1943a). Effect of 180-degree rotation of the retinal field on visuomotor coordination. *J. Exp. Zool.* 92:263−279.

Sperry, R.W. (1943b). Visuomotor coordination in the newt (*Triturus viridescens*) after regeneration of the optic nerve. *J. Comp. Neurol.* 79:33−55.

Sperry, R.W. (1944). Optic nerve regeneration with return of vision in anurans. *J. Neurophysiol.* 7:57−69.

Sperry, R.W. (1945). Restoration of vision after crossing of optic nerves and after contralateral transplantation of eye. *J. Neurophysiol.* 8:15−28.

Sretavan, D.W., Shatz, C.J., and Stryker, M.P. (1988). Modification of retinal ganglion cell axon morphology by prenatal infusion of tetrodotoxin. *Nature* 336:468−471.

Stone, L.S. (1948). Functional polarization in developing and regenerating retinae of transplanted eyes. *Ann. N.Y. Acad. Sci.* 49:856−865.

Stone, L.S. (1953). Normal and reversed vision in transplanted eyes. *Arch. Ophthalmol.* 49:28−53.

Stone, L.S. (1957). Further experiments on lens regeneration from retina pigment cells in adult newt eyes. *J. Exp. Zool.* 134:69−84.

Stroeva, O.G., and Mitashova, V.J. (1983). Retinal pigment epithelium: Proliferation and differentiation during development and regeneration. *Int. Rev. Cytol.* 83:221−293.

Stryker, M.P., and Harris, W.A. (1986). Binocular impulse blockage prevents the formation of ocular dominance columns in cat visual cortex. *J. Neurosci.* 6:2117−2133.

Tsunematsu, Y., and Coulombre, A.J. (1981). Demonstration of transdifferentiation of neural retina from pigmented retina in culture. *Dev. Growth Differ.* 23:297−311.

Turner, J.E., Blair, J.R., Seiler, M., Aramant, R., Laedtke, T.W., Chappell, E.T., and Clarkson, L. (1988). Retinal transplants and optic nerve bridges: Possible strategies for visual recovery as a result of trauma of disease. *Int. Rev. Neurobiol.* 29:281−307.

Udin, S.B., and Scherer, W.J. (1990). Restoration of the plasticity of binocular maps by NMDA after the critical period in *Xenopus*. *Science* 249:669−672.

Valverde, F. (1967). Apical dendritic spines of the visual cortex and light deprivation in the mouse. *Exp. Brain Res.* 3:337−352.

Wiesel, T.N., and Hubel, D.H. (1963a). Effects of visual deprivation on morphology and physiology of cells in the cat's lateral geniculate body. *J. Neurophysiol.* 26:978−993.

Wiesel, T.N., and Hubel, D.H. (1963b). Single-cell responses in striate cortex of kittens deprived of vision in one eye. *J. Neurophysiol.* 26:1003−1017.

Wiesel, T.N., and Hubel, D.H. (1965). Comparison of the effects of unilateral and bilateral eye closure on cortical unit responses in kittens. *J. Neurophysiol.* 28:1029−1040.

II Cells and Molecules that Influence Neuronal Survival

2   The Nerve Growth Factor Receptors

Susan O. Meakin and Eric M. Shooter

The last few years have produced several important developments in the nerve growth factor (NGF) field. Among these, the characterization of several new members of the family of NGF proteins, and of a second family of receptors for these proteins, is especially interesting. The partial amino acid sequencing of purified brain-derived neurotrophic factor (BDNF) activity and the subsequent molecular cloning of its complementary DNA (cDNA) revealed the significant homology between NGF and BDNF, particularly in the location of the six common cysteine residues (Leibrock et al., 1989). With these two homologous sequences in hand the search for further members of the NGF family using the polymerase chain reaction (PCR) method quickly identified the third member, neurotrophin-3 (NT-3) (Hohn et al., 1990; Maisonpierre et al., 1990). A fourth member, neurotrophin-4 (NT-4), has just been identified in *Xenopus* ovary (Hallböök et al., 1991). In spite of the homology between NGF, BDNF, and NT-3, significant differences in their biological activities are apparent (Barde, 1989). For example, NGF but not BDNF supports survival and neurite outgrowth from embryonic sympathetic neurons while the converse is true for embryonic sensory nodose neurons. In the central nervous system (CNS), BDNF promotes retinal ganglion and dopaminergic neuronal survival while NGF does not (Hyman et al., 1991). Both, however, support the survival of basal forebrain cholinergic neurons (Alderson et al., 1990). The differences of expression of NGF, BDNF, and NT-3 during development as well as their different (but sometimes overlapping) distribution in brain also emphasize their potentially different functions (Ernfors et al., 1990a; Wetmore et al., 1991; Hofer et al., 1990; Phillips et al., 1990; Maisonpierre et al., 1990). The neurotrophic factors are among the most conserved proteins known; the amino acid sequences of BDNF and NT-3 from several different mammalian species, for example, are identical (Maisonpierre et al., 1991; Hallböök et al., 1991). One of the important questions that arises is how these several homologous proteins generate their specific biological actions, and the first clues to this question come from an examination of the neurotrophin receptors.

THE BINDING AND KINETIC PROPERTIES OF THE NGF RECEPTORS

Two different classes of NGF receptors are recognized on primary sensory (Sutter et al., 1979) and sympathetic (Godfrey and Shooter, 1986) neurons by steady-state binding, a major population with a dissociation constant (K_d) of 10^{-9}M and a minor population with a K_d of 10^{-11}M. These receptors have been referred to as the low (LNGFR) and high (HNGFR) affinity receptors, respectively. Both classes of receptors are observed in binding experiments at 0 or 37°C. Since the dose response curve for NGF-induced neurite outgrowth on sensory neurons has a half-maximal response below 10^{-12}M, it appears that relative low occupancy of the HNGFR is responsible for this biological activity of NGF (Sutter et al., 1979). The major difference between the two receptors is in their rate of NGF dissociation, being relatively slow from the HNGFR ($t_{1/2} = 10$ minutes) and fast from the LNGFR ($t_{1/2}$ approximately 3 seconds). Indeed, an easy way to distinguish the two receptors experimentally is to wash the cells with ice-cold NGF for 5 minutes after binding ^{125}I at 0 or 37°C; the ^{125}I-NGF is completely released from the LNGFR but retained in the HNGFR (Vale and Shooter, 1984). The K_d's measured by the ratio of the rates of dissociation and association agree well with those determined by steady-state binding. Scatchard analyses of NGF binding to PC12 cells at 37°C shows a curvilinear plot (Bernd and Greene, 1984; Woodruff and Neet, 1986) indicating that the K_d's of the two classes of NGF receptors on these cells are close together. Nevertheless, dissociation experiments on PC12 cells define the same two classes, slow dissociating (HNGFR) and fast dissociating (LNGFR), seen on primary neurons (Landreth and Shooter, 1980; Schechter and Bothwell, 1981). The presence of a slowly dissociating NGF component on PC12 cells at 0°C indicates that internalization of NGF in these cells does not account for the appearance of HNGFR. The biological response of PC12 cells to NGF is also mediated at very low NGF concentrations where low occupancy of the HNGFR is achieved. The two receptor classes also differ importantly in susceptibility in trypsin (HNGFRs are stable, LNGFRs are labile) (Landreth and Shooter, 1980; Hosang and Shooter, 1985).

MOLECULAR PROPERTIES OF THE NGF RECEPTORS

Following the initial demonstration by cross-linking that the NGF receptors on sympathetic neurons are of two different sizes (140 and 80 kD respectively), Hosang and Shooter (1985) showed that the lower-molecular-weight species on PC12 cells display some of the properties of the LNGFR (fast dissociation and trypsin instability) while the higher-molecular-weight species display some of the properties of the HNGFR (slow dissociation and trypsin stability) (figure 2.1). The latter also efficiently internalize ^{125}I-NGF while the former do not (Bernd and Greene, 1984; Hosang and Shooter, 1987). The molecular cloning and expression of the 80-kD-species confirmed that it is the

    Cells and Molecules that Influence Neuronal Survival

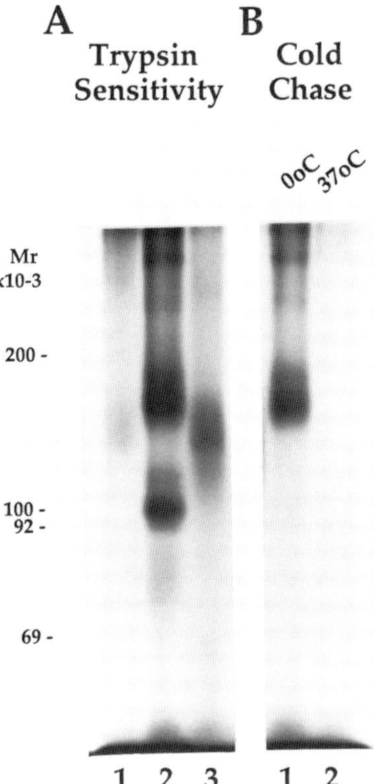

Figure 2.1 The two NGF receptors are of different size and have different sensitivities to trypsin and to cold chase with NGF. *A*, Effects of trypsin (0.5 mg/ml, 30 min, 37°C) digestion on the stability of the NGFR complexes. PC12 cells were labeled with 1nM^{125}I-NGF either before or after trypsin digestion, as described, and chemically cross-linked with DSS. *Lane 1*: trypsin digestion prior to NGF binding and cross-linking. *Lane 2*: normal NGF binding and cross-linking. No trypsin treatment. *Lane 3*: trypsin digestion after NGF binding and cross-linking. *B*, Cold chase properties of the NGF-receptor complexes. PC12 cells were labeled with ^{125}I-NGF and then treated with 1μM unlabeled NGF for 30 minutes prior to cross-linking. *Lane 1*: cold chase performed at 0°C. *Lane 2*: cold chase performed at 37°C. (Reproduced with permission from Meakin and Shooter, 1991a.)

LNGFR. The cloning of the LNGFR was achieved for both the rat and human species by gene transfer and subsequent rescue of the receptor cDNA by differential library screening (Radeke et al., 1987; Johnson et al., 1986). In the isolation of the rat LNGFR, amplification of the expression of the LNGFR gene in the recipient L cells produced a stable cell line expressing approximately 2×10^{6} LNGFR per cell. The isolation of these cells, in turn, by fluorescent-activated cell sorting was made possible by the use of the monoclonal antibody MC-192, which interacts with, and increases binding of NGF to, the LNGFR (Chandler et al., 1984). The LNGFR is a single peptide chain of approximately 400 amino acid residues with a single membrane-spanning domain separating a slightly longer extracellular domain from a shorter cytoplasmic domain. This receptor, when expressed in L cells, has a K_d of 10^{-4}M,

NGF dissociates from it rapidly, and it is trypsin-labile, all properties of the LNGFR (Radeke et al., 1987). A comparison of the amino acid sequences of rat, human, and chick LNGFR shows significant conservation in the extracellular domain around the four cysteine-rich repeats which make up the NGF binding domain, in the membrane-spanning domain, and at the C-terminus in the cytoplasmic domain (Large et al., 1989). The cytoplasmic domain also contains a consensus sequence that binds G proteins (Feinstein and Larhammer, 1990), raising the possibility that the LNGFRs may generate their own signal transduction mechanism.

The LNGFRs bind not only NGF but also BDNF (Rodriguez-Tebar et al., 1990) and NT-3 (Rodriguez-Tebar et al., 1991; Squinto et al., 1991; Ernfors et al., 1990b) with the same K_d of 10^{-9}M. This receptor may therefore be more accurately referred to as gp80^{NTR} indicating its property of binding all the neurotrophins. BDNF and NT-3 do display small, but significant differences in kinetic properties for gp80^{NTR} suggesting that their three-dimensional structures differ in detail from that of NGF. In contrast, BDNF and NT-3 can only displace NGF from the HNGFR at concentrations well above its K_d showing that HNGFR is specific for binding NGF (Rodriguez-Tebar et al., 1990).

The ratio of the high- and low-molecular-weight receptor species which appear after cross-linking with the lipophilic agent HSAB (hydroxy succinimydyl-4-azidobenzoate) does not change over a wide range of cross-linker concentrations (Hosang and Shooter, 1985). Although this was thought to be due to sequestering of HSAB in the membrane and the maintenance of a rather constant concentration in the membrane, the same effect is observed with hydrophilic cross-linkers such as DTSSP (3,3'-dithio-*bis*-sulfosuccinimidyl-proprionate) (Radeke and Feinstein, 1991). This result suggests that there is only a single peptide chain receptor in the high-molecular-weight cross-linked complex and recent work has shown this to be true. Cross-linked or uncross-linked LNGFRs, but not HNGFRs, are immunoprecipitated with the MC-192 monoclonal antibody. Both NGF-occupied receptors are immunoprecipitated with anti-NGF antibody (Meakin and Shooter, 1991a). The cross-linked high-molecular-weight complex is also specifically recognized and immunoprecipitated by antibodies against phosphotyrosine, indicating that it contains one or more of these residues (Meakin and Shooter, 1991a) (figure 2.2). This finding immediately suggested that the high-molecular-weight complex might possess tyrosine kinase activity; this was tested using the ability of anti-NGF antibody to immunoprecipitate both NGF-occupied, but not cross-linked molecular-weight receptor complexes. This immunoprecipitate was effective in phosphorylating enolase and in particular the artificial substrate, poly(glu$_4$tyr$_1$) but not poly(glu$_1$tyr$_1$) (figure 2.3). Since the first, but not the second, artificial substrate is an excellent substrate for tyrosine kinases, it is clear that one or both NGF-occupied molecular-weight receptor complexes possess tyrosine kinase activity (Meakin and Shooter, 1991b). Given that the LNGFR does not possess the appropriate sequences or a tyrosine kinase, a fact that was proved by the failure of the immunoprecipit-

     Cells and Molecules that Influence Neuronal Survival

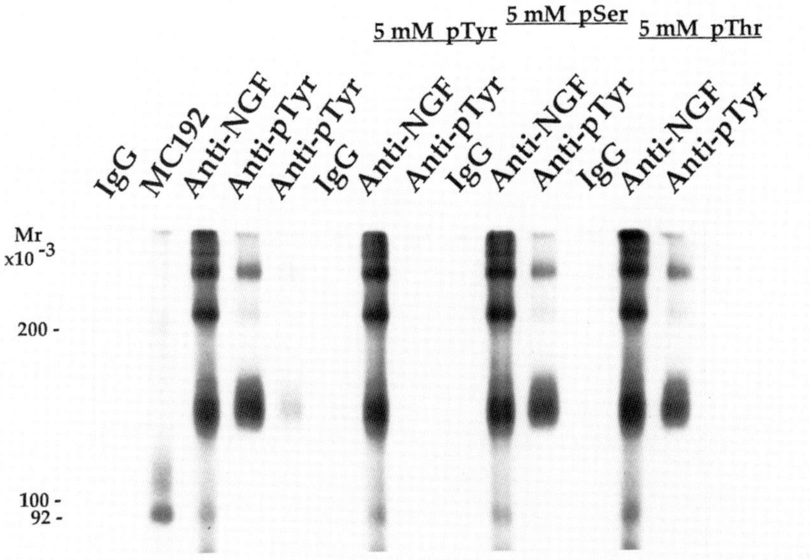

Figure 2.2 The high-molecular-weight NGF-NGFR complex contains phosphotyrosine (*pTyr*) residues. The precipitation of this complex by antiphosphotyrosine antibodies is blocked by phosphotyrosine but not by phosphoserine (*pSer*) or phosphothreonine (*pThr*). ^{125}I-NGF– labeled and DSS-cross-linked PC12 cells were lysed (300mM NaCl, 20mM Tris [pH 7.4], 1mM EDTA, 1% NP-40, 0.5% deoxycholate) and assayed with the indicated antibodies. *Lanes 1, 6, 9, and 12*: normal rabbit IgG. *Lane 2*: MC192. *Lanes 3, 7, 10, and 13*: rabbit anti-NGF antiserum. *Lanes 4, 5, 8, 11, and 14*: rabbit antiphosphotyrosine antiserum. Free phosphotyrosine, phosphoserine, or phosphothreonine (5mM) was added prior to immunoprecipitation in *lanes 6–8, lanes 9–11,* and *lanes 12–14*, respectively. The sample in *lane 5* was pretreated with 20 units of calf intestinal alkaline phosphatase for 30 minutes at 37°C. (reproduced with permission from Meakin and Shooter, 1991a.)

ate of the LNGFR obtained with MC-192 to phosphorylate any of the above substrates, the tyrosine kinase activity resides in the high-molecular-weight receptor complex. The kinase activity is blocked by 5′-S-methyladenosine, an inhibitor which also blocks the NGF-induced differentiation of PC12 cells. The inhibitor has no effect on the binding of NGF but it does prevent the tyrosine phosphorylation of the complex (figure 2.4). The high-molecular-weight receptor complex phosphorylates its own tyrosine residues in the absence of an exogenous substrate. Although these data suggest that the high-molecular-weight receptor complex is a tyrosine kinase, it cannot distinguish between this conclusion and the possibility that the kinase activity is in a receptor-associated protein.

The situation has been clarified, however, by concurrent reports from two different groups of investigators who have identified the high-molecular-weight NGF receptor as the proto-oncogene *trk* (Kaplan et al., 1991a,b; Klein et al., 1991). This proto-oncogene (referred to here as trkA), first identified as

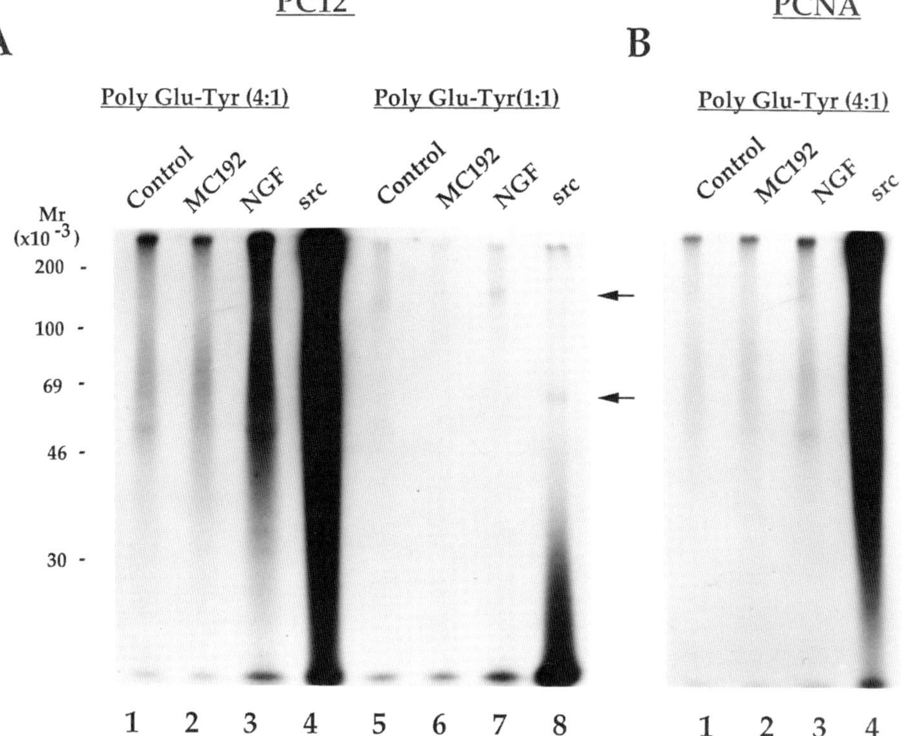

Figure 2.3 The high-molecular-weight NGF-NGFR complex has tyrosine kinase activity and phosphorylates poly(glu$_4$tyr$_1$) polymers but not poly(glu$_1$tyr$_1$) polymers. PC12 cells express both HNGFR and LNGFR, PCNA cells only LNGFR. Poly(glu$_4$tyr$_1$) was used as substrate in *lanes 1–4* of panels *A* and *B* and poly(glu$_1$tyr$_1$) in *lanes 5–8* of panel *A*. *Src lanes* contained five times less reaction product. Gels were soaked in 1N NaOH as described above. *A*, PC12 cells. *Lanes 1 and 5*: normal rabbit IgG. *Lanes 2 and 6*: MC192. *Lanes 3 and 7*: rabbit anti-NGF IgG. *Lanes 5 and 8*: Mb327. *B*, PCNA cells. *Lane 1*: normal rabbit IgG. *Lane 2*: MC192. *Lane 3*: rabbit anti-NGF IgG. Lane 4: Mb327. (Reproduced with permission from Meakin and Shooter, 1991b.)

an oncogenic fusion protein with tropomyosin (Martin-Zanca et al., 1986), has a molecular weight of 135 kD and its distribution in the nervous system parallels that of NGF-responsive neurons (Martin-Zanca et al., 1989) . Like LNGFR, trkA is a single peptide chain with a single membrane-spanning domain. Its cytoplasmic domain, however, encompasses a tyrosine kinase. Antibodies to trk specifically immunoprecipitate the NGF cross-linked—high-molecular-weight complex (Hempstead et al., 1991; Klein et al., 1991; Meakin et al., 1992). It is clear from these data that the 100 kD-cross-linked complex contains only LNGFR and the 160 kD-cross-linked complex only trkA.

A small family of trk receptors are known. BDNF shows a preference for binding to trkB and NT-3 for binding to trkC (Squinto et al., 1991), although it should be noted that the absolute specificities of the trks have not yet been firmly established.

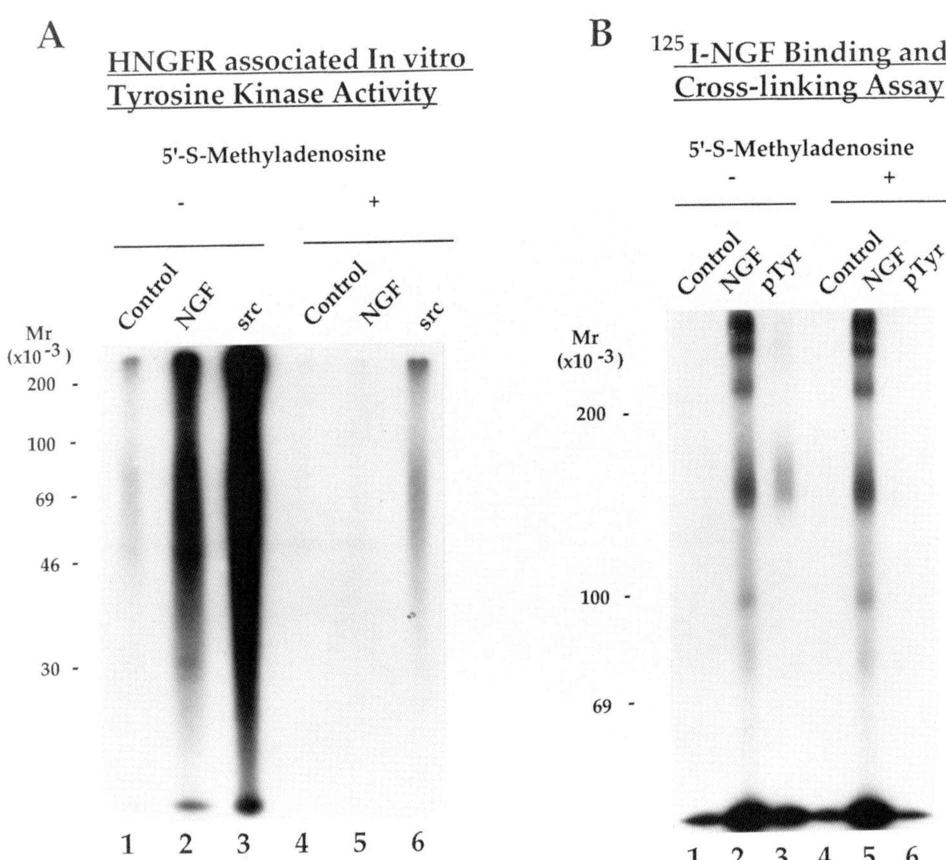

Figure 2.4 The tyrosine kinase inhibitor 5'-S-methyladenosine blocks the tyrosine kinase activity of the huge-molecular-weight NGF-NGFR complex and its phosphorylation on tyrosine residues but has no effect on NGF binding. *A, In vitro* tyrosine kinase assay. PC12 cells were assayed for HNGFR kinase activity, using poly(glu$_4$tyr$_1$) as substrate, in the absence (*lanes 1–3*) and presence (*lanes 4–6*) of 3mM 5'-*S*-methyladenosine. Gels were soaked in 1N NaOH as described above. *Lanes 1 and 4*: normal rabbit IgG. *Lanes 2 and 5*: rabbit anti-NGF IgG. *Lanes 3 and 6*: Mb327. *B,* ^{125}I-NGF binding and cross linking assay. PC12 cells were labeled with ^{125}I-NGF, cross-linked, and immunoprecipitated as described. *Lanes 1 and 4*: normal rabbit IgG. *Lanes 2 and 5*: rabbit anti-NGF IgG. *Lanes 3 and 6*: affinity purified rabbit anti-pTyr IgG. (reproduced with permission from Meakin and Shooter, 1991.)

        Meakin & Shooter: Nerve Growth Factor Receptors

WHAT IS THE HIGH AFFINITY NGF RECEPTOR?

Because the high-molecular-weight–NGF cross-linked complex displayed some of the properties of the HNGFR, a slow dissociation rate for NGF, and trypsin stability, it was assumed that it represented the HNGFR (Hosang and Shooter, 1985). For a variety of reasons, it was thought that this complex contained the LNGFR and a second protein of approximately 60 kD, which would be responsible for the signal transduction mechanism of the HNGFR (Hosang and Shooter, 1987). The finding that the high-molecular-weight complex contains only trkA disproves this idea. In turn, it raises the question whether trkA is the high affinity, biologically active NGF receptor (table 2.1). The alternative model views the high affinity receptor as a combination of LNGFR and trkA, therefore having a molecular weight of approximately 220 kD (Thoenen, 1991; Bothwell, 1991). This is an attractive model, particularly in view of the finding that the LNGFR (gp80^{NTR}) binds all three known neurotrophins with the same equilibrium K_d (Rodriguez-Tebar et al., 1990). The different specificities of the three neurotrophins in this model would be achieved by interacting the LNGFR with the appropriate trk. Evidence in support of such a model was originally obtained from experiments which reintroduced the LNGFR into a PC12 mutant lacking the LNGFR and high affinity NGF binding (Hempstead et al., 1989). It was argued that if the transfection of LNGFR into this cell line, NR18, reestablished an NGF-induced biological response, then LNGFR was a component of the high affinity NGF receptor. In the actual experiment, the LNGFR-transfected NR18 cells recovered an NGF-induced c-fos induction, a reasonable indication of an NGF-induced biological response, but failed to display NGF-induced neurite outgrowth. While Scatchard analysis of the NGF binding to the original NR18 cells showed only one component of binding, the analysis of the transfected NR18 cell showed two components, the new component having a higher affinity for NGF than the original component. It was assumed that this was high affinity NGF binding. The NR18 cell line that was obtained by chemical mutagenesis, however, expresses very low levels of trkA (Hempstead et al., 1991; Meakin et al., 1992).

The above experiment was repeated using membrane fusion instead of transfection (Hempstead et al., 1991). When NR18 membranes, which expressed no NGF binding (indicative of the very low levels of trkA), were fused

Table 2.1 The Neurotrophin Receptors

Neurotrophin	Low Affinity Receptor	High Affinity Receptor*
NGF	LNGFR	LNGFR + trkA *or* trkA
BDNF	LNGFR	LNGFR + trkB *or* trkB
NT-3	LNGFR	LNGFR + trkC *or* trkC

* Two possible models for the high affinity NGF receptor are described. For simplicity, the table assumes an absolute specificity for neurotrophin binding to the trks.

Cells and Molecules that Influence Neuronal Survival

with fibroblasts expressing LNGFR, approximately 300 receptors with a K_d of 2.5×10^{-11}M were produced. Transient expression of LNGFR and trkA in Cos cells resulted in membranes expressing approximately 2,000 receptors with a K_d of 3×10^{-11}M (as well as many receptors with a K_d of 5×10^{-9}M), while membranes from cells transfected with either trkA or LNGFR alone expressed only receptors with K_d's of 3.3×10^{-9}M and 1.1×10^{-9}M, respectively. Transfection of trkA into the human melanoma Hs 294 cell line, which expresses many hundreds of thousands of LNGFRs, also produced approximately 3,000 receptors with a K_d of 3.1×10^{-11}M. These data suggest that both LNGFR and trkA are required to generate a receptor with the K_d approximating that of HNGFR in primary neurons. Given that the HNGFRs in PC12 cells, as opposed to membranes, do not produce a distinct second clear component of NGF binding, it would be advantageous to determine if the membrane binding components with a K_d of approximately 10^{-11}M characterized in these experiments possess any of the other known properties of HNGFR. A different line of investigation has also produced evidence in favor of the model and is based on the knowledge that the high affinity NGF receptor is necessary for a biological response such as neurite outgrowth (Eveleth et al., 1988). Several polyclonal antibodies were raised against peptide segments of the LNGFR. Several of these partially inhibited NGF binding to LNGFR and at the same time partially inhibited NGF-induced neurite outgrowth. This result would be expected only if the high affinity NGF receptors contained LNGFR. In contrast, another polyclonal antibody to the extracellular domain of LNGFR fully inhibited NGF binding to LNGFR, but still permitted NGF-induced neurite outgrowth (Weskamp and Reichardt, 1991). The reasons for these differing results are not clear.

Other experiments favor the idea that the HNGFR does not contain LNGFR. In one of the original cross-linking experiments (Hosang and Shooter, 1985), ^{125}I-NGF was removed from LNGFR on PC12 cells by washing with unlabeled NGF. The ^{125}I-NGF was then cross-linked to the cells to, in effect, label only the HNGFR. If the HNGFRs were a complex of LNGFR and trkA, then cross-linking should result in the formation of a tertiary complex (LNGFR + trkA + ^{125}I-NGF—which may not be observed if its concentration is low), as well as the binary complexes of LNGFR + ^{125}I-NGF and trkA + ^{125}I-NGF. Only the last complex (160kb) was observed, suggesting that trkA alone is the HNGFR. This result contrasts with the finding of Green and Greene (1986) who, using the cross-linker EDAC (ethyldimethylaminopropyl carbodiimide) which only cross-links ^{125}I-NGF to LNGFR, observed the LNGFR + ^{125}I-NGF complex even under conditions where binding was only to HNGFR. Further evidence that trkA is the HNGFR comes from its observed slow rate of NGF dissociation and trypsin stability when transiently expressed in Cos cells (Meakin et al., 1992). On the basis that the K_d for NGF binding to trkA is significantly lower than the K_d for NGF binding to HNGFR, Klein et al. (1991) also concluded that trkA is the HNGFR.

     Meakin & Shooter: Nerve Growth Factor Receptors

It is also clear that a second trk, trkB, can initiate a biological response by itself to the neurotrophin BDNF. In a 3T3 cell line which is dependent on fibroblast growth factor (FGF) for survival and growth, expression of trkB allows BDNF to substitute for FGF. Similar results have been found for trkA expressed in NIH 3T3 cells. These cells proliferate and are morphologically transformed by NGF (and NT-3) in the absence of LNGFR (Cordon-Cardo, et al., 1991). It is likely that the final answer to this question of the identity of the HNGFR will only come from a comparison of the binding properties of LNGFR, trkA, and the two in combination when expressed in a neuron or neuronal cell line.

Acknowledgment

Original work described in this paper was supported by grants from the (NINDB) (NS04270) and the American Cancer Society (BE47J) and by a Damon Runyon–Walter Winchell Cancer Fellowship (DRG-984) to S.O.M.

REFERENCES

Alderson, R.F., Alterman, A.L., Barde, Y.-A., and Lindsay, R.M. (1990). Brain-derived neurotrophic factor increases survival, and differentiated functions of rat septal cholinergic neurons in culture. *Neuron* 5:297–306.

Barde, Y.-A. (1989). Trophic factors and neuronal survival. *Neuron* 2:1525–1534.

Bernd, P., and Greene, L.A. (1984). Association of ^{125}I-NGF with PC12 cells. Evidence for internalization via high affinity receptors only and for long-term regulation by NGF of both high- and low-affinity receptors. *J. Biol. Chem.* 259:15509–15516.

Bothwell, M. (1991). Keeping track of neurotrophin receptors. *Cell* 65:915–918.

Chandler, C.E., Parsons, L.M., Hosang, M., and Shooter, E.M. (1984). A monoclonal antibody modulates the interaction of nerve growth factor with PC12 cells. *J. Biol. Chem.* 259:6882–6889.

Cordon-Cardo, C., Tapley, P., Jing, S., Nanduri, V., O'Rourke, E., Lamballe, F., Kovary, K., Klein, R., Jones, K.R., Reichardt, L.F., and Barbacid, M. (1991). The trk tyrosine protein kinase mediates the mitogenic properties of nerve growth factor and neurotrophin-3. *Cell* 66:173–183.

Ernfors, P., Wetmore, C., Olson, L. and Persson, H. (1990a). Identification of cells in rat brain and peripheral tissues expressing mRNA for members of the nerve growth factor family. *Neuron* 5:511–526.

Ernfors, P., Ibanez, C.F., Ebendal, T., Olson, L., and Persson, H. (1990b). Molecular cloning and neurotrophic activities of a protein with structural similarities to nerve growth factor: developmental and topographical expression in the brain. *Proc. Natl. Acad. Sci. U.S.A.* 87:5454–5458.

Eveleth, D.D., Gillespie, L.S. and Bradshaw, R.A. (1988). Identification of rat growth factor receptor species using antipeptide antibodies. *J. Cell Biol.* 107:69a.

Feinstein, D.L., and Larhammer, D. (1990). Identification of a conserved protein motif in a group of growth factor receptors. *FEBS Letters* 272:7–11.

Godfrey, E.W., and Shooter, E.M. (1986). Nerve growth factor receptors on chick sympathetic ganglion cells: Binding characteritics and development. *J. Neurosci.* 6:2543–2550.

   Cells and Molecules that Influence Neuronal Survival

Green, S.H., and Greene, L.A. (1986). A single Mr 103,000 ^{125}I-nerve growth factor affinity labeled species represents both the high and low affinity forms of the nerve growth factor receptor. *J. Biol. Chem.* 261:15316–15326.

Hallböök, F., Ibanez, C.F., and Persson, H. (1991). Evolutionary studies of the nerve growth factor family reveal a novel member abundantly expressed in *Xenopus* ovary. *Neuron* 6:845–858.

Hempstead, B.L., Martin-Zanca, D., Kaplan, D.R., Parada, L.F., and Chao, M.V. (1991). High affinity NGF binding requires coexpression of the trk proto-oncogene and the low affinity NGF receptor. *Nature* 350:678–683.

Hempstead, B.L., Schleifer, L.S., and Chao, M.V. (1989). Expression of functional nerve growth factor receptors after gene transfer. *Science* 243:373–375.

Hofer, M., Pagliusi, S.R., Hohn, A., Leibrock, J., and Barde, Y.-A. (1990). Regional distribution of brain-derived neurotrophic factor mRNA in the adult mouse brain. *EMBO J.* 9:2459–2464.

Hohn, A., Leibrock, J., Bailey, K., and Barde, Y.-A. (1990). Identification and characterization of a novel member of the nerve growth factor/brain-derived neurotrophic factor family. *Nature* 344:339–341.

Hosang, M., and Shooter, E.M. (1985). Molecular characteristics of nerve growth factor receptors in PC12 cells. *J. Biol. Chem.* 260:655–662.

Hosang, M., and Shooter, E.M. (1987). The internalization of nerve growth factor by high affinity receptors on pheochromocytoma PC12 cells. *EMBO J.* 6:1197–1202.

Hyman, C., Hofer, M., Barde, Y.-A., and Lindsay, R.M. (1991). BDNF is a neurotrophic factor for dopaminergic neurons of the substantia nigra. *Nature* 350:230–232.

Johnson, D., Lanahan, A., Buck, C.R., Seghal, A., Morgan, C., Mercer, E., Bothwell, M., and Chao, M. (1986). Expression and structure of the human NGF receptor. *Cell* 47:545–554.

Kaplan, D.R., Martin-Zanca, D., and Parada, L.F. (1991a) Tyrosine phosphorylation and tyrosine kinase activity of the trk protooncogene product induced by NGF. *Nature* 350:158–160.

Kaplan, D.R., Hempstead, B.L., Martin-Zanca, D., Chao, M.V., and Parada, L.F. (1991b). The trk proto-oncogene product: A signal transducing receptor for nerve growth factor. *Science* 252:554–557.

Klein, R., Jing, S., Nanduri, V., O'Rourke, E., and Barbacid, M. (1991). The trk proto-oncogene encodes a receptor for nerve growth factor. *Cell* 65:189–197.

Landreth, G.E., and Shooter, E.M. (1980). Nerve growth factor receptors on PC12 cells: ligand-induced conversion from low- to high-affinity states. *Proc. Natl. Acad. Sci. U.S.A.* 77:4751–4755.

Large, T.H., Weskamp, G., Helder, J.C., Radeke, M.J., Misko, T.P., Shooter, E.M., and Reichardt, L.F. (1989). Structure and developmental expression of the nerve growth factor receptor in the chicken central nervous system. *Neuron* 2:1123–1134.

Leibrock, J., Lottspeich, F., Hohn, A., Hofer, M., Hengerer, B., Masiakowski, P., Thoenen, H., and Barde, Y.-A. (1989). Molecular cloning and expression of brain-derived neurotrophic factor. *Nature* 341:149–152.

Maisonpierre, P.C., Belluscio, L., Squinto, S., Ip, N.Y., Furth, M.E., Lindsay, R.M., and Yancopoulos, G.D. (1990). NT-3, BDNF, and NGF in the developing rat nervous system: Parallel as well as reciprocal patterns of expression. *Science* 5:501–509.

Maisonpierre, P.C., LeBeau, M.M., Espinosa, R., Ip, N.Y., Belluscio, L., De La Monte, S.M., Squinto, S.P., Furth, M.E., and Yancopoulos, G.D. (1991). Human and rat brain-derived neurotrophic factor and neurotrophin-3: Gene structures, distributions, and chromosomal localizations. *Genomics* 10:558–568.

Martin-Zanca, D., Hughes, S.H., and Barbacid, M. (1986). A human oncogene formed by the fusion of truncated tropomyosin and protein tyrosine kinase sequences. *Nature* 319:743–748.

Martin-Zanca, D., Oskam, R., Mitra, G., Copeland, T., and Barbacid, M. (1989). Molecular and biochemical characterization of the human trk proto-oncogene. *Mol. Cell. Biol.* 9:24–33.

Meakin, S.O., and Shooter, E.M. (1991a). Molecular investigations on the high-affinity nerve growth factor receptor. *Neuron* 6:153–163.

Meakin, S.O., and Shooter, E.M. (1991b). Tyrosine kinase activity coupled to the high-affinity nerve growth factor-receptor complex. *Proc. Natl. Acad. Sci. U.S.A.* 88:5862–5866.

Meakin, S.O., Suter, U., Drinkwater, C.C., Welcher, A.A., and Shooter, E.M. (1992). The rat trk-protooncogene product exhibits properties characteristic of the slow nerve growth factor receptor. *Proc. Natl. Acad. Sci. U.S.A.* 89:2374–2378.

Phillips, H.S., Hains, J.M., Laramee, G.R., Rosenthal, A., and Winslow, J.W. (1990). Widespread expression of BDNF but not NT3 by target areas of basal forebrain cholinergic neurons. *Science* 250:290–294.

Radeke, M.J., and Feinstein, S. (1991). Analytical purification of the slow, high affinity NGF receptor; identification of a novel 135 Kd polypeptide. *Neuron* 7:141–150.

Radeke, M.J., Misko, T.P., Hsu, C., Herzenberg, L.A., and Shooter E.M. (1987). Gene transfer and cloning of the rat nerve growth factor receptor: a new class of receptors. *Nature* 325:593–597.

Rodriguez-Tebar, A., Dechant, G., and Barde, Y.-A. (1990). Binding of brain-derived neurotrophic factor to the nerve growth factor receptor. *Neuron* 4:487–492.

Rodriguez-Tebar, A., Dechant, G., and Barde, Y.-A. (1991). Neurotrophins: Structural relatedness and receptor interactions. *Philos. Trans. R. Soc. Lond. [Biol.]* 331:255–258.

Schechter, A.L., and Bothwell, M.A. (1981). Evidence for two receptor classes with differing cytoskeletal association. *Cell* 24:867–874.

Squinto, S.S., Stitt, T.N., Aldrich, T.H., Davis, S., Bianco, S.M., Radziejewski, C., Glass, D.J., Masiakowski, P., Furth, M.E., Valenzuela, D.M., DiStefano, P.S., and Yancopoulos, G.D. (1991). trkB encodes a functional receptor for brain-derived neurotrophic factor but not nerve growth factor. *Cell* 65:1–20.

Sutter, A., Riopelle, R.J., Harris-Warwick R.M., and Shooter, E.M. (1979). Nerve growth factor receptors. Characterization of two distinct classes of binding sites on chick embryo sensory ganglia cells. *J. Biol. Chem.* 25:5972–5982.

Thoenen, H. (1991). The changing scene of neurotrophic factors. *Trends Neurosci.* 14:165–170.

Vale, R.D., and Shooter, E.M. (1984). Assaying binding of nerve growth factor to cell surface receptors. *Methods Enzymol.* 109:21–39.

Weskamp, G., and Reichardt, L.F. (1991). Evidence that biological activity of NGF is mediated through a novel subclass of high affinity receptors. *Neuron* 6:1–20.

Wetmore, C., Ernfors, P., Persson, H., and Olson, L. (1991). Localization of brain-derived neurotrophic factor mRNA to neurons in the brain by in situ hybridization. *Exp. Neurol.* 109:141–152.

Woodruff, N.R., and Neet, K.E. (1986). Nerve growth factor binding to PC 12 cells. Association kinetics and cooperative interactions. *Biochemistry* 25:7956–7966.

3 Death and Survival of Axotomized Retinal Ganglion Cells

Garth M. Bray, Maria-Paz Villegas-Pérez, Manuel Vidal-Sanz, and Albert J. Aguayo

In addition to interrupting neural connectivity, axotomy has major retrograde effects on proximal axons and neuronal perikarya, including the death of the affected neurons (Lieberman, 1974), a phenomenon that contributes to the limited axonal regeneration and reconnectivity that occurs in mammals after the interruption of central nervous system (CNS) pathways such as the optic nerve or tract. Among the several experimental variables that are known to influence the survival of axotomized neurons (Lieberman, 1974), the greater extent of cell loss that occurs with lesions near the perikaryon than with more distal lesions is particularly striking. For some groups of neurons, this difference might be explained by the existence of intact axon collaterals (Fry and Cowan, 1972) but in other situations, such as the optic nerve in rodents, there are few, if any, such axon collaterals. In an attempt to understand the basis for the loss of axotomized retinal ganglion cells (RGCs), we have reviewed the possible mechanisms that might lead to such devastating effects on injured neurons and have summarized some of the short- and long-term quantitative studies on the effects of time and lesion site on the survival of axotomized RGCs in adult rodents (Grafstein and Ingoglia, 1982; Misantone et al., 1984; Allcutt et al., 1984: Barron et al., 1986; Villegas-Pérez et al., 1988a,b).

MECHANISMS OF NEURON DEATH

Cell death can be a physiological process as well as a response to injury or disease. During the past few years, much has been learned about the phenomenon of "natural" or "spontaneous" death of neurons and other cells that occurs during development and in response to special physiological situations. Some of these current issues concerning various types of cell death are relevant to the loss of axotomized neurons.

During development, cell death occurs at several stages of embryonic life and probably affects most cell types (reviewed by Oppenheim, 1991). Here we emphasize the death of neurons that occurs relatively late in development when connections with target structures are forming, because this phase of neuron death appears to be particularly relevant to the study of axotomy. Synaptic connections have important influences on the developmental death of neurons. Firstly, the numbers of neurons that survive in the developing nervous system can be manipulated experimentally by increasing or decreasing the size of their target fields (Hamburger and Levi-Montalcini, 1949; Oppenheim, 1991). Secondly, developmental neuronal death is increased by reducing the number of afferent connections or by blocking electrical activity (Lipton, 1986; for review, see Oppenheim, 1991).

The survival of sympathetic (Levi-Montalcini and Angeletti, 1968; Oppenheim et al., 1982) or dorsal root ganglion (DRG) (Hamburger et al., 1981) neurons during development can also be influenced by nerve growth factor (NGF), while other groups of neurons appear to be critically dependent on different trophic factors such as brain-derived neurotrophic factor (BDNF) (Hofer and Barde, 1988). Thus, the concept has evolved that developing neurons compete for limited amounts of target-derived neurotrophic molecules, a dependency that develops when axons are forming synapses in the target regions that are the source of their trophic factors (reviewed by Barde, 1989). Although the mechanisms whereby afferent connections influence neuron survival have not been determined, growth factors from sources other than neuron targets might be involved. For example, fibroblast growth factor (FGF), which can enhance the survival of neurons in vitro (e.g., Walicke, 1989) and in vivo (Sievers et al., 1987), has been shown to be transported anterograde from the eye to RGC targets in the brain (Ferguson et al., 1990).

Gene Regulation of Neuron Death

Most neurons whose survival in vivo appears to depend on specific growth factors also require these molecules to support their survival in vitro. Thus, for example, sympathetic or DRG neurons require NGF (for review, see Barde, 1989) while placode-derived sensory neurons (Davies et al., 1986) or RGCs (Johnson et al., 1986) depend on BDNF; the survival of other classes of neurons presumably depends on different factors, as yet unidentified. The death of neurons caused by trophic factor deprivation in vitro can be prevented by certain experimental manipulations: (1) inhibiting protein or RNA synthesis (Martin et al., 1988, 1990; Scott and Davies, 1990), suggesting that this type of cell death requires the activation of genes; or (2) adding cyclic adenosine monophosphate (cAMP) analogues (Rydel and Greene, 1988), suggesting that NGF affects cell function through this second messenger. The developmental death of motoneurons and DRG neurons in vivo also requires protein and RNA synthesis (Oppenheim et al., 1990). As a corollary to these observations, it has been suggested that trophic factors such as NGF influence neuron survival by suppressing genes that generate "killer" proteins (Martin et al., 1990).

In invertebrates such as *Caenorhabditis elegans*, certain neurons undergo a process during development that has been designated "programmed" cell death. Studies of mutations in *C. elegans* have identified several genes that cause the death of these cells as well as their engulfment by phagocytic cells and the degradation of their DNA (Ellis and Horvitz, 1991).

     Cells and Molecules that Influence Neuronal Survival

"Physiological" cell death that is the result of gene expression also occurs in cells other than neurons. Examples of this phenomenon include the terminal differentiation of specialized cells such as erythrocytes and the lens (Counis et al., 1989), the death of hormone-dependent cells in the prostate or mammary gland, and the responses of lymphocytes or thymocytes to various stimuli (reviewed by Bursch et al., 1990). Such cell death, which shows several common morphological and biochemical features in these different tissues, has been termed *apoptosis* to distinguish it from necrosis, the type of cell death that occurs in response to injuries that cause the failure of cellular energy metabolism or the loss of osmoregulation, leading to cell swelling, disruption of plasma membranes, dissolution of cell structure, and the late degradation of DNA by lysosomal enzymes (Wyllie et al., 1980). Many of these examples of apoptosis share common biochemical features (for review, see Bursch et al., 1990); these include: early increases of intracellular Ca^{2+}; the activation of endogenous endonucleases that lead to the characteristic nuclear condensation and fragmentation; the induction of transglutaminases and other degrading enzymes and activation of protein kinases; the expression of surface molecules, such as the vitronectin receptor (Savill et al., 1990), that promote phagocytosis by macrophages; and the prevention of cell death by inhibitors of RNA or protein synthesis. Although these morphological and biochemical features are common to apoptosis in many types of cells, the process may be initiated by distinct stimuli in different experimental systems of susceptible cells, and the sequence of biochemical changes may vary among tissues (Bursch et al., 1990). For example, the death of sympathetic neurons in vitro by NGF deprivation is associated with *decreased* intracellular levels of Ca^{2+} (Koike and Tanaka, 1991) and can be prevented by depolarization with K^+ or cholinergic stimulation (Koike et al., 1989).

Developmental Death of Retinal Ganglion Cells

Large numbers of RGCs die during development (e.g., Fawcett et al., 1984). The death of these neurons in vitro can be prevented by co-culture with target tissues (Armson and Bennett, 1983) or by BDNF (Johnson et al., 1986), which is synthesized in the superior colliculus (Hofer et al., 1990). RGC death in vitro can be augmented by blockade of synaptic activity (Lipton, 1986), an effect that can be reversed by cAMP induction (Kaiser and Lipton, 1990). Thus, the mechanisms for the death or survival of developing RGCs appear to be analogous to those of other neurons.

Excitotoxic Neuron Death

Although various types of injury and disease can cause the death of neurons, the mechanism(s) underlying most of these pathological situations is poorly understood. However, in vitro and in vivo studies have demonstrated that several types of injury, such as anoxia or trauma, can affect neurons through the excessive release of excitatory amino acids (for review, see Choi and

Rothman, 1990). Although many of the features of excitotoxic injury to neurons suggest that the cell death caused by this mechanism is due to impaired osmoregulation, and therefore would be classified as necrosis rather than apoptosis, the delayed phase of postanoxic loss of neurons in the rat hippocampus presumably involves gene activation because it can be reduced by inhibiting protein synthesis with cycloheximide (Goto et al., 1990).

Neuronal populations differ in their susceptibility to excitotoxic neurotransmitters. For example, some neurons that contain calbindin-D_{28k} are relatively resistant to excitotoxic injury (Mattson et al., 1991) while others that contain somatostatin or parvalbumin are particularly sensitive to the excitotoxic effects of kainate or α-amino-3-hydroxy-5-methyl-4-isoxazole-propionate (AMPA) but are relatively insensitive to N-methyl-D-aspartate (NMDA) (Weiss et al., 1990). Although the neurotransmitter of RGCs is probably an excitatory amino acid (Tsai et al., 1990), it has not been shown that axotomy or other lesions that affect the retina have excitotoxic effects on RGCs.

Axotomy and Neuron Death

For susceptible neurons, axotomy is presumed to initiate processes that lead to cell death by disconnecting neurons from their source of target-derived trophic factors (Barde, 1989). This concept, which has its genesis in the studies of developmental neuronal death and target-derived trophic factors summarized above, is also supported by experimental evidence for the "rescue" of axotomized neurons by certain trophic factors. Administration of NGF prevents the death of axotomized neurons in peripheral sympathetic (Hendry, 1975) and dorsal root ganglia (Yip et al., 1984) as well as the cholinergic neurons of the basal forebrain (e.g., Williams et al., 1986); it is postulated that the mechanism for this effect involves the "desuppression" of genes whose products are lethal to the cell (Martin et al., 1990). The survival of other classes of axotomized neurons can be enhanced by BDNF and other homologous neurotrophins (NT) such as NT-3 (for review, see Thoenen, 1991). Although a detailed understanding of the molecular interactions involved is still incomplete, it has recently been determined that these members of the neurotrophin family exert their effects through receptor complexes that interact with specific proto-oncogenes (see chapter 2). Finally, other populations in neurons are sustained after axotomy by nontarget-derived trophic factors such as FGF (Sievers et al., 1987) and ciliary neuronotrophic factor (CNTF) (Sendtner et al., 1990).

The extensive evidence that young animals of many species are more vulnerable to retrograde neuron death after axotomy (e.g., Allcutt et al., 1984) is taken as strong evidence for the dependence of immature neurons on target-derived trophic molecules (reviewed by Barde, 1989). Moreover, the effect of axotomy on target-dependent neurons in ova can be ameliorated by inhibiting protein or RNA synthesis (Oppenheim et al., 1990). However, the effects of NGF, and presumably other trophic factors, on the survival of dependent neurons are not limited to development; for example, the administration of NGF antibodies to adult mice causes the loss of nearly one half of the neurons in the superior cervical ganglion over 3 months (Gorin and Johnson, 1980; Ruit et al., 1990). However, sensory neurons derived from adult animals, in contrast to those obtained from fetal or neonatal animals, can survive in vitro without added NGF or BDNF (Lindsay, 1988).

METHODS FOR ASSESSING NEURON SURVIVAL AFTER AXOTOMY

Using standard histological stains for qualitative studies of cell survival in the CNS of adult mammals, other investigators reported a greater loss with axonal lesions near the neuronal somata (Leinfelder, 1938; Mantz and Klein, 1951; Liu, 1955; Glover, 1967; Loewy and Schader, 1977; Fry and Cowan, 1972; Radius and Anderson, 1978). Biochemical or cytochemical indicators of neurotransmitter expression have further substantiated these observations; for example, a greater cell loss occurs when dopaminergic neurons of the substantia nigra pars compacta (Reis et al., 1978) or the cholinergic neurons of the basal forebrain (Sofroniew and Isacson, 1988) are axotomized near their cell bodies than when the injury is more distal. While there can be a correspondence between the presence of neurotransmitter-related markers and estimates of cell numbers based on retrograde neuronal labeling (Tuszynski et al., 1990; O'Brien et al., 1990), such markers may not be totally suitable for detailed long-term quantitative studies of cell populations because neurotransmitter expression and that of other labile phenotypes can be altered in injured cells that survive axotomy (Lams et al., 1988; Hagg et al., 1988). Moreover, the size and shape of nerve cells are often altered after axotomy. Neuronal atrophy can be particularly troublesome in the retina (Misantone et al., 1984, Villegas-Pérez et al., 1988a) where RGCs share the same layer with many small interneurons, the displaced amacrine cells (Cowey and Perry, 1979, Perry, 1981). The dendritic arrangement of otherwise viable RGCs can also be altered by injury (Cho and So, 1989; Thanos and Aguayo, 1988), further contributing to the difficulty of differentiating classes of cells by their morphology alone.

RGCs can be identified more specifically by labeling with tracers transported retrograde. For this purpose, we have used a carbocyanine dye, diI, to label RGCs for periods of time that range from 2 weeks to 20 months. This labeling technique (Vidal-Sanz et al., 1988), which avoids dependence on phenotypic markers such as neurotransmitter expression or neuron size, was validated by comparing the densities of diI-labeled cells in the retina with the results of other quantitative techniques. In control rats, 98% of retinal neurons labeled retrograde with diI for periods up to 9 months were also labeled with Fast blue for 2 days, while for RGCs axotomized intracranially for up to 3 months, the correlation was 80% to 90% (Vidal-Sanz et al., 1988). Furthermore, in retinas examined 15 days to 12 months after axotomy, there was a close correspondence between the densities of diI-labeled neurons and the

Bray et al.: Axotomized Retinal Ganglion Cells

Table 3.1 Retinal Ganglion Cell Survival* after Axotomy in Adult Rodents

	Intraorbital	Intracranial
Mice	Allcutt et al., 1984 (crush)	Grafstein and Ingoglia, 1982 (cut)
Early	20 days: 20%–40%	15 days: 70%
Late	80 days: 0%–20%	90 days: 60%
Rats	Barron et al., 1986 (crush)	Misantone et al., 1982 (crush)
Early	7 days: 65%	90 days: no loss detected
Late	180 days: 32%	230 days: 60%

* Expressed as approximate percentage of control values.

population of methylene blue–stained cells in the ganglion cell layer that are estimated to be RGCs (Villegas-Pérez et al., unpublished observations).

RGC LOSS AFTER OPTIC NERVE TRANSECTION

Earlier qualitative studies suggested that the distance between the axotomy site and the RGC cell body influenced the amount of cell death (Leinfelder, 1938; Mantz and Klein, 1951; Radius and Anderson, 1978). Subsequently, other investigators used standard histological staining techniques to quantitate the changes in RGC numbers after axotomy (table 3.1). Although these studies used different animal species, axotomy techniques (cut or crush), and observation times, their results, when considered together, show trends which suggest that intraorbital optic nerve (ON) lesions cause greater RGC death than intracranial lesions and that additional RGCs may be lost subsequently.

Prompted by observations that ON transection near the eye caused the loss of more than 90% of RGCs identified by retrograde labeling with diI applied at the lesion site (Villegas-Pérez et al., 1988a; fig 3.1), we have used the labeling of RGCs with diI retrogradely transported from the main targets of these axons—the superior colliculus and dorsolateral geniculate nucleus (Vidal-Sanz et al., 1988), to determine the densities of surviving RGCs after intraorbital (0.5 or 3.0 mm from the eye) or intracranial (8 or 10 mm) lesions of the ON in adult rats. By 1 month after such lesions, RGC densities were reduced to 18% to 31% with intraorbital transection of the ON but only to 55% to 71% with intracranial ON lesions (Villegas-Pérez et al., 1988b). Following this early rapid loss of RGCs, which varied with the distance of the lesion from the eye, there was a less marked but protracted loss of RGCs in all groups of experimental animals which could not be explained by age-related changes or loss of diI labeling (Villegas-Pérez et al., unpublished observations).

POSSIBLE CAUSES OF DIFFERENT RATES OF RGC DEATH

Several mechanisms, acting singly or in combination, could potentially cause the loss of RGCs after ON transection near the eye. These include: injury effects such as the influx of Ca^{2+} or the actions of excessive excitotoxin

     Cells and Molecules that Influence Neuronal Survival

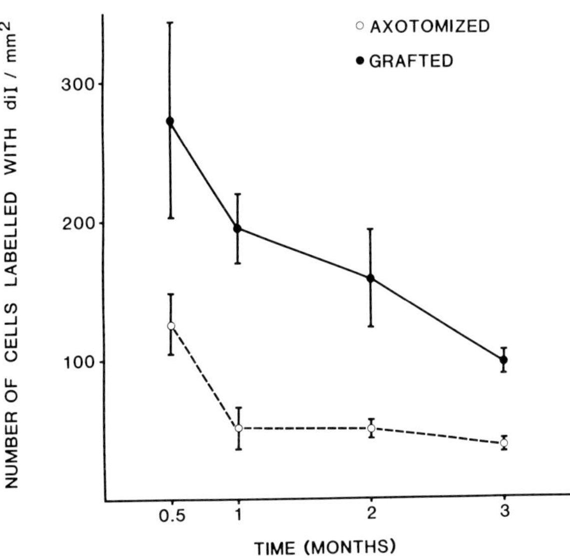

Figure 3.1 Survival of axotomized retinal ganglion cells (RGCs) in adult rats. At the time of optic nerve transection, RGCs were labeled with diI, a retrograde-transported tracer that persists for many months. Surviving RGCs were counted in standard areas of each retina and expressed as numbers of cells per square millimeter. By 1 month, RGC densities in the retinas without peripheral nerve (PN) grafts (*open circles*) had decreased to less than 10% of control values. In the retinas with attached PN grafts (*solid circles*), there was an enhancement of RGC densities, but this effect diminished with time. (Reproduced with permission from Villegas-Pérez et al., 1988a).

release; limited or ineffective trophic support from the ON stump; and the interruption of trophic support from target regions in the brain.

"Injury" effects of axotomy could include Ca^{2+} influx, which can extend along the axon for several millimeters (Strautman et al., 1990), or depolarization with release of excitotoxic quantities of neurotransmitter (for review, see Choi and Rothman, 1990). Either mechanism could lead to intracellular perturbations, disruptions of plasma membranes, Ca^{2+} influxes, and the activation of proteolytic enzymes. Although such graded changes would be more likely to affect RGCs with lesions closer to the perikarya, it remains to be determined if these mechanisms contribute to the greater losses of RGCs that occur with intraorbital ON lesions than do intracranial interruptions of the same nerve. However, the RGCs lost by 2 weeks after axotomy near the eye may not die immediately; many continue to express messenger RNAs (mRNAs) for cytoskeletal proteins for several days after injury (McKerracher, Essagian, and Aguayo, unpublished observations).

Trophic Support from the Environment of Injured Axons

When peripheral nerves are transected, there is increased synthesis of NGF (Heumann et al., 1987), NGF receptor (Taniuchi et al., 1986), and BDNF (H. Thoenen, personal communication, 1991) in the distal nerve stump. These

     Bray et al.: Axotomized Retinal Ganglion Cells

growth factors are presumed to contribute to the survival of responsive neurons as their axons regrow along the peripheral nerve (PN) stump. After lesions in the brain, neurotrophic substances (Nieto-Sampedro et al., 1983; Gage et al., 1984), including NGF and acidic FGF (aFGF) (Ishikawa et al., 1991), are released into the wound cavity. Thus, it is possible that such trophic molecules are produced in the distal segments of lesioned ONs. Indeed, after interruption of the ON in adult rats, there is enhanced expression of NGF mRNA although it is not sustained (Lu et al., 1991). However, it has not been determined if after such ON lesions there is increased synthesis of BDNF, a growth factor that would presumably be more likely to promote the survival of injured RGCs (Johnson et al., 1986). Although it is unlikely that the distal stumps of transected ONs would provide trophic support for RGCs because of the failure of their axons to regrow in this CNS milieu, it is possible that such interactions are effective in the proximal (ocular) stumps of the transected ONs. Furthermore, more extensive interactions between RGC axons and molecular components in the longer ON stumps might contribute to the greater survival of RGCs axotomized at a distance from the retina.

Target-Derived Trophic Influences

The dependence of adult RGCs on their targets was suggested by the losses of RGCs that occur in primates or cats after removal or retrograde degeneration of the RGC targets (reviewed by Cowan, 1970). In neonatal rats, the removal of the superior colliculus or its destruction with injections of kainic acid causes marked RGC death (Perry and Cowey, 1979; Carpenter et al., 1986) but in adult rats, such lesions do not cause RGC loss (Perry and Cowey, 1979), perhaps because their terminals establish contacts with other neurons (Campbell and Frost, 1988; Zwimpfer et al., 1989).

There is substantial evidence to indicate that BDNF is the probable trophic factor for RGCs. BDNF mRNA (Hofer et al., 1990) is present in the superior colliculus, which, in rodents, is the target of more than 95% of RGCs, and the survival of fetal (Johnson et al., 1986) or adult (Thanos et al, 1989) RGCs in vitro is enhanced by BDNF. Thus, the deprivation of RGCs of this target-derived trophic molecule is an attractive explanation for the slow, protracted losses of RGCs that follow the earlier rapid losses of axotomized RGCs, which cannot be explained solely by this mechanism. With 50% survival times ranging from 5.2 to 6.7 months (Villegas-Pérez et al., unpublished observations), the time course of this RGC loss after distal transections of the adult rat ON approximated that reported when the vagus nerve was severed in guinea pigs and its regrowth was mechanically blocked (Laiwand et al., 1987). Under such conditions, the 50% survival time of neurons in the dorsal motor nucleus of the vagus was 8.6 months. Such data suggest that the slow rates of cell death may reflect a general pattern of degeneration that affects nerve cells that have lost, or are chronically prevented from making connections with, their targets in either the peripheral nervous system (PNS) or CNS.

Several experimental strategies have been used to increase neuronal survival after axotomy. In vitro, RGC survival can be enhanced by co-culture with fetal explants of RGC target regions of brain (e.g., Armson and Bennett, 1983). In vivo, the placement of embryonic thalamic and tectal tissue at the site of axotomy 2 to 3 mm from the eye led to a threefold enhancement in the survival of RGCs at 1 month (Sievers et al., 1989). Similar effects were observed after the positioning of fetal retina adjacent to retinal lesions in adult rats (Laedtke and Turner 1989). The extent of RGC loss that follows ON transection close to the eye can also be reduced in adult rats, at least temporarily, by the apposition of a segment of PN to the ocular stump of the transected ON. One month after attaching such grafts, Berry et al. (1986) observed a 10% increase in RGC survival. Using a different method to identify RGCs, Villegas-Pérez et al. (1988a) reported that the survival of these neurons was enhanced nearly four fold 1 month after the placement of PN grafts (see figure 3.1). However, with these grafts, which did not permit terminal connectivity, the beneficial effects on RGC survival decreased with time after axotomy and graft placement (see fig 3.1; Villegas-Pérez, Vidal-Sanz, Aguayo, and Bray, unpublished observations). The apposition of PN segments to small retinal lesions that interrupted RGC axons also delayed the onset of RGC death by 2 weeks (Turner et al., 1987). Finally, it has been reported that the introduction of Schwann cells into the eye enhances the viability of axotomized RGCs (Maffei et al., 1990). Each of these experimental manipulations presumably enhances RGC survival by providing trophic factors that mimic or replace, at least temporarily, those target-derived molecules that ordinarily sustain the intact neurons. Moreover, the administration of large amounts of NGF (Carmignoto et al., 1989) or FGF (Sievers et al., 1987) has been shown to increase the survival of axotomized RGCs.

Although the RGC loss that follows ON transection near the eye was diminished by the grafting of PN segments to the stumps of the ON, this effect declined after 2 months (see figure 3.1). In addition, electrophysiological studies of blind-ended PN grafts attached to the ocular stump of the ON, but not to the superior colliculus, documented a progressive decrease in the number of light-responsive units in the grafts between 2 and 12 months after grafting (Keirstead et al., 1985). On the other hand, regenerated RGC arbors persisted in the superior colliculus of rats with PN bridges linking the retina and the tectum for periods of up to 18 months in rats (Vidal-Sanz et al., 1991) and 10 months in hamsters (Carter et al., 1989). Thus, while growth of the RGC axons along PN grafts only appears to enhance the survival of axotomized RGCs transiently, the restoration of terminal connections with CNS targets may assure the persistent survival of the injured neurons.

Future efforts to minimize the effects of axonal damage on cell survival may require a combination of different approaches that include measures to overcome the early effects of axotomy and increase the number of cells capable of regenerating axons that restore connections within the time frame allowed by the more protracted phase of cell degeneration that follows axotomy.

REFERENCES

Allcutt, D., Berry, M., and Sievers, J. (1984). A quantitative comparison of the reactions of retinal ganglion cells to optic nerve crush in neonatal and adult mice. *Dev. Brain. Res.* 15:219–230.

Armson, P.F., and Bennett, M.R. (1983). Neonatal retinal ganglion cell cultures of high purity: Effect of superior colliculus on their survival. *Neurosci. Lett.* 38:181–186.

Barde, Y.-A. (1989). Trophic factors and neuronal survival. *Neuron* 2:1525–1534.

Barron, K.D., Dentinger, M.P., Krohel, G., Easton, S.K., and Mankes, R. (1986). Qualitative and quantitative ultrastructural observations on retinal ganglion cell layer of rat after intraorbital optic nerve crush. *J. Neurocytol.* 15:345–362.

Berry, M., Rees, L., and Sievers, J. (1986). Regeneration of axons in the mammalian visual system. *Exp. Brain Res.* 13(suppl.):18–33.

Bursch, W., Kleine, L., and Tenniswood, M. (1990). The biochemistry of cell death by apoptosis. *Biochem. Cell Biol.* 68:1071–1074.

Campbell, G., and Frost, D.O. (1988). Synaptic organization of anomalous retinal projections to the somatosensory and auditory thalamus: Target controlled morphogenesis of axon terminals and synaptic glomeruli. *J. Comp. Neurol.* 272:383–408.

Carmignoto, G., Maffei, L., Candeo, P., Canella, R., and Comelli, C. (1989). Effect of NGF on the survival of rat retinal ganglion cells following optic nerve section. *J. Neurosci.* 9:1263–1272.

Carpenter, P., Sefton, A.J., Dreher, B., and Lim, W.-L. (1986). Role of target tissue in regulating the development of retinal ganglion cells in the albino rat: Effects of kainate lesions in the superior colliculus. *J. Comp. Neurol.* 251:240–259.

Carter, D.A., Bray, G.M., and Aguayo A.J. (1989). Extension and persistence of regenerated retinal ganglion cell axons in the superior colliculus of adult hamsters. *Soc. Neurosci. Abstr.* 15:872.

Cho, E.Y.P., and So, K.F. (1989). De novo formation of axon-like processes from axotomized retinal ganglion cells which exhibit long distance growth in a peripheral nerve graft in adult hamsters. *Brain Res.* 484:371–377.

Choi, D.W., and Rothman, S.M. (1990). The role of glutamate neurotoxicity in hypoxic-ischemic neuronal death. *Annu. Rev. Neurosci.* 13:171–182.

Counis, M.F., Chaudun, E., Courtois, Y., and Allinquant, B. (1989). Lens differentiation correlated with activation of two different DNAases in lens embryonic cells. *Cell Differ. Dev.* 27:137–146.

Cowan, W.M. (1970). Anterograde and retrograde transneuronal degeneration in the central and peripheral nervous system. In *Contemporary Research Methods in Neuroanatomy* ed. W.J.H. Nauta and Ebbeson S.O.E., 217–249, New York: Springer-Verlag.

Cowey, A., and Perry, V.H. (1979). The projection of the temporal retina in rats studied by retrograde transport of horseradish peroxidase. *Exp. Brain Res.* 35:457–464.

Davies, A.M., Thoenen, H., and Barde, Y.-A. (1986). The response of chick sensory neurons to brain-derived neurotrophic factor. *J. Neurosci.* 6:1897–1904.

     Cells and Molecules that Influence Neuronal Survival

Ellis, R.E., and Horvitz, H.R. (1991). Two *C. elegans* genes control the programmed deaths of specific cells in the pharynx. *Development* 112:591–603.

Fawcett, J.W., O'Leary, D.D.M., and Cowan, W.M. (1984). Activity and the control of ganglion cell death in the rat retina. *Proc. Natl. Acad. Sci. U.S.A.* 81:5589–5593.

Ferguson, I.A., Schweitzer, J.B., and Johnson, E.M., Jr. (1990). Basic fibroblast growth factor: Receptor-mediated internalization, metabolism, and anterograde axonal transport in retinal ganglion cells. *J. Neurosci.* 10:2176–2189.

Fry, F.J., and Cowan, W.M. (1972). A study of retrograde cell degeneration in the lateral mammillary nucleus of the cat, with special reference to the role of axonal branching in the preservation of the cell. *J. Comp. Neurol.* 144:1–24.

Gage, F.H., Björklund, A., and Stenevi, U. (1984). Denervation releases a neuronal survival factor in adult rat hippocampus. *Nature* 308:637–639.

Glover, R.A. (1967). Sequential cellular changes in the nodosal ganglion following section of the vagus nerve at two levels. *Anat. Rec.* 157:248.

Gorin, P.D., and Johnson, E.M. (1980). Effects of long-term nerve growth factor deprivation on the nervous system of the adult rat: An experimental autoimmune approach. *Brain Res.* 198:27–42.

Goto, R., Ishige, A., Sekiguchi, K., Iizuka, S., Sugimoto, A., Yuzurihara, M., Aburada, M., Hosoya E., and Kogure, K. (1990). Effects of cycloheximide on delayed neuronal death in rat hippocampus. *Brain Res.* 534:299–302.

Grafstein, B., and Ingoglia, N.A. (1982). Intracranial transection of the optic nerve in adult mice: Preliminary observations. *Exp. Neurol.* 76:318–330.

Hagg, T., Manthorpe, M., Vahlsing, H.L., and Varon, S. (1988). Delayed treatment with nerve growth factor reverses the apparent loss of cholinergic neurons after acute brain damage. *Exp. Neurol.* 101:303–312.

Hamburger, V., Brunso-Bechtold, J.K., and Yip, J. (1981). Neuronal death in the spinal ganglia of the chick embryo and its reduction by nerve growth factor. *J. Neurosci.* 1:60–71.

Hamburger, V., and Levi-Montalcini, R. (1949). Proliferation, differentiation and degeneration of the spinal ganglia of the chick. *J. Exp. Zool.* 111:457–501.

Hendry, I.A. (1975). The response of adrenergic neurons to axotomy and nerve growth factor. *Brain Res.* 94:87–97.

Heumann, R., Korsching, S., Bandtlow, C., and Thoenen, H. (1987). Changes in nerve growth factor synthesis in non-neuronal cells in response to sciatic nerve transection. *J. Cell Biol.* 104:1623–1631.

Hofer, M., Pagliusi, S.R., Hohn, A., Leibrock, J., and Brade, Y.-A. (1990). Regional distribution of brain-derived neurotrophic factor mRNA in the adult mouse brain. *EMBO J.* 9:2459–2464.

Hofer, M.M., and Barde, Y.-A. (1988). Brain-derived neurotrophic factor prevents neuronal death in vivo. *Nature* 331:261–262.

Ishikawa, R., Nishikori, K., and Furukawa, S. (1991). Appearance of nerve growth factor and acidic fibroblast growth factor with different time courses in the cavity-lesioned cortex of the rat brain. *Neurosci. Lett.* 127:70–72.

Johnson, J.E., Barde, Y.-A., Schwab, M., and Thoenen, H. (1986). Brain-derived neurotrophic factor supports the survival of cultured retinal ganglion cells. *J. Neurosci.* 6:3031–3038.

Kaiser, P.K., and Lipton, S.A., (1990). VIP-mediated increase in cAMP prevents tetrodotoxin-induced retinal ganglion cell death in vitro. *Neuron* 5:373–381.

Keirstead, S.A., Vidal-Sanz, M., Rasminsky, M., Aguayo, A.J., Levesque, M., and So, K.F. (1985). Responses to light of retinal neurons regenerating axons into peripheral nerve grafts in the rat. *Brain Res.* 359:402–406.

Koike, T., and Tanaka, S. (1991). Evidence that nerve growth factor dependence of sympathetic neurons for survival in vitro may be determined by levels of cytoplasmic free Ca^{2+}. *Proc. Natl. Acad. Sci. U.S.A.* 88:3892–3898.

Koike, T., Martin, D.P., and Johnson, E.M. (1989). Role of Ca^{2+} channels in the ability of membrane depolarization to prevent neuronal death induced by trophic factor deprivation: Evidence that levels of internal Ca^{2+} determine nerve growth factor dependence of sympathetic ganglion cells. *Proc. Natl. Acad. Sci. U.S.A.* 86:6421–6425.

Laedtke, T.W., and Turner, J.E. (1989). Embryonic grafts have a beneficial effect on the damaged host retina. *Brain Res.* 500:61–66.

Laiwand, R., Werman, R., and Yarom, Y. (1987). Time course and distribution of motoneuronal loss in the dorsal motor vagal nucleus of the guinea pig after cervical vagotomy. *J. Comp. Neurol.* 256:527–537.

Lams, B.E., Isacson, O., and Sofroniew, M.V. (1988). Loss of transmitter-associated staining following axotomy does not indicate death of brainstem cholinergic neurons. *Brain Res.* 475:401–406.

Leinfelder, P.J. (1938). Retrograde degeneration in the optic nerves and retinal ganglion cells. *Trans. Am. Ophthalmol. Soc.* 36:307–315.

Levi-Montalcini, R., and Angeletti, P.U. (1968). Nerve growth factor. *Physiol. Rev.* 48:534–565.

Lieberman, A.R. (1974). Some factors affecting retrograde neuronal responses to axonal lesions. In *Essays on the Nervous System*, ed. (R. Bellairs and Gray E.G., 71–105, Oxford England: Clarendon.

Lindsay, R.M. (1988). Nerve growth factors (NGF, BDNF) enhance axonal regeneration but are not required for survival of adult sensory neurons. *J. Neurosci.* 8:2394–2405.

Lipton, S.A. (1986). Blockade of electrical activity promotes the death of mammalian retinal ganglion cells in culture. *Proc. Natl. Acad. Sci. U.S.A.* 83:9774–9778.

Liu, C.-N. (1955). Time pattern in retrograde degeneration after trauma of central nervous system of mammals. In *Regeneration in the Central Nervous System*, ed. W.F., Windle 84–93, Springfield, Ill, Charles C Thomas.

Loewy, A.D., and Schader, R.E. (1977). A quantitative study of retrograde neuronal changes in Clarke's column. *J. Comp. Neurol.* 171:65–82.

Lu, B., Yokoyama, M., Dreyfus, C., Black, I. (1991). NGF gene expression in actively growing brain glia. *J. Neurosci.* 11:318–326.

Maffei, L., Carmignoto, G., Perry, V.H., Candeo P., and Ferrari, G. (1990). Schwann cells promote the survival of rat retinal ganglion cells after optic nerve section. *Proc. Natl. Acad. Sci. U.S.A.* 87:1855–1859.

Mantz, J., and Klein, M. (1951). Recherches expérimentales sur la section et la ligature du nerf optique chez le rat. *C. R. Soc. Biol. (Paris)* 145:920–924.

Martin, D.P., Schmidt, R.E., DiStefano, P.S., Lowry, O.H., Carter, J.G., and Johnson, E.M. (1988). Inhibitors of protein synthesis prevent neuronal death caused by nerve growth factor deprivation. *J. Cell Biol.* 106:829–844.

Martin, D.P., Wallace, T.L., and Johnson, E.M. (1990). Cytosine arabinoside kills postmitotic neurons in a fashion resembling trophic factor deprivation: Evidence that a deoxycytidine-

    Cells and Molecules that Influence Neuronal Survival

dependent process may be required for nerve growth factor signal transduction. *J. Neurosci.* 10:184–193.

Mattson, M.P., Rychlik, B., Chu, C., and Christakos, S. (1991). Evidence for calcium-reducing and excito-protective roles for the calcium-binding protein calbindin-D28k in cultured hippocampal neurons. *Neuron* 6:41–51.

Misantone, L.J., Gershembaum, M., and Murray, M. (1984). Viability of retinal ganglion cells after optic nerve crush in adult rats. *J. Neurocytol.* 13:449–465.

Nieto-Sampedro, M., Manthorpe, M., Barbin, G., Varon, S., and Cotman, C.W. (1983). Injury-induced neuronotrophic activity in adult rat brain; correlation with survival of delayed implants in the wound cavity. *J. Neurosci.* 2:2219–2229.

O'Brien, T.S., Svendsen, C.N., Isacson, O., and Sofroniew, M.V. (1990). Loss of True Blue labelling from the medial septum following transection of the fimbria-fornix: evidence for the death of cholinergic and non-cholinergic neurons. *Brain Res.* 598:249–256.

Oppenheim, R.W. (1991). Cell death during development of the nervous system. *Annu. Rev. Neurosci.* 14:453–501.

Oppenheim, R.W., Maderdrut, J.L., and Wells, D.J. (1982). Cell death of motoneurons of the chick embryo spinal cord. VI. Reduction of naturally occurring cell death in the thoracolumbar column of Terni by nerve growth factor. *J. Comp. Neurol.* 210:174–179.

Oppenheim, R.W., Prevette, D., Tytell, M., and Homma, S. (1990). Naturally occurring and induced neuronal death in the chick embryo in vivo requires protein and RNA synthesis: Evidence for the role of cell death genes. *Dev. Biol.* 138:104–113.

Perry, V.H. (1981). Evidence for an amacrine cell system in the ganglion cell layer of the rat retina. *Neuroscience* 6:931–944.

Perry, V.H., and Cowey, A. (1979). The effects of unilateral cortical and tectal lesions on retinal ganglion cells in rats. *Exp. Brain Res.* 35:97–108.

Radius, R.L., and Anderson, D.R. (1978). Retinal ganglion cell degeneration in experimental optic atrophy. *Am. J. Ophthalmol.* 86:673–679.

Reis, D.J., Gilad, G., Pickel, V.M., and Joh, T.H. (1978). Reversible changes in the activities and amounts of tyrosine hydroxylase in dopamine neurons of the substantia nigra in response to axonal injury as studied by immunochemical and immunocytochemical methods. *Brain Res.* 144:325–342.

Ruit, K.G., Osborne, P.A., Schmidt, R.E. Johnson, E.M., Jr., and Snider, W.D. (1990). Nerve growth factor regulates sympathetic ganglion cell morphology and survival in the adult mouse. *J. Neurosci.* 10:2412–2419.

Rydel, R.E., and Greene, L.A. (1988). Cyclic AMP analogues promote survival and neurite outgrowth in cultures of rat sympathetic and sensory neurons independently of nerve growth factor. *Proc. Natl. Acad. Sci. U.S.A.* 85:1257–1261.

Savill, I., Dransfield, I., Hogg, N., and Haslett, C. (1990). Vitronectin receptor-mediated phagocytosis of cells undergoing apoptosis. *Nature* 343:170–173.

Scott, S.A., and Davies, A.M. (1990). Inhibition of protein synthesis prevents cell death in sensory and parasympathetic neurons deprived of neurotrophic factor in vitro. *J. Neurobiol.* 21:630–638.

Sendtner, M., Kreutzberg G.W., and Thoenen, H. (1990). Ciliary neurotrophic factor prevents the degeneration of motor neurons after axotomy. *Nature* 345:440–441.

Sievers J., Hausmann, B., Unsicker, K., and Berry, M. (1987). Fibroblast growth factors promote the survival of adult rat retinal ganglion cells after transection of the optic nerve. *Neurosci. Lett.* 76:157–162.

Sievers J., Hausmann, B., and Berry, M. (1989). Fetal brain grafts rescue adult retinal ganglion cells from axotomy-induced cell death. *J. Comp. Neurol.* 281:467–478.

Sofroniew, M.V., and Isacson, O. (1988). Distribution of degeneration of cholinergic neurons in the septum following axotomy in different portions of the fimbria-fornix: A correlation between degree of cell loss and proximity of neuronal somata to the lesion. *J. Chem. Neuroanat.* 1:327–337.

Strautman, A.F., Cork, R.J., and Robinson, K.R. (1990). The distribution of free calcium in transected spinal axons and its modulation by applied electrical fields. *J. Neurosci.* 10:3564–3575.

Taniuchi, M., Clark, H.B., Johnson, E.M. Jr. (1986). Induction of nerve growth factor receptor in Schwann cells after axotomy. *Proc. Natl. Acad. Sci. U.S.A.* 83:4094–4098.

Thanos, S., and Aguayo, A.J. (1988). Changes in dendrites of adult rat ganglion cells regenerating axons into peripheral grafts. In *Post-Lesion Neural Plasticity*, ed. H. Flohr, 129–138, Berlin: Springer-Verlag.

Thanos, S., Bahr, M., Barde, Y.-A., and Vanselow, J. (1989). Survival and axonal elongation of adult rat retinal ganglion cells. In vitro effects of lesioned sciatic nerve and brain-derived neurotrophic factor. *Eur. J. Neurosci.* 1:19–26.

Thoenen, H. (1991). The changing scene of neurotrophic factors. *Trends Neurosci.* 14:165–170.

Tsai, G., Stauch, B.L., Vornov, J.J., Deshpande, J.K., and Coyle, J.T. (1990). Selective release of N-acetylaspartylglutamate from rat optic nerve terminal in vivo. *Brain Res.* 518:313–316.

Turner, J.E., Blair, J.R., and Chappel, E.T. (1987). Peripheral nerve implants effects on survival of retinal ganglion layer cells after axotomy initiated by a penetrating lesion. *Brain Res.* 419:46–54.

Tuszynski, M.H., Armstrong, D.M., and Gage, F.H. (1990). Basal forebrain cell loss following fimbria/fornix transection. *Brain Res.* 508:241–248.

Vidal-Sanz, M., Villegas-Pérez, M.P., Bray, G.M., and Aguayo, A.J. (1988). Persistent retrograde labelling of adult rat retinal ganglion cells with the carbocyanine dye, diI. *Exp. Neurol.* 102:92–101.

Vidal-Sanz, M., Bray, G.M., and Aguayo, A.J., (1991). Regenerated synapses persist in the superior colliculus after the regrowth of retinal ganglion cell axons. *J. Neurocytol.* 20:940–952.

Villegas-Pérez, M.P., Vidal-Sanz, M., Bray, G.M., and Aguayo, A.J. (1988a). Influences of peripheral nerve grafts on the survival and regrowth of axotomized retinal ganglion cells in adult rats. *J. Neurosci.* 8:265–280.

Villegas-Pérez, M.P., Vidal-Sanz, M., Bray, G.M., and Aguayo, A.J. (1988b). Retinal ganglion cell (RGC) death after axotomy is influenced by the distance between the lesion and the neuronal somata. *Soc. Neurosci. Abstr.* 14:673.

Walicke, P.A. (1989). Novel neurotrophic factors, receptors, and oncogenes. *Annu. Rev. Neurosci.* 12:103–126.

Weiss, J.H., Koh, J.-Y., Baimbridge, K.G., and Choi, D.W. (1990). Cortical neurons containing somatostatin- or parvalbumin-like immunoreactivity are atypically vulnerable to excitotoxic injury in vitro. *Neurology* 40:1288–1292.

Williams, L.R., Varon, S., Peterson, G.M., Wictorin, K., Fischer, W., Björklund, A., and Gage, F. (1986). Continuous infusion of nerve growth factor prevents basal forebrain neuronal death after fimbria fornix transection. *Proc. Natl. Acad. sci. U.S.A.* 83:9231–9235.

Wyllie, A.H., Kerr, J.F.R., and Currie, A.R. (1980). Cell death: The significance of apoptosis. *Int. Rev. Cytol.* 68:251–306.

Yip, H.K., Rich, K.M., Lampe, P.A., and Johnson, E.M. (1984). The effects of nerve growth factor and its antiserum on the postnatal development and survival after injury of sensory neurons in rat dorsal root ganglia. *J. Neurosci.* 4:2986–2992.

Zwimpfer, T.J., Aguayo, A.J., and Bray, G.M. (1992). Synapse Formation and preferential distribution in the granule cell layer by regenerating vetinal ganglion cell axons guided to the cerebellum of adult hamsters. *J. Neurosci.* 12:1144–1159.

4 Role of Neurotrophic Factors in the Plasticity of the Mammalian Visual System

Lamberto Maffei, Nicoletta Berardi, Giorgio Carmignoto, Alessandro Cellerino, Luciano Domenici, Adriana Fiorentini, and Tommaso Pizzorusso

The classic investigations of Wiesel and Hubel (1963) demonstrated many years ago that binocularity of cortical striate neurons is very vulnerable. Monocular deprivation in mammals during early life (critical period) renders neurons of the striate cortex largely unresponsive to visual stimulation of the deprived eye, shifting ocular dominance distribution in favor of the eye receiving normal visual input. In addition, the deprived eye becomes amblyopic, i.e., visual acuity is dramatically impaired and contrast sensitivity depressed. The eye which sees wins and dominates the cortical input and the eye which does not loses and its input to the cortical cell becomes permanently negligible or ineffective.

The effects of monocular deprivation have usually been ascribed to competition between the visual inputs from the two eyes on the cortical binocular cells (Wiesel and Hubel, 1963). At the level of the cortical neuron, competition is between incoming trains of electrical nervous impulses. Synapses that receive stronger or better organized electrial messages become functionally and structurally stronger.

It is not yet well known how a stronger electrical message achieves this effect. Structural synaptic changes are expected to occur. The synaptic strengthening as an activity-dependent reward is a notion introduced by the Canadian psychologist D.O. Hebb (Hebb, 1949). He also favored a structural explanation of this effect, writing, "When one cell repeatedly assists in firing another, the axon of the first cell develops synaptic knobs (or enlarges them if they already exist) in contact with the ... second cell" (Hebb, 1949, p. 63).

The strengthening of synaptic contacts could be based on the acquisition of a trophic factor from the target cell. According to this hypothesis the lateral geniculate input to the cortical cell driven by the deprived eye could be insufficient or inappropriate for the production or release of a trophic factor from the cortical cell or uptake by the afferent fibers. The synapses driven by the deprived input would lose anatomical or functional grip on the cortical cell and eventually become ineffective, causing two main consequences: (1) a large percentage of cells become monocular, and (2) the cells that remain responsive to the deprived eye strongly deteriorate in visual resolution and contrast sensitivity.

Previous experiments (Carmignoto et al., 1989; Maffei et al., 1990) of our group had shown that nerve growth factor (NGF) is effective in partly preventing degeneration of axotomized retinal ganglion cells in the rat. In addition, the presence of NGF and NGF receptors in the visual system of the rat, particularly during early life, has been described. Thus NGF was taken as the neurotrophic factor to be tested. We supplied it exogenously in monocularly deprived (MD) rats or cats during the critical period, either intraventricularly or by local application onto the striate binocular visual cortex, with the idea that the large availability of NGF would prevent competition between the two visual inputs, and therefore hinder the effects of monocular deprivation. The following results have been obtained:

1. Application of NGF prevents the shift in ocular dominance distribution in the neurons of the visual cortex of the MD rat.

2. Application of NGF prevents the loss in visual acuity and contrast sensitivity in the deprived eye of rats as tested by visual evoked potentials in response to gratings of various spatial frequencies and contrasts.

3. Application of NGF prevents the shrinkage of lateral geniculate cells which usually follows monocular deprivation in rats.

4. Application of NGF injected intraventricularly during the critical period of MD kittens largely preserves visual acuity of the deprived eye, as tested with behavioral experiments.

METHODS

Forty-two Long Evans hooded rats were used. Eight rats served as controls. Thirty-four rats were monocularly deprived for 1 month by means of eyelid sutures starting immediately after eye opening (postnatal day 14, P14). In 17 rats only monocular deprivation was performed. Deprivation was combined with intraventricular injection of a solution containing β-NGf (1.0–1.6 $\mu g/\mu l$ in buffered saline). Injections were repeated every 2 days for a period of 1 month with a standard method (Vantini et al., 1989). The volume injected was 2 μl. Eyelid suture and intraventricular injections were performed under ether anesthesia.

Electrophysiology

At the end of the critical period we recorded single units and visual evoked potentials (VEPs) with a glass micropipette inserted in the binocular portion of area 17 of the visual cortex. Two of the NGF-treated rats were recorded during the treatment (P42) to evaluate possible transient effects of NGF on neuronal electrical activity. All rats were anesthetized in urethane (6 ml/kg, 20% solution, Sigma Chemical, St. Louis) by peritoneal injection.

In single cell recording visual stimuli consisted of light bars projected on a reflecting tangent screen. On isolating a cell, the location of the receptive field

    Cells and Molecules that Influence Neuronal Survival

in the visual field and the optimal stimulus orientation were determined. Only cells with receptive fields within the binocular visual field were included in our sample. The ocular dominance and the receptive field type were then assessed with bars of optimal orientation according to standard criteria.

In VEP experiments, the visual stimuli were vertical gratings of different spatial frequencies generated on a display (HP 1300A, mean luminance 12 cd/m^2). The gratings were alternated in phase with a fixed temporal frequency (2–4 Hz). The signals were filtered and amplified in a conventional manner, computer-averaged, and analyzed. For each condition (visual cortex, viewing eye, spatial frequency, contrast), at least 400 responses were averaged. For the temporal frequency employed, the signals consisted mainly of the second harmonic. For this reason, the amplitude of the second harmonic (one half of the peak-to-trough amplitude) was taken as the amplitude of VEP for that condition.

To assess the spatial resolution value (visual acuity), gratings of maximum available contrast were used (70%); the spatial frequency was increased progressively until the signal was indistinguishable from background. The visual acuity was taken as the highest spatial frequency still evoking a reliable response.

Anatomy

In the lateral geniculate nucleus (LGN) of the rat there is no obvious lamination apparent in the cytoarchitecture. To reveal the ipsilateral LGN laminae which project exclusively to the binocular portion of the rat visual cortex, a tracer transported anterograde (horseradish peroxidase, HRP) was injected into one eye of MD rats. At the end of the critical period, in four MD untreated and four MD treated rats, 10 μl of a 30% HRP solution (HRP grade I, dissolved in 2% solution of dimethyl sulfoxide, DMSO) was injected through a pipette into the deprived eye. The animals were perfused after 24 to 36 hours' survival with a solution of 1.2% formaldehyde (from freshly prepared paraformaldehyde) and 2% glutaraldehyde (in 0.1M phosphate buffer, pH 7.4). The brain was removed and postfixed for 4 hours in the same solution. Coronal sections were cut by a vibratome and reacted using phenylenediamine as a chromogen (Cowey and Perry, 1979). The sections were successively counterstained with cresyl violet. Following this protocol, the LGN lamina ipsilateral to the injected deprived eye resulted in a patch of terminals surrounding stained perikarya, while the LGN lamina ipsilateral to the nondeprived eye contained cresyl violet–stained cells without HRP-labeled terminals. Cell soma sizes were calculated by a computer program from drawings of the cell soma outline made on a graphic tablet and fed into the computer. For each rat brain, we measured the soma size of cells in the LGN lamina ipsilateral to each eye. For each LGN lamina, the median of the soma size distribution was calculated.

Behavioral Experiments

Three kittens were treated intraventricularly with NGF and monocularly deprived for 2 weeks during their critical period (days 40–55 or 55–70). One kitten was monocularly deprived (days 58–73) and left untreated. Soon after the beginning of monocular deprivation, the kittens were trained using the jumping stand procedure (Mitchell et al., 1977) to make forced choice discriminations of a high contrast grating from a uniform gray of the same mean luminance, using their undeprived eye. Daily measures of visual acuity were then performed using high contrast gratings of increasing spatial frequency. After opening the eyelids of the deprived eye, visual acuity was measured monocularly with the undeprived eye and with the previously deprived eye on alternate days.

RESULTS

1. *Intraventricular injections of NGF prevent the shift in ocular dominance of cortical cells induced by monocular deprivation.* In the rat, the binocular visual cortex covers an area of the upper visual field which extends approximately 40 degrees from the vertical meridian. The ocular dominance distribution for normal rats is reported in figure 4.1,A. The percentage of binocular cells is quite high (80%) and comparable to that described for cats or monkeys. There is a clear dominance of the contralateral eye (classes 1, 2, and 3) which is due to the predominance in the rat of the crossed optic fibers. In rats monocularly deprived for the whole critical period, which extends up to P45, the number of binocular cells is reduced (43% of the total). The proportion of cells driven by the contralateral eye falls to 16% while the nondeprived (ipsilateral) eye dominates exclusively or predominantly (65% of the cells in our sample) (figure 4.1,B).

By contrast, the ocular dominance distribution of MD rats treated with NGF (figure 4.1,C) is practically indistinguishable from the ocular dominance distribution of normal rats.

Figure 4.1 Ocular dominance distribution compiled from single neuron responses recorded in the primary visual cortex of normal rats (*A*, 110 cells), monocularly deprived (MD) rats (*B*, 117 cells), and MD rats treated with intraventricular injections of NGF (*C*, 119 cells). Recordings were made in the hemisphere contralateral to the deprived eye. Neurons in ocular dominance class 1 were driven only by the stimulation of the contralateral eye; neurons in ocular dominance classes 2 and 3 were binocular and driven preferentially by the contralateral eye; neurons in ocular dominance class 4 were driven equally by the two eyes; neurons in ocular dominance classes 5 and 6 were binocular and driven preferentially by the ipsilateral eye, and neurons in ocular dominance class 7 were driven only by the ipsilateral eye. The category labeled *NC* contains those neurons that could not be classified using visual stimuli. A χ^2 test, 4 df, was used to evaluate the differences between the ocular dominance distributions. The distributions for the deprived untreated animals and for the deprived cytochrome *c*–treated animals differed significantly from the distribution in normal rats ($p < .001$) and in MD NGF-treated rats ($p < .001$). No significant difference was found between the ocular dominance distribution in normal and in MD NGF-treated rats ($p < .005$).

Cells and Molecules that Influence Neuronal Survival

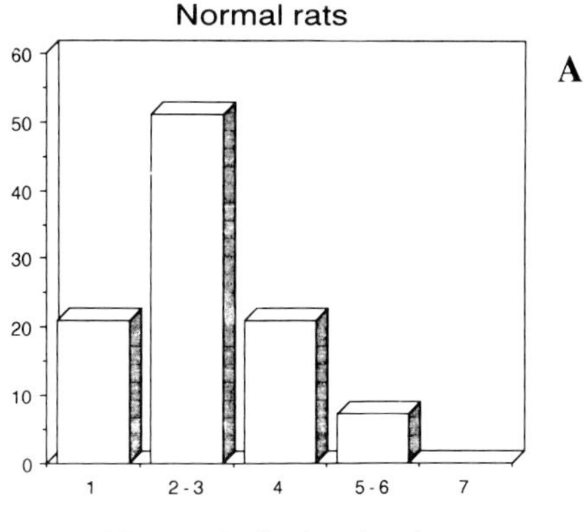

Normal rats
A
60
50
40
30
20
10
0
1
2 - 3
4
5 - 6
7

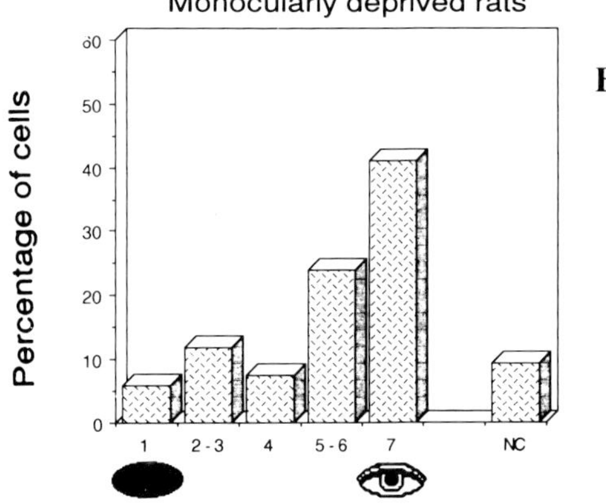

Monocularly deprived rats
B
60
50
40
30
20
10
0
Percentage of cells
1
2 - 3
4
5 - 6
7
NC

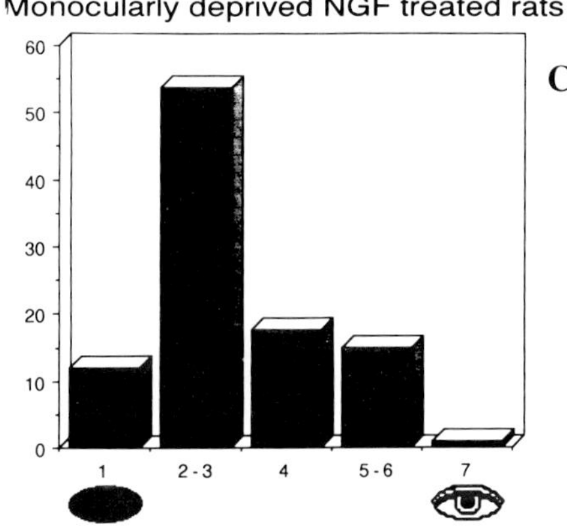

Monocularly deprived NGF treated rats
C
60
50
40
30
20
10
0
1
2 - 3
4
5 - 6
7
Class of ocular dominance

The ocular dominance distribution of MD rats treated with cytochrome C during the critical period does not differ from that of untreated MD rats.

2. NGF prevents the amblyopic effects due to monocular deprivation. Monocular deprivation during the critical period, in addition to shifting ocular dominance of cortical cells, also prevents a normal development of contrast sensitivity and visual acuity in the deprived eye. A way of assessing contrast sensitivity and visual acuity in man and in animals is to use the technique of evoked potentials (VEP) introduced by Campbell and Maffei (1970), in response to gratings of various spatial frequency and contrast.

The curve relating VEP amplitude to stimulus spatial frequency in the rat is shown in figure 4.2. The visual acuity estimated from evoked potentials is 1.2 cycles per degree, in keeping with visual acuity estimated with behavioral methods (Silveira et al., 1987). The dramatic effects of 1 month of monocular deprivation are shown in figure 4.2, where the mean VEP amplitudes for both the deprived and the nondeprived eye are shown as a function of the stimulus spatial frequency. Data for the ipsilateral and contralateral cortex are plotted separately. For the MD eye, visual acuity is reduced to approximately one third. In rats with intraventricular NGF injections the effects of monocular

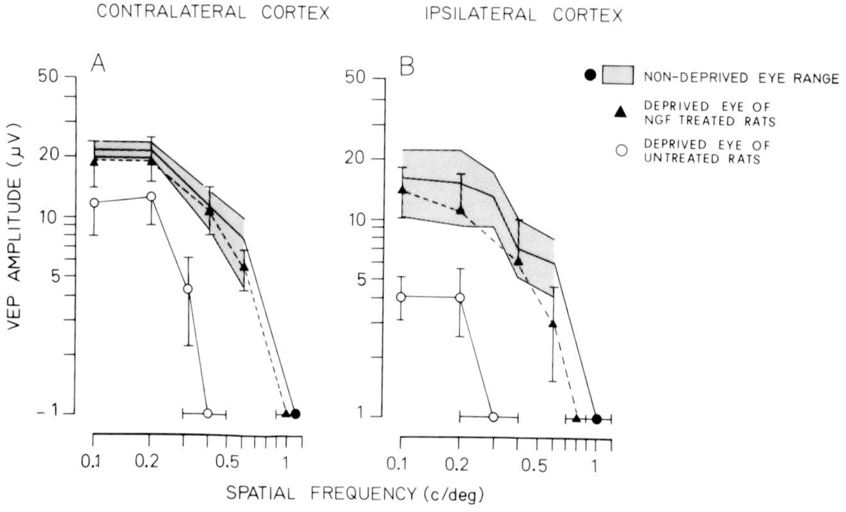

Figure 4.2 Effects of monocular deprivation on visual evoked potentials (VEPs) recorded in untreated rats and NGF-treated rats. The mean VEP amplitude is reported as a function of the stimulus spatial frequency in cycles per degree. The contrast of the visual stimuli was 30% to 40% but in the monocularly deprived (MD) rats it was 40% to 50%. *A*, VEPs recorded in the cortex contralateral to the stimulated eye. *B*, VEPs recorded in the cortex ipsilateral to the stimulated eye. The *shaded area* is the range found for the VEP amplitude in response to stimulation of the nondeprived eye (n = 7) in mean values (*inner solid line*) plus 1 SD. *Solid triangles* = mean VEP amplitude for the deprived eyes of NGF-treated rats (n = 8); *open circles,* mean VEP amplitude for the deprived eyes of untreated rats (n = 8); *Vertical bars,* standard deviation. The symbols on the abscissa correspond to the mean visual acuity, i.e., the highest spatial frequency still able to evoke a reliable signal with maximum contrast. *Solid circles,* normal eyes; *solid triangles,* deprived eyes of NGF-treated rats; *open circles,* deprived eyes of untreated rats; *horizontal bars,* standard deviation. The mean noise level was 2 µV, SD-1.

   Cells and Molecules that Influence Neuronal Survival

deprivation are clearly weaker, and even absent in some cases (see figure 4.2) (Domenici et al., 1991).

Control experiments in which cytochrome C was injected intraventricularly during monocular deprivation showed that the injection of this protein, which has some biochemical characteristics similar to NGF, has no effect in preventing the amblyopia induced by monocular deprivation.

The NGF treatment also prevents the loss in contrast sensitivity resulting from monocular deprivation. The contrast threshold for various spatial frequencies was measured in two MD rats and in two MD rats treated with NGF. The contrast thresholds estimated electrophysiologically using evoked potentials and behavioral methods are very similar. In the deprived eye the contrast thresholds, by any estimation, are markedly depressed. In MD animals treated with NGF, the contrast thresholds are practically normal.

3. Intraventricular injections of NGF prevent the shrinkage of the neurons in the deprived laminae of the LGN. One month of monocular deprivation causes a clear change in the neuronal soma size distribution of the LGN-deprived lamina. Most of the cells shift toward smaller sizes and the averaged median of the soma size distribution is significantly decreased with respect to the averaged median of the LGN-undeprived lamina (n-4; two-tailed *t*-test for paired observations *p*-.01). This is documented in figure 4.3, A, which plots the mean soma size distribution for the ipsilateral deprived LGN lamina (open columns).

By contrast, 1 month of NGF treatment completely prevents the shrinkage of neurons in the LGN-deprived lamina. Indeed, the soma size distributions for the deprived and undeprived LGN lamina overlap extensively (figure 4.3, B) and the difference between the averaged medians is not significant (two-tailed *t*-test for paired observations, *P*-.05).

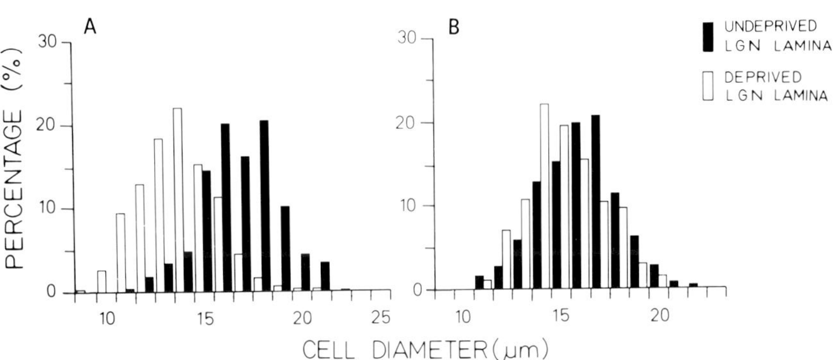

Figure 4.3 Cell soma size distribution in the lateral geniculate nucleus (LGN) of monocularly deprived rats untreated *(A)* and treated *(B)* with NGF. The percentage (%) of cells has been plotted as a function of cell diameter (µm) for the LGN-deprived laminae (*open columns*) and the LGN-undeprived laminae (*solid columns*). A, Data from 700 cells (320 in the deprived and 380 in the undeprived laminae). B, Data from 650 cells (320 in the deprived and 330 in the undeprived laminae).

The protocol employed does not differentiate the effect of monocular deprivation on LGN relay neurons from those on interneurons. In the rat the latter only represent 20% of the LGN neurons. To fill this gap we performed a double labeling experiment. The outcome of this experiment together with the previous data allows the conclusion that NGF treatment rescues from atrophy the neurons of those parts of LGN-deprived laminae which project to the binocular portion of the visual cortex.

Control Experiments

To make sure that the effects of NGF were not due to irritative phenomena or pathological processes, the following observations were collected.

• The behavior of NGF-treated rats was in no way different from that of normal animals. The same was true for the NGF-treated kittens used in the behavioral experiments.

• Spontaneous activity of visual cortical neurons was measured at various times after injection of NGF in rats. No significant variation in spontaneous activity was found. In experimental NGF-treated and control animals and in both normal and MD animals, the spontaneous discharge was always on the average of the order of seven impulses per second.

• The orientation tuning curve of cortical cells in rats in response to stimuli of various orientations was also measured. No change was observed under the influence of NGF. The width of the orientation tuning curve was, on average $\pm$ 50 to 60 degrees.

• A possible interaction of exogenous NGF with the cholinergic input to the visual cortex was examined by measuring choline acetyltransferase (ChAT) activity in the visual cortices of MD rats treated either with NGF ($n = 10$) or cytochrome c ($n = 5$). With the amount of NGF supply we employed, the ChAT activity in the visual cortex of NGF-treated rats was not significantly different from that found in cytochrome C–treated rats or in normal rats (Domenici et al., 1991).

4. *Behavioral visual acuity in MD kittens treated with NGF.* These experiments were performed in MD kittens treated with NGF or with cytochrome C. In two of the MD NGF-treated kittens monocular deprivation did not appreciably affect the visual acuity of the deprived eye. During the training period following eye opening, the acuity of the deprived eye (open circles in figure 4.4) improved progressively, approximately at the same rate as the acuity of the normal eye (solid circles), though lagging somewhat behind it. But at the end of the testing period the acuity of the deprived eye had reached the same level as the normal eye. This contrasts with the behavior of untreated MD kittens: in these animals the acuity of the deprived eye remains lower than that of the undeprived eye during a testing period of 1 month or longer following eye opening. We confirmed this finding in the untreated MD kitten, in which monocular deprivation from 58 to 73 days from birth resulted in a 39% reduction in acuity of the deprived eye with respect to the normal eye.

   Cells and Molecules that Influence Neuronal Survival

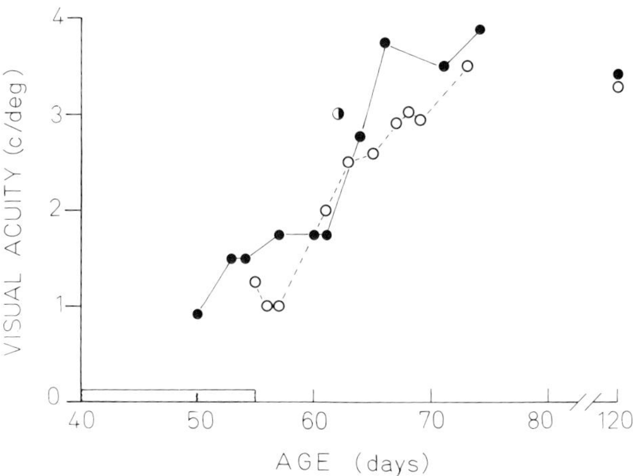

Figure 4.4 Visual acuity in cycles per degree measured in daily sessions in a kitten treated intraventricularly with NGF and monocularly deprived from 40 to 55 days of age. Training with the behavioral technique began during the treatment, using the undeprived eye. Monocular visual acuities of the normal eye (*solid circles*) and of the deprived eye (*open circles*) were measured daily for 20 days after the end of treatment, and again 2 months after eye opening. The *half-solid circle* indicates binocular acuity.

One of the three NGF-treated animals, however, showed a clear reduction (29%) of acuity in its deprived eye, not dissimilar to that found in untreated MD animals. This kitten was from the same litter as another NGF-treated cat, and received exactly the same treatement and the same behavioral training. Although we have no explanation for this difference, the positive results obtained in two NGF-treated kittens prove that a plentiful supply of this neurotrophic factor in the visual cortex during the critical period can prevent the deterioration of behavioral visual acuity otherwise expected in the deprived eye.

DISCUSSION

The electrophysiological and anatomical results that we have reported for the rat and the behavioral experiments in the cat converge to the conclusion that local application of NGF on the visual cortex or an intraventricular injection of NGF largely prevents the amblyopic effects of monocular deprivation and their underlying neuronal events. A tacit assumption of our working hypothesis is that NGF is produced in the target structure. Indeed, NGF and NGF receptors are present in the rat and in the primate visual cortex both in newborns and in adults (Large et al., 1986; Hayashi et al., 1990; Pioro and Cuello, 1990). The content of NGF in the visual cortex is higher during the first part of the critical period, and then decreases to adult values that are of the order of less than 1 ng/g of nervous tissue.

Whether the source of NGF is neuronal or glial is not known. Astrocytes are known to produce NGF in vitro (Vige and Wise, 1990; Lindsay, 1979). In

   Maffei et al.: Role of Neurotrophic Factors

the hippocampus kainic acid lesions, which spare glial cells, abolish the content of messenger RNA for NGF (Ayer-Lalièvre et al., 1988).

For the moment we cannot speculate on the mechanism of action of NGF at the cellular level, nor can we be confident that NGF is *the* neurotrophic factor or the *only* neurotrophic factor in question. The presence of NGF is not *in itself* evidence that NGF is the only neurotrophic factor. The NGF receptors can be distinguished by low and high affinity binding classes. It is the high affinity receptor which is thought to mediate NGF responses. It has been shown that brain-derived neurotrophic factor (BDNF) and neurotrophin-3 (NT-3) at high concentrations can interact with NGF high affinity receptor, and vice versa (Rodriguez-Tébar et al., 1990). (It has to be noted, however, that NT-3 is highly expressed only in the early stages of development [Maisonpierre et al., 1990a]). The amounts of NGF that we have used are very large, of the order of 1 μg. It may well be that these large amounts of NGF have mimicked the action of other neurotrophic factors of the NGF family such as the BDNF or NT-3 which have a rather similar structure at the DNA and protein level (Maisonpierre et al., 1990b; Ernfors et al., 1990).

We emphasize that the aim of our experiments was not to elucidate the precise nature of the neurotrophic factor, but rather to investigate whether the neurotrophic hypothesis (namely the theory that during development the patterns of neural connections are regulated, at least in part, by neurotrophic signals that derive from the targets) is appropriate for explaining the effects of monocular deprivation.

The hypothesis that the two visual inputs could compete for a neurotrophic factor, the production of which is activity-dependent, is not a theory in a mathematical sense but rather, as Purves writes, "A word that is used in its primary sense of a contemplation of what might be the case" (Purves, 1988). The aim of the hypothesis is to draw attention to this important biological strategy—neurotrophic interaction at the level of the visual system—and possibly to dismiss it experimentally with a more suitable working hypothesis.

So far what we have tried to show is that the effects that we have observed are physiological in nature and not due to irritation or possible direct or indirect pathological actions of NGF. The fact that the spontaneous activity and the responses of cortical cells remain within normal physiological ranges, together with the results of the behavioral experiments in the cat showing that visual performance remains normal, seem to make this possibility rather unlikely.

There are two other hypotheses for the mechanism of action of NGF, which also turn out to be rather unlikely.

1. Treatment with NGF could interfere with the normal development of the visual system, particularly of the visual cortex. To test this point we have studied the functional properties of visual cortical cells at the beginning and at the end of the critical period of control and NGF-treated rats. It has been found that the ocular dominance distribution, orientation tuning, and spatial

     Cells and Molecules that Influence Neuronal Survival

frequency properties of cortical visual neurons are not affected by NGF provided exogenously.

2. The effects of NGF could be indirect, mediated via cholinergic neurons. The visual cortex receives a cholinergic input from the basal forebrain (NBM) (Dinopoulos et al., 1989), and NGF receptor immunoreactivity in the visual cortex (as determined with antibody IgG192) is consistent with the pattern of cholinergic afferents (Pioro and Cuello, 1990). NGF could activate the cholinergic system and thus increase the cholinergic input onto visual neurons. It has been shown that NGF intraventricular injections increase ChAT activity in the basal ganglia (Gnahn et al., 1983).

An increase of the cholinergic input onto visual neurons, however, is not necessarily expected to decrease cortical plasticity and thus prevent ocular dominance shift. Indeed, the contrary has been reported in the literature: a lesion to cholinergic afferents to visual cortical neurons is required to decrease visual cortical plasticity (Bear and Singer, 1986). In addition, variation in the cholinergic input to cortical cells, either excitatory or inhibitory, is expected to affect the spontaneous discharge and the responsiveness and orientation selectivity of visual cortical neurons (Sato et al., 1987). We have failed to observe these effects.

To assess further the point of action of NGF on visual cortical plasticity through the cholinergic input, ChAT activity was measured in the visual cortex of NGF-treated rats. We found that ChAT activity is not significantly changed by NGF treatment.

Unfortunately, we cannot offer any clear and conclusive explanation of the mechanism of NGF in the plasticity of the visual system. The possibility that NGF, or a neurotrophic factor of the NGF family, preserves the functional input from the deprived eye through a specific direct trophic action on visual neurons remains a valid working hypothesis. The specific trophic action and the mechanism of NGF at the cellular level remain open questions.

REFERENCES

Ayer-Lelièvre, C., Olson, L., Ebendal, T., Seiger A. and Persson, H. (1988). Expression of the β-nerve growth factor gene in hippocampal neurons. *Science 240*: 1339–1441.

Bear, M.F. and Singer, W. (1986). Modulation of visual cortical plasticity by acetylcholine and noradrenaline. *Nature 320*: 172–176.

Campbell, F.W., and Maffei, L. (1970). Electrophysiological evidence for the existence of orientation in size detectors in the human visual system. *J. Physiol. (Lond.) 207*: 635–652.

Carmignoto, G., Candeo, C., Canella, R., Comelli, C, and Maffei, L. (1989). Effect of NGF on the survival of retinal ganglion cells after section of the optic nerve. *J. Neurosci. 9*: 1263–1273.

Cowey, A., and Perry, V.H. (1979). The projection of the temporal retina in rats, studied by retrograde transport of horseradish peroxidase. *Exp. Brain Res. 35*: 457–464.

Dinopoulos, A., Eadie, L.A., Dori, I., and Parnavelas, J.G. (1989). The development of basal projections to the rat visual cortex. *Exp. Brain Res. 76*: 563–571.

Domenici, L., Berardi, N., Carmignoto, G., Vantini, G., and Maffei, L. (1991). Nerve growth factor prevents the amblyopic effects of monocular deprivation *Proc. Natl. Acad. Sci.* 88:8811–8815.

Ernfors, P., Ibanez C.F., Ebendal, T., Olson, L., and Persson, H. (1990). Molecular cloning and neurotrophic activities of a protein with structural similarities to nerve growth factor: Developmental and topographical expression in the brain. *Proc. Natl. Acad. Sci. U.S.A.* 87:5454–5458.

Gnahn, H., Hefti, F., Heumann, R., Schwab, M.E., and Thoenen, H. (1983). NGF-mediated increase of choline acetyltransferase (ChAT) in the neonatal rat forebrain: Evidence for a physiological role of NGF in the brain?. *Dev. Brain Res.* 9:45–52.

Hayashi, M., Yamashita, A., and Shimizu K. (1990). Nerve growth factor in the primate central nervous system: Regional distribution and ontogeny. *Neuroscience* 36:683–689.

Hebb, D.O. (1949). *Organization of Behavior.* New York: John Wiley & Sons.

Large, T.H., Bodary, S.C., Clegg, D. O., Weskamp, G., Otten, U., and Reichardt, L.F. (1986). Nerve growth factor gene expression in the developing rat brain. *Science* 234:252–255.

Lindsay, R.M. (1979). Adult brain astrocytes support survival of both NGF-dependent and NGF-insensitive neurons. *Nature* 282:80–82.

Maffei, L., Carmignoto, G., Perry, V.H., Candeo, P., and Ferrari G. (1990). Schwann cells promote the survival of rat retinal ganglion cells after optic nerve section. *Proc. Natl. Acad. Sci. U.S.A.* 87:1855–1859.

Maisonpierre, P.C., Belluscio, L., Friedman, B., Alderson, R.F., Wiegand, S.J., Furth, M.E., Linday, R.M., and Yancopoulos, G.D. (1990a). NT-3, BDNF, and NGF in the developing rat nervous system: Parallel as well as reciprocal patterns of expression. *Neuron* 5:501–509.

Maisonpierre, P.C., Belluscio, L., Squinto, S., Ip, N.Y., Furth, M.E., Lindsay, R.M., and Yancopoulos, G.D. (1990b). Neurotrophin-3: A neurotrophic factor related to NGF and BDNF. *Science* 247:1446–1451.

Mitchell, D.E., Giffin, F., and Timney, B. (1977). A behavioural technique for the rapid assessment of the visual capabilities of kittens. *Perception* 6:181–193.

Pioro, E.P., and Cuello, A.C. (1990). Distribution of Nerve Growth Factor receptor-like immunoreactivity in the adult rat central nervous system. Effect of colchicine and correlation with the cholinergic system-I. Forebrain. *Neuroscience* 34:57–87.

Purves D. (1988). *Body and Brain.* Cambridge, Mass.: Harvard University Press.

Rodriguez-Tébar, A., Dechant, G., and Barde, Y.-A. (1990). Binding of brain-derived neurotrophic factor to the nerve growth factor receptor. *Neuron* 4:487–492.

Sato, H., Hata, Y., Masui, H., and Tsumoto, T. (1987). A functional role of cholinergic innervation to neurons in the cat visual cortex. *J. Neurophysiol.* 58:765–780.

Silveira, L.C.L., Heywood, C.A., and Cowey, A. (1987). Contrast sensitivity and visual acuity of the pigmented rat determined electrophysiologically. *Vision Res.* 27:1719–1731.

Vantini, G., Schiavo N., Di Martino, A., Polato, P., Triban, C., Callegaro, L., Toffano, G. and Leon, A. (1989). Evidence for a physiological role of nerve growth factor in the central nervous system of neonatal rats. *Neuron* 3:267–273.

Vige, X., and Wise, B.C., (1990). Mechanism of NGF mRNA regulation by interleukin 1 and basic FGF in rat astrocyte. *Soc. Neurosci. Abstr.* 16:132.10.

Wiesel, T.N., and Hubel, D.H. (1963). Single cell responses in striate cortex of kittens deprived of vision in one eye. *J. Neurophysiol.* 26:1003–1007.

   Cells and Molecules that Influence Neuronal Survival

III Molecular Mechanisms of Axonal Regeneration

5 Neuronal Interactions with the Extracellular Matrix that Regulate Axon Growth

Louis F. Reichardt

Extrinsic molecules regulate the differentiation of neurons and other cells in the embryonic nervous system. Among those are several classes of molecules that direct the establishment of specific axonal pathways early in development and regulate regeneration after neural injury. As illustrated in figure 5.1, these include neurotrophic factors, chemotrophic factors, Ca^{2+}-dependent and -independent cell adhesion molecules, extracellular matrix (ECM) constituents, and incompletely characterized glycoproteins that inhibit neurite outgrowth. The number of molecules in each of these classes has expanded dramatically in recent years (Yancopoulos et al., 1990; Hallbook et al., 1991; Placzek et al., 1990; O'Leary et al., 1990; Takeichi, 1991; Edelman and Cunningham, 1990; Grenningloh et al., 1990; Furley et al., 1990; Reichardt and Tomaselli, 1991; Schwab, 1990; Keynes and Cook, 1990).

Progress has been made recently in characterizing receptors for many of these molecules. Thus, the nerve growth factor (NGF)–related neurotrophic factors have been shown to utilize tyrosine kinases (trkA, trkB, or trkC) as ligand-binding, signal-transducing subunits (reviewed in Bothwell, 1991). Another class of trophic factors, including cholinergic differentiation factor (CDF) and ciliary neurotrophic factor, appear to be structurally similar to several interleukins and most likely utilize receptors and signal transduction pathways similar to those employed by these lymphokines (Bazan, 1991). Cell adhesion molecules interact in large part, but not exclusively, with other cell adhesion molecules (Takeichi, 1991; Edelman and Cunningham, 1990). Integrins have been identified as a large, prominent family of receptors for ECM constituents (Reichardt and Tomaselli, 1991). Progress has also been made in characterizing both chemotropic molecules and motility-inhibiting glycoproteins (Placzek et al., 1990; Keynes and Cook, 1990), making it seem probable that receptors for these molecules will be identified and characterized in the near future. At this point, it is clear that subclasses of neurons differ dramatically in their responses to individual members of each of these classes of molecules. Thus the expression patterns of these receptors seem likely to play critical roles in determining individual neuronal phenotypes. Clearly, characterizing these morphogenetic molecules and their receptors is important for understanding development of the nervous system.

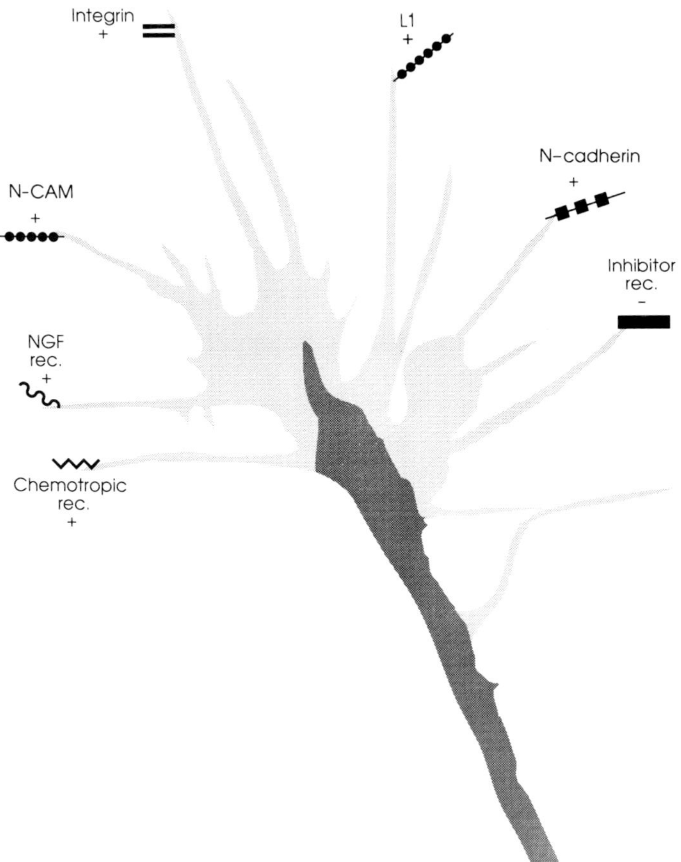

Figure 5.1 Schematic of examples of the major receptors that regulate growth cone movements. In a clockwise direction, a putative receptor for a chemotropic agent is depicted at lower left. There is convincing evidence that several proteins function as *chemotropic* molecules to direct growth cones (Placzek et al., 1990; O'Leary et al., 1990). While none of these have yet been completely purified, they must act by interaction with specific receptors. The nerve growth factor (*NGF*) receptor is illustrated as an example of a trophic factor receptor. Trophic factors regulate neuronal survival and differentiation. Evidence is reasonably convincing that they can both promote and direct growth cone movements. Recent work has shown that the tyrosine kinase (*trk*) family of proto-oncogenes are ligand-binding, signal-transducing subunits for NGF and related neurotrophins (Bothwell, 1991). The neural cell adhesion molecule (*N-CAM*) and *L1* are examples of a large number of Ca^{2+}-independent cell adhesion molecules expressed by neurons (Edelman and Cunningham, 1990). The *integrin* heterodimer is an example of the large number of distinct receptors of this class expressed by neurons (Reichardt and Tomaselli, 1991). *N-cadherin* is an example of the Ca^{2+}-dependent adhesion molecules expressed by neurons (Takeichi, 1991). To date, all Ca^{2+}-independent adhesion molecules, integrins, and cadherins appear to promote growth cone motility. The receptor depicted at *lower right* is a putative receptor for one of the proteins that inhibits growth cone movements, none of which has yet been completely characterized molecularly (Schwab, 1990; Keynes and Cook, 1990). *rec*, receptor; plus sign indicates that receptor activation promotes growth cone motility; minus sign indicates that receptor activation inhibits growth cone motility.

     Molecular Mechanisms of Axonal Regeneration

A major target for extrinsic molecules that regulate axon pathway formation is the growth cone, which constitutes the leading edge of the axon. Cell culture has been an important experimental tool for understanding how individual molecules affect growth cone behavior. In culture systems, neurotrophic factors have been shown to promote and direct axon growth (Campenot, 1977; Gundersen and Barrett, 1980). It has been possible to show that virtually all ECM glycoproteins and cell adhesion molecules promote growth by responsive axons (Reichardt et al., 1990). Cell culture has been essential for identifying chemotropic factors (Placzek et al., 1990; O'Leary et al., 1990) and glycoproteins that inhibit the motility of all or subsets of growth cones (Keynes and Cook, 1990; Schwab, 1990). Individual regulators of axon growth have been shown to have specific, developmentally regulated patterns of expression and localization within embryos. Several are localized at positions appropriate for exerting the same effects on growth cone behavior in vivo that are observed in vitro. It seems likely that the expression patterns of these molecules determine much of the circuitry of the nervous system. This chapter focuses on a subset of these, the constituents of the ECM.

THE EXTRACELLULAR MATRIX

Most nonneural cells secrete proteins that form an ECM (Sanes, 1989; Reichardt and Tomaselli, 1991). Recently, neurons have been shown to be a major source of at least one ECM glycoprotein, agrin (Rupp et al., 1991). Outside the central nervous system (CNS), the ECM typically includes one or more collagens, which helps organize the ECM into a morphologically visible entity. Additional constituents include adhesion-promoting glycoproteins. proteoglycans, and many growth or differentiation-promoting factors, such as fibroblast growth factor (FGF) and transforming growth factor β (TGF-β). Collagens do not appear to be present in the CNS, but several adhesion-promoting glycoproteins and proteoglycans have been detected there (O'Shea and Dixit, 1988; Neugebauer et al., 1991; Edelman and Cunningham, 1990; Hockfield et al., 1990; Herndon and Lander, 1990). These observations suggest that the ECM is comparatively poorly organized in the CNS, but functions to direct development there as well as in the peripheral nervous system.

ECM glycoproteins are typically large, multidomain proteins that span several hundred nanometers. Many potentially adhesive domains are found in these proteins, often in multiple copies, including fibronectin type I, II, and III repeats, epidermal growth factor (EGF) repeats, complement regulatory repeats, hyaluronic acid–binding motifs, Ca^{2+}-dependent lectinlike domains, and other structures (see Reichardt and Tomaselli, 1991). Single ECM glycoproteins or proteoglycans typically have domains representing several of these motifs. Major constituents of the ECM that stimulate neurite growth in vitro and are encountered by peripheral neurons in vivo include fibronectin, laminin, tenascin, thrombospondin and several collagens. While perturbation studies on neurite outgrowth in vivo are rare, antibodies to a laminin isoform clearly inhibit peripheral nerve regeneration in vivo (Sandrock and Matthew,

1987) and antibodies to each of these, with the exception of the collagens, have been shown to inhibit migration of neural crest cells (Perris and Bronner-Fraser, 1989). Fibronectin, tenascin, thrombospondin, and other adhesion-promoting glycoproteins are also detected within the CNS, where the major source of these molecules appears to be neuroepithelial cells in the early embryo and astroglia at later stages. Again, studies in vivo on neurite outgrowth are rare, but antibodies to tenascin and thrombospondin inhibit strongly the migration of granule cells across the molecular layer of the embryonic cerebellum (Edelman and Cunningham, 1990; O'Shea et al., 1990). The differential localizations of these molecules in vivo and observed responses of neurons to these same molecules in vitro suggest a role for each in establishing axon pathways and directing other events in development of neurons and glia (reviewed in Reichardt and Tomaselli, 1991).

NEURONAL RECEPTORS FOR THE EXTRACELLULAR MATRIX

Potential neuronal receptors for ECM constituents include integrin heterodimers, cell surface associated hyaluronic acid–binding proteins, proteoglycans, and galactosyltransferases. Integrins are a large family of receptors with noncovalently associated α- and β- subunits that form receptors for ECM glycoproteins, collagens, and some cell adhesion molecules. To date, seven β-subunits and 12 α-subunits have been characterized. Individual integrin heterodimers, many of which are present in the nervous system, are listed with their ligands in table 5.1 (Hemler, 1990). To date, only one cell surface receptor for hyaluronic acid, the homing-cell adhesion molecule-H-CAM (also named the Hermes antigen and CD-44), has been identified in the nervous system (Picker et al., 1989). H-CAM is localized on CNS glia and peripheral Schwann cells. It is uncertain whether it is expressed on embryonic neurons. Large numbers of proteoglycans, some of which are membrane-associated, are present in the nervous system (Hokfield et al., 1990; Herndon and Lander, 1990). There is unambiguous evidence that at least one proteoglycan, syndecan, can function as an ECM receptor, utilizing glycosaminoglycan side chains to bind cells to the ECM (Saunders et al., 1989). It is not yet certain whether syndecan is present in the nervous system. Evidence suggests, in particular, that proteoglycans may be one class of neuronal receptor for thrombospondin (Neugebauer et al., 1991). Galactosyltransferases are present on surfaces of many cells and functional evidence implicates them as receptors that regulate neuronal and neural crest cell responses to laminin (Begovac and Shur, 1990; Begovac et al., 1991).

Experiments in vitro using antibodies that inhibit the functions of integrin heterodimers have localized these proteins to the surfaces of neurons and provided convincing evidence that they are major receptors used by neurons to interact with the ECM (reviewed in Reichardt and Tomaselli, 1991). For example, interactions of embryonic chick retinal neurons with laminin, fibronectin, and several collagens are virtually eliminated by antibodies to the integrin β_1-subunit (Hall et al., 1987). Receptors containing the β_1-subunit

     Molecular Mechanisms of Axonal Regeneration

Table 5.1 Summary of Integrin Heterodimers and Their Ligands

Class	Mr	α Subunit	Mr	I domain	Ca/Mg sites	Cleaved	Ligands
β_1	115k	α_1	200k	+	3	−	COL, LN (E1)
		α_2	150k	+	3	−	COL, LN*
		α_3	150k	−	3	+	LN (E8), FN (RGD), col*
		α_4	140k	−	3	+/−	FN (CS-1), VCAM-1
		α_5	150k	−	4	+	FN (RGD)
		α_6	150k	−	3	+	LN (E8)
		α_7	150k	−	3	+	LN
		α_8	150k	−	3	+	?
		α_{VN}	150k	−	4	+	FN (RGD)*, VN*
β_2	90k	α_{LFA-1}	170k	+	3	−	ICAM-1, ICAM-2
		α_{Mac-1}	180k	+	3	−	C3bi, FG
		α_{p150}	150k	+	3	−	?
β_3	95k	α_{IIb}	136k	−	4	+	FN, VN, VWF, FG
		α_{VN}	150k	−	4	+	VN, TS, VWF, FG
β_4	205k	α_6	150k	−	3	+	?
β_5	90k	α_{VN}	150k	−	4	+	VN
β_6	95k	α_{VN}	150k	−	4	+	FN (RGD)
β_p	95k	α_4	140k	−	3	+/−	?
β_8	90k	α_{VN}	150k	−	4	+	?

Six integrin classes, distinguished by distinct but homologous β subunits, are shown. Each β subunit can associate noncovalently with a subgroup of homologous α subunits (see Hemler, 1990). The relative molecular weight (Mr) of each subunit is indicated. These values reflect relative mobilities compared to standards of the different subunits in SDS-polyacrylamide gel electrophoresis in nonreducing conditions. The I domain is a motif of approximately 200 amino acids that is present in many collagen-binding proteins and in a subset of integrin α subunits (see Hemler, 1990). Integrin α subunits contain three of four sites with homology to the Ca^{2+}-binding sites in calmodulin. The function of individual integrin heterodimers depends on the presence of Ca^{2+} or Mg^{2+}. The number of potential Ca^{2+}/Mg^{2+} binding sites identified in each α subunit is indicated. Some integrin α subunits are proteolytically cleaved during maturation. Both uncleaved and cleaved forms of the integrin α_4 subunit exist on the cell surface. For references, see Hemler (1990), Reichardt and Tomaselli (1991), Moyle et al. (1991), Bossy et al. (1991), and Song et al. (1992). Abbreviations: COL, collagen; (CS-1), CS-1 site in FN; c3bi, fragment b1 of complement component 3; (E1) and (E8), elastase fragments of LN; FG, fibrinogen; FN, fibronectin; ICAM, intercellular adhesion molecule; LN, laminin; (RGD), the cell attachment site with the sequence RGDS (arginine-glycine-aspartic acid-serine) in FN; TS, thrombospondin; VCAM, vascular cell adhesion molecule; VN, vitronectin; VWF, von Willebrand factor.
* Indicates ligands recognized by an integrin when the integrin is expressed in some, but not all cells.

  Reichardt: Neuronal Interactions with Extracellular Matrix

also help mediate interactions of these neurons with vitronectin and thrombospondin (Neugebauer et al., 1991). Other integrins not containing this subunit appear to mediate additional interactions of these neurons with vitronectin. In studies using peripheral neurons, including sensory, sympathetic, and ciliary neurons, integrins have also been shown to function as prominent ECM receptors (Bozyczko and Horwitz, 1986; Tomaselli et al., 1986; Tomaselli and Reichardt, 1988). Anti-integrin β_1-subunit–specific antibodies strongly inhibit adhesion and neurite outgrowth responses on laminin, fibronectin, and the collagens. In addition, the same antibodies virtually eliminate neurite outgrowth on several intact ECMs, including those deposited by Schwann cells, skeletal myotubes, and endothelial cells (Tomaselli et al., 1986). Thus integrins appear to be major receptors used by both central and peripheral neurons to interact with complex ECMs. While direct evidence is lacking, localization patterns suggest that some will prove to interact also with cell adhesion molecules (Bossy et al., 1991).

IDENTIFICATION OF INDIVIDUAL INTEGRIN RECEPTORS FOR PURIFIED ECM CONSTITUENTS

Since the integrin β_1-subunit associates with many distinct α-subunits, results utilizing β_1-subunit–specific antibodies are not sufficient to identify the expression patterns or functions of individual heterodimeric receptors on neurons. Three distinct assays have been used to identify functions of individual receptors on neuronal and non-neural cells. In one approach, α-subunit–specific antibodies have been used to detect expression and inhibit cellular interactions with purified ECM glycoproteins. With these reagents, we have identified two heterodimers—$\alpha_1\beta_1$ and $\alpha_3\beta_1$—as receptors used by PC12 cells and embryonic sensory neurons to interact with laminin (Tomaselli et al., 1990; Tomaselli et al., unpublished data). The two other known laminin receptors in the β_1-family, $\alpha_2\beta_1$ and $\alpha_6\beta_1$ do not appear to function on these cells, probably because they are not expressed at high levels. In similar studies on embryonic retinal neurons, significantly different results have been obtained. On these cells, the $\alpha_6\beta_1$- and $\alpha_3\beta_1$-heterodimers are both expressed as potential laminin receptors (de Curtis et al., 1991; de Curtis and Reichardt, unpublished data). Function-blocking antibodies to the α_6-subunit inhibit neurite outgrowth by these neurons on laminin. The $\alpha_1\beta_1$- and $\alpha_2\beta_1$-heterodimers do not appear to be expressed at significant levels on these neurons. Thus separate populations of neurons utilize different receptors to interact with the same ECM glycoprotein.

As a second approach, individual integrin heterodimers have been purified by affinity chromatography on single ECM glycoproteins. Exploiting the observation that integrin functions depend upon the presence of divalent cations (Ca^{2+} or Mg^{2+}), it has been possible to purify the $\alpha_1\beta_1$-heterodimer from neuroblastoma cells on laminin columns, showing directly that it is a receptor for this protein (Ignatius and Reichardt, 1988). Using other cells as sources for integrins, it has been possible to obtain similar, direct biochemical

     Molecular Mechanisms of Axonal Regeneration

evidence that the $\alpha_2\beta_1$- and $\alpha_3\beta_1$-heterodimers can interact directly with laminin (Gehlsen et al., 1989). It is intriguing that, the $\alpha_2\beta_1$-heterodimer's ability to bind laminin is regulated by cell-specific factors (Languino et al., 1989; Elices and Hemler, 1989). On some cells it functions as a dual laminin-collagen receptor; on others as a collagen receptor only. The ligand-binding specificity of the $\alpha_1\beta_1$-heterodimer, a close relative structurally to the $\alpha_2\beta_1$-heterodimer, may be regulated by similar factors. Results to date suggest that it may be a dual receptor for laminin and collagen in PC12 cells and sensory neurons, but only a collagen receptor in sympathetic neurons (Tomaselli et al., 1990 and unpublished data; Lein et al., 1991). For unknown reasons, affinity chromatography has not provided direct evidence that the $\alpha_6\beta_1$-heterodimer interacts with laminin. As a third approach, localization of individual hetero-dimers in the adhesion plaques of cells cultured on ECM substrates has provided results consistent with the ligand specificities of the same receptors as characterized in other assays. For example, the vitronectin receptor, but not the fibronectin receptor, is localized in adhesion plaques on vitronectin-coated substrates (Singer et al., 1988). Many integrins co-localize with basement membranes in vivo, indicating that they have ligands in these ECM structures (Sonnenberg et al., 1991). While not utilized to date, this approach may be useful in future studies on integrins in the nervous system.

REGULATION OF INTEGRIN RECEPTOR FUNCTIONS IN NEURONS

With cell adhesion and neurite outgrowth assays, it has been possible to show that neuronal interactions with several ECM constituents are regulated during development. Typically, integrin functions are down-regulated at approxi-mately the same time as a class of neurons innervates its targets. Some evidence suggests that manipulations that prevent or disrupt target contact prolong or reinduce, respectively, integrin functions. As one example, embry-onic chick ciliary neurons progressively lose functional laminin receptors between embryonic days 8 and 14 (Tomaselli and Reichardt, 1988). This correlates closely with the time course of functional innervation of the iris by these same neurons. When explanted for 2.5 days in vitro, ciliary neurons recover substantial integrin function. The results suggest that target contact may regulate integrin receptor expression or activity on these neurons.

In embryonic chick retina, neuronal interactions with fibronectin and laminin are strongly down-regulated during development between embryonic days 6 and 12 (Cohen et al., 1986; 1989; Hall et al., 1987). This occurs in retinal ganglion cells, which innervate the tectum during this same period (Cohen et al., 1986; 1989). Ablation of the optic tectum in early embryos has been reported to reduce subsequent down-regulation of integrin receptor function in the retinal ganglion cells (Cohen et al., 1989). We have had difficulty reproducing this result. If confirmed, though, it again would suggest that integrin functions can be regulated by target contact.

Mechanisms of integrin receptor regulation have been examined in detail in the retina. In the ganglion cells, there is at least a fivefold reduction in expression of the $\alpha_6\beta_1$-integrin, which is a functionally important laminin receptor on these cells (de Curtis et al., 1991). This reflects a similar reduction in α_6–messenger RNA (mRNA) levels in these source cells. Loss of laminin receptor function correlates with loss of receptors detected in binding assays, using ^{125}I-laminin (Cohen et al., 1989). To date, we have obtained no evidence that tectal ablation in early embryos enhances expression of α_6-mRNA or $\alpha_6\beta_1$-protein in older retinal ganglion cells, so it has not been possible to obtain more direct evidence that a signal from the optic tectum inhibits α_6-gene expression in the retinal ganglion cells.

The functions of laminin-binding integrins on other neuronal cells in the embryonic chick retina are down-regulated during development by distinct mechanisms. In binding assays using ^{125}I-labeled laminin, Cohen et al. (1989) detected a change in receptor affinity, but not number, in this neuronal population. In protein and mRNA assays, we have seen continued high expression of the α_6-gene's mRNA product and of the $\alpha_6\beta_1$-heterodimer on the surface of these cells (de Curtis et al., 1991). In quantitative assays, no significant differences could be detected in either assay. Since older neurons no longer bind laminin efficiently in attachment assays (Hall et al., 1987), receptor function must be lost by a posttranslational mechanism. Thus, unknown factors appear to be able to regulate the activities of surface integrins.

To obtain more direct evidence that integrins exist in more than one activity state on neuronal cell surfaces, we have isolated a monoclonal antibody, named TASC, that binds the β_1-subunit and activates the ligand-binding functions of many integrins containing this β_1-subunit (Neugebauer and Reichardt, 1991). The TASC antibody restores the ability of older (E12) chick retinal neurons to attach to the laminin. Thus they clearly have laminin receptors on their surfaces that can be activated by this antibody. It is not yet certain whether the comparatively few laminin receptors present on older (E12) retinal ganglion cells are in an active state. The activities of integrins on lymphccytes, macrophages, and platelets can also be regulated on a rapid posttranslational level (Shaw et al., 1990; Dustin and Springer, 1989; Phillips et al., 1991).

DISCUSSION

One of our objectives has been to identify the major classes of molecules that regulate axon outgrowth in in vitro assays. Previous work from our laboratory has shown that both ECM glycoproteins and cell adhesion molecules promote axon extension (reviewed in Reichardt et al., 1990). Integrins appear to be the major class of receptors used for interactions with the ECM. In recent studies, the ligand specificities of individual heterodimers have been determined and progress has been made in identifying the functions of these receptors on selected neuronal subpopulations. On cellular substrates, such as Schwann cells, myotubes, or astroglia, neurons have been shown to utilize cell adhesion molecules in addition to integrins. On different cell substrates, distinct cell adhesion molecules are important. The importance of individual cell adhesion molecules or integrins also depends on the identity and age of the neurons. On most cells, multiple interactions need to be blocked to see dramatic effects on axon growth in vitro, suggesting that combinations of cues may often direct axon growth in vitro. Consistent with this possibility, antibodies to single neurite-promoting molecules reduce the rate, but do not prevent regeneration in vivo (Sandrock and Matthew, 1987). In *Drosophila*, antibodies to similar adhesion-promoting molecules and genetic ablations also do not always have dramatic inhibitory effects on establishment of the axon tracts (Grenningloh et al., 1990).

One major future challenge is to understand the roles of the receptors and ligands described above in directing axon growth in vivo. A second is to understand what signals are transduced by binding of integrins and other adhesion-promoting molecules. A third is to identify the physiological regulations of their expression and function. Since activators of platelets and lymphocytes have been shown to regulate adhesive functions (Dustin and Springer, 1989; Phillips et al., 1991), it seems possible that neurotrophic factors and chemotrophic agents, which have dramatic and rapid effects on growth cone activity and guidance, may act in part by modulating the functions of neuronal repertoires of adhesion-promoting receptors.

Acknowledgments

We thank Marion Meyerson for help in preparing this manuscript and members of the laboratory for useful discussions that have shaped much of this work. Work in this laboratory has been supported by the Howard Hughes Medical Institute and U. S. Public Health Service (NIH grants NS19090 and NS16033). L.F.R. is an investigator of the Howard Hughes Medical Institute.

REFERENCES

Bazan, J.F. (1991). Neuropoietic cytokines in the hematopoietic fold. *Neuron* 7:197–208.

Begovac, P.C., Shur, B.D. (1990). Cell surface galactosyltransferase mediates the initiation of neurite outgrowth from PC12 cells on laminin. *J. Cell. Biol.* 110:461–470.

Begovac, P.C., Hall, D.E., and Shur, B.D. (1991). Laminin fragment E8 mediates PC12 cell neurite outgrowth by binding to cell surface β1, 4 galactosyltransferase. *J. Cell Biol.* 113:637–644.

Bossy, B., Bossy-Wetzel, E., and Reichardt, L.F. (1991). Characterization of the integrin α_8 subunit: A new integrin β_1-associated subunit, which is prominently expressed on axons and on cells in contact with basal laminae in chick embryos. *EMBO J.* 10:2379–2389.

Bothwell, M. (1991). Keeping track of neurotrophin receptors. *Cell* 65:915–918.

Bozyczko, D., and Horwitz, A. (1986). The participation of a putative cell surface receptor for laminin and fibronectin in peripheral neurite extension. *J. Neurosci.* 6:1241–1251.

Campenot, R.B. (1977). Local control of neurite development by nerve growth factor. *Proc. Natl. Acad. Sci. U. S. A.* 74:4516–4519.

Cohen, J., Burne, J.F., Winter, J., and Bartlett, P. (1986). Retinal ganglion cells lose response to laminin with maturation. *Nature* 322:465–467.

Cohen, J., Nurcombe, V., Jeffrey, P., and Edgar, D. (1989). Developmental loss of functional laminin receptors on retinal ganglion cells is regulated by their target tissue, the optic tectum. *Development* 107:381–387.

de Curtis, I., Quaranta, V., Tamura, R.N., and Reichardt, L.F. (1991). Laminin receptors in the retina: Sequence analysis of the chick integrin α_6 subunit; evidence for transcriptional and posttranslational regulation. *J Cell Biol* 113:405–416.

Dustin, M.L., and Springer, T.A. (1989). T-cell receptor cross-linking transiently stimulates adhesiveness through LFA-1. *Nature* 341:619–624.

Edelman, G.M., and Cunningham, B.A. (1990) Place-dependent cell adhesion, process retraction, and spatial signaling in neural morphogenesis. *Cold Spring Harbor Symp. Quant. Biol.* 55:303–318.

Elices M.J., and Hemler, M.E. (1989). The human integrin VLA-2 is a collagen receptor on some cells and a collagen/laminin receptor on others. *Proc. Natl. Acad. Sci. U. S. A.* 86:9906–9910.

Furley, A.J., Morton, S.B., Manalo, D., Karagogeos, D., Dodd, J., Jessell, T. (1990). The axonal glycoprotein TAG-1 is an immunoglobulin superfamily member with neurite outgrowth–promoting activity. *Cell* 81:157–170.

Gehlsen, K., Dickerson, K., Argraves, W.S., Engvall, E., Ruoslahti, E. (1989). Subunit structure of a laminin-binding integrin and localization of its binding site on laminin. *J. Biol. Chem.* 264:19034–19038.

Grenningloh, G., Bieber, A.J., Rehm, E.J., Snow, P.M., Traquina, Z.R., Hortsch, M., Patel, N.H., and Goodman, C.S. (1990). Molecular genetics of neuronal recognition in *Drosophila*: Evolution and function of immunoglobulin superfamily cell adhesion molecules. *Cold Spring Harbor Symp. Quant. Biol.* 55:327–340.

Gundersen, R.W., and Barrett, J.N. (1980). Characterization of the turning response of dorsal root neurites toward nerve growth factor. *J. Cell Biol.* 87:546–554.

Hall, D.E., Neugebauer, K.M., and Reichardt, L.F. (1987). Embryonic neural retinal cell response to extracellular matrix proteins: Developmental changes and effects of the CSAT antibody. *J. Cell Biol.* 104:623–634.

Hallbook, F., Ibanez, C.F., and Persson, H. (1991). Evolutionary studies of the nerve growth factor family reveal a novel member abundantly expressed in *Xenopus* ovary. *Neuron* 6:845–858.

Hemler, M.E. (1990). VLA proteins in the integrin family: Structure, functions, and their role on leukocytes. *Annu. Rev. Immunol.* 8:365–400.

Herndon, M.E., and Lander, A.E. (1990). A diverse set of developmentally regulated proteoglycans is expressed in rat central nervous system. *Neuron* 4:949–961.

Hockfield, S., Kalb, R.G., Zaremba, S., and Fryer, H. (1990). Expression of neural proteoglycans correlates with the acquisition of mature neuronal properties in the mammalian brain. *Cold Spring Harbor Symp. Quant. Biol.* 55:505–514.

Ignatius, M.J., Reichardt, L.F. (1988). Identification and characterization of a neuronal laminin receptor: An integrin heterodimer that binds laminin in a divalent cation-dependent manner. *Neuron* 1:713–725.

Keynes, R., and Cook, G. (1990). Review: Cell-cell repulsion: Clues from the growth cone? *Cell* 62:609–610.

Languino, R.R., Gehlsen, K.R., Wayner, E., Carter, W.G., Engvall, E., and Ruoslahti, E. (1989). Endothelial cells use $\alpha_2\beta_1$ integrin as a laminin receptor. *J. Cell Biol.* 109:2455–2462.

Molecular Mechanisms of Axonal Regeneration

Lein, P.J., Higgins, D., Turner, D.C., Flier, L.A., and Terranova, V.P. (1991). The NC1 domain of type IV collagen promotes axonal growth in sympathetic neurons through interaction with the $\alpha_1\beta_1$ integrin. *J. Cell Biol.* 113:417–428.

Moyle, M., Napier, M.A., and McLean, J.W. (1991). Cloning and expression of a divergent integrin subunit β_8. *J. Biol. Chem.* 266:19650–19658.

Neugebauer, K.M., and Reichardt, L.F. (1991). Cell surface regulation of β_1-integrin activity on developing retinal neurons. *Nature* 350:68–71.

Neugebauer, K.M., Emmett, C.J., Venstrom, K.A., and Reichardt, L.F. (1991). Vitronectin and thrombospondin promote retinal neurite outgrowth: Developmental regulation and role of integrins. *Neuron* 6:345–358.

O'Leary, D.D.M., Bicknese, A.R., De Carlos, J.A., Heffner, C.D., Doester, S.E., Kutka, L.J., and Terashima, T. (1990). Target selection by cortical axons: Alternative mechanisms to establish axonal connections in the developing brain. *Cold Spring Harbor Symp. Quant. Biol.* 55:453–468.

O'Shea, K.S., and Dixit, V.M. (1988). Unique distribution of the extracellular matrix component thrombospondin in the developing mouse embryo. *J. Cell Biol.* 107:2737–2748.

O'Shea, K.S., Rheinheimer, J.S.T., and Dixit, V.M. (1990). Deposition and role of thrombospondin in the histogenesis of the cerebellar cortex. *J. Cell Biol.* 110:1275–1284.

Perris, R., and Bronner-Fraser, M. (1989). Recent advances in defining the role of the extracellular matrix in neural crest development. *Comments Dev. Neurobiol.* 1:61–83.

Phillips, D.R., Charo, I.F., and Scarborough, R.M. (1991). GPIIb-IIIa: The responsive integrin. *Cell* 65:359–362.

Picker, L.J., Nakache, M., Butcher, E.C. (1989). Monoclonal antibodies to human lymphocyte homing receptors define a novel class of adhesion molecules on diverse cell types. *J. Cell. Biol.* 109:927–937.

Placzek, M., Tessier-Lavigne, M., Yamada, T., Dodd, J., and Jessell, T.M. (1990). Guidance of developing axons by diffusible chemoattractants. *Cold Spring Harbor Symp. Quant. Biol.* 55:279–290.

Reichardt, L.F., and Tomaselli, K.J. (1991). Extracellular matrix molecules and their receptors: Functions in neural development. *Annu. Rev. Neurosci.* 14:531–570.

Reichardt, L.F., Bossy, B., Carbonetto, S., de Curtis, I., Emmett, C., Hall, D.E., Ignatius, M.T., Large, T., Lefcort, F., Napolitano, E., Neugebauer, K.M., and Tomaselli, K.J. (1990). Neuronal receptors that regulate axon growth. *Cold Spring Harbor Symp. Quant. Biol.* 55:341–350.

Rupp F., Payan, D.G., Magill-Solc, C., Cowan, D.M., and Scheller, R.H. (1991). Structure and expression of a rat agrin. *Neuron* 6:811–823.

Sandrock, A.W. and Matthew, W.D. (1987). An *in vitro* neurite-promoting antigen functions in axonal regeneration *in vivo. Science* 237:1605–1608.

Sanes, J.R. (1989). Extracellular matrix molecules that influence neural development. *Annu. Rev. Neurosci.* 12:491–516.

Saunders, S., Jalkanen, M., O'Farrell, S., and Bernfield, M. (1989). Molecular cloning of syndecan, an integral membrane proteoglycan. *J. Cell Biol.* 108:1547–1556.

Schwab, M.E. (1990). Myelin-associated inhibitors of neurite growth. *Exp. Neurol.* 109:2–5.

Shaw, L.M., Messier, J.M., and Mercurio, A.M. (1990). The activation dependent adhesion of macrophages to laminin involves cytoskeletal anchoring and phosphorylation of the $\alpha_6\beta_1$ integrin. *J. Cell Biol.* 110:2167–2174.

Singer, I.I., Scott, S., Kawka, D.W., Kazazis, D.M., Gailit, J., and Ruoslahti, E. (1988). Cell surface distribution of fibronectin and vitronectin receptors depends on substrate composition and extracellular matrix accumulation. *J. Cell. Biol.* 106:2171–2182.

Song, W.K., Wang, W., Foster, R.F., Bielser, D.A., and Kaufman, S.J. (1992). H36-α_7 is a novel integrin α chain that is developmentally regulated during skeletal myogenesis. *J. Cell Biol.,* in press.

Sonnenberg, A., Calafat, J., Janssen, H., Daama, H., van der Raaij-Helmer, L.M.H., Falcioni, R., Kennel, S.J., Aplin, J.D., Baker, J., Loizidou, M., and Garrod, D. (1991). Integrin $\alpha_6\beta_4$ complex is located in hemidesmosomes, suggesting a major role in epidermal cell–basement membrane adhesion. *J. Cell Biol* 113:907–917.

Takeichi, M. (1991). Cadherin cell adhesion receptors as a morphogenetic regulator. *Science* 251:1451–1455.

Tomaselli, K.J., and Reichardt, L.F. (1988). Peripheral motoneuron interactions with laminin and Schwann cell–derived neurite-promoting molecules: Developmental regulation of laminin receptor function. *J. Neurosci. Res.* 21:275–285.

Tomaselli, K.J., Reichardt, L.F., and Bixby, J.L. (1986). Distinct molecular interactions mediate neuronal process outgrowth on non-neuronal cell surfaces and extracellular matrices. *J. Cell Biol.* 103:2659–2672.

Tomaselli, K.J., Hall, D.E., Flier, L.A., Gehlsen. K,R,, Turner, D.C., Carbonetto, S., and Reichardt, L.F. (1990). A neuronal cell line (PC12) expresses two β_1-class integrins—$\alpha_1\beta_1$ and $\alpha_3\beta_1$—that recognize different neurite outgrowth–promoting domains in laminin. *Neuron* 5:651–662.

Yancopoulos, G.D., Maisonpierre, P.C., Ip, N.Y., Aldrich, T.H., Belluscio, L., Boulton, T.G., Cobb, M.H., Squinto, S.P., and Furth, M.E. (1990). Neurotrophic factors: Their receptors and the signal transduction pathways they activate. *Cold Spring Harbor Symp. Quant. Biol.* 55:371–380.

Molecular Mechanisms of Axonal Regeneration

6 Transcriptional Control in Glial Development and Regeneration

Greg E. Lemke, Rainer Kuhn, and Edwin S. Monuki

Schwann cells, the principal glial cells of the peripheral nervous system (PNS), exhibit a remarkable developmental plasticity that is controlled almost entirely through a contact-dependent interaction with axons. Both in normal development, and in nerve degeneration and regeneration, it is the presence or absence of axons that specifies the differentiated fate of these cells (Bray et al., 1981). We have examined this cellular interaction at the molecular level, and have used a set of cloned marker genes to identify three separate stages in Schwann cell differentiation. These include an early phase in which a subpopulation of neural crest cells becomes committed to the glial lineage, a transitional "blast" phase during which Schwann cell progenitors rapidly divide, and a differentiated phase marked by the elaboration of the best-known organelle of Schwann cells, the myelin sheath. (Differentiated Schwann cells may also assume a non-myelinating phenotype.)

Several genes are uniquely expressed at high levels by the early neural crest progenitors. These include the low affinity nerve growth factor (NGF) receptor, the voltage-sensitive Na^+ and K^+ channel, and the L1 cell adhesion molecule genes. We have routinely used NGF receptor expression to mark early Schwann cell progenitors (Yan and Johnson, 1988). To identify fully differentiated, myelinating Schwann cells we have monitored expression of a set of glial-specific genes that encode essential structural proteins of the myelin sheath. The most abundant of these myelin proteins are protein zero (P_0), an immunoglobulin-related adhesion molecule, and myelin basic protein (MBP) (Lemke, 1988). Interposed between the commitment of a subpopulation of neural crest cells and the eventual differentiation of these cells into myelinating Schwann cells is a transitional or blast phase marked by rapid Schwann cell division. This proliferative blast phase is marked by elevated expression of a specialized transcription factor, called SCIP, which has been the focus of work in our laboratory over the past 2 years.

IDENTIFICATION AND COMPLEMENTARY DNA (cDNA) CLONING OF SCIP

SCIP is a member of a large family of DNA-binding proteins called the POU domain transcription factors. POU is an acronym for *Pil-1, Oct-1* and *-2*, and *unc-86*, the first four members of the family that were identified. These proteins share a highly conserved, bipartite DNA-binding domain—the POU domain—made up of a class-specific homeobox (related to but distinct from the DNA-binding domains of homeobox proteins in *Drosophila*) and an immediately upstream region called the POU-specific domain, which regulates the specificity of DNA binding (Herr et al., 1988). Many additional members of the POU domain family have recently been described in both vertebrates and invertebrates.

Several POU domain transcription factors are known to play essential roles in the regulation of cell-specific gene expression in higher vertebrates. Pit-1 (also known as GHF-1), for example, is stably expressed by a restricted set of cells in the pituitary, including lactotrophs and somatotrophs. In these cells, it acts as an important transactivator of the prolactin and growth hormone genes, respectively (Bodner et al., 1988; Ingraham et al., 1988). Similarly, Oct-2 is expressed by B lymphocytes, where it recognizes the "octamer" motif of immunoglobulin enhancers, and thereby serves as a cell-specific transactivator of immunoglobulin genes (Müller et al., 1988). In *Caenorhabditis elegans*, mutational analyses have also demonstrated that POU proteins play determinative roles in development. Loss-of-function mutations in the *unc-86* gene, for example, result in specific cellular deficits in neural development (Finney et al., 1988).

We asked whether a POU domain gene is expressed during glial differentiation in the PNS and central nervous systems (CNS). We used degenerate oligonucleotides reverse-transcribed from highly conserved regions of Pit-1, Oct-1 and -2, and *unc-86* to screen a rat Schwann cell cDNA library, and isolated two nonoverlapping sets of cDNAs. One of these encoded rat Oct-1 and the other encoded SCIP (Monuki et al., 1989). The latter is a 451-amino-acid nuclear protein that carries the highly conserved POU domain (157 amino acids) near its C-terminus (Monuki et al., 1990). We used SCIP cDNA clones as hybridization probes and demonstrated that SCIP is primarily expressed in neural tissues. SCIP messenger RNA (mRNA) can be detected in both the developing CNS and PNS, and in the neonatal testes, but not in neonatal liver, kidney, heart, lung, or spleen (Monuki et al., 1989). Among cultured cells, SCIP mRNA is, under appropriate conditions (see below), present in Schwann cells and Schwann cell lines, but not in cultured astrocytes or non-neural cells (Monuki et al., 1989).

CYCLIC ADENOSINE MONOPHOSPHATE (cAMP) REGULATION OF THE SCIP GENE IN CULTURED SCHWANN CELLS

Like the major myelin genes, expression of the SCIP gene in cultured Schwann cells is strongly induced by agents that raise the intracellular concentration of AMP (Lemke and Chao, 1988; Monuki et al., 1989). Up-regulation in the steady-state level of SCIP mRNA is seen with concentrations of the drug forskolin (1–10 μM) that result in physiologically significant elevations of cAMP (Monuki et al., 1989). In order to assess its potential regulatory influence over major myelin gene expression, we compared the time course of cAMP induction of SCIP expression to cAMP induction of major myelin gene expression in cultured Schwann cells. We first detected an increase in the steady-state level of SCIP mRNA at 1 hour after the addition of forskolin; this was followed by a substantial rise between 1 and 6 hours, and relatively constant levels (in the continued presence of the drug) thereafter (Monuki et al., 1989). Upon forskolin withdrawal, the level of SCIP mRNA rapidly returned to baseline (within 6 hours). In these same experiments, cAMP induction of the SCIP gene preceded cAMP induction of myelin-specific gene expression by approximately 12 hours.

cAMP does not induce SCIP expression through the prior induction of a transcriptional activator of the SCIP gene, since co-application or prior application of the protein synthesis inhibitor cycloheximide does not block induction by forskolin. Indeed, such treatments significantly potentiate cAMP induction, and cycloheximide acts as a moderate inducer of SCIP mRNA even in the absence of cAMP elevation (Monuki et al., 1989). Together, these results indicate that the SCIP gene is, at some level, suppressed in the absence of cAMP elevation, and that this elevation serves to relieve suppression. We have not yet determined whether suppression is exercised through transcriptional repression, or through selective destabilization of the SCIP mRNA. The regulation and structure of SCIP provide the basis for its name, which is an acronym for *suppressed cAMP-inducible POU*.

SCIP EXPRESSION DURING DEVELOPMENT AND REGENERATION

If SCIP acts as a regulator of myelin gene expression during normal glial development, then its appearance should precede transcriptional activation of myelin-specific genes. We examined this question by isolating RNA from rat sciatic nerves at various postnatal days and examining these RNA populations for expression of the SCIP and major myelin mRNAs. These studies demonstrated that peak SCIP expression does precede myelin-specific gene expression during normal development. In contrast to genes such as Oct-2 and Pit-1, however, which are stably expressed in fully differentiated cells, SCIP expression is transient. Peak SCIP mRNA levels are observed at 1 day after birth, fall to less than 50% of this level by 7 days after birth, and to less than 10% of this level by day 21. At the same time major myelin mRNAs rise to a peak around postnatal day 7 and remain high for the next several weeks (Monuki et al., 1989). The SCIP developmental expression profile is thus not consistent with the protein functioning as a direct transactivator of myelin-specific genes, since these genes continue to be transcribed at a time when SCIP expression has fallen to low basal levels. The phase of Schwann cell development with which this profile *is* well correlated is the period of rapid cell division that immediately precedes differentiation. Indeed, the relative time courses of SCIP mRNA expression, as measured by Northern blot, and Schwann cell proliferation, as measured by tritiated thymidine incorporation, are nearly superimposable (Monuki et al., 1989, 1990).

     Lemke et al.: Transcriptional Control

If a peripheral nerve is damaged such that axons distal to the site of injury degenerate, Schwann cells in this distal region dedifferentiate in response to the loss of axon contact (Bray et al., 1981; Trapp et al., 1988)). This unusual developmental plasticity can be monitored using the same set of genes whose expression is regulated during the course of normal Schwann cell differentiation. We measured SCIP mRNA levels at 2, 5, 10, and 20 days after permanent sciatic nerve transection and found that while SCIP expression was very low in the intact nerve, this expression was transiently up-regulated at 2 days after the nerve was cut (Monuki et al., 1990). This pattern differed markedly from those of genes that mark myelinating Schwann cells and early Schwann cell progenitors. The genes encoding the myelin-specific proteins P_0 and MBP were stably down-regulated in response to transection (Trapp et al., 1988; Monuki et al., 1990) at the same time that the NGF receptor gene, whose expression marks early progenitors, was stably reinduced (Taniuchi et al., 1986). As in normal Schwann cell differentiation, the transient activation of SCIP gene expression that we observed during dedifferentiation was well correlated with a transient burst of Schwann cell proliferation previously described by others as a response to nerve transection (Lemke et al., 1991). The relative time course of expression of the NGF receptor, SCIP, and major myelin genes is summarized diagramatically in figure 6.1.

TRANSCRIPTIONAL REGULATION BY SCIP

We investigated the regulatory properties of SCIP by cotransfecting (into cultured Schwann cells) SCIP expression plasmids together with plasmids in which transcription of the bacterial chloramphenicol acetyltransferase (CAT) reporter gene was driven by different eukaryotic promoters. In accordance with its Schwann cell expression pattern during both normal nerve development and degeneration, SCIP functioned as a transcriptional repressor of the major myelin promoters in these experiments (Monuki et al., 1990). For example, cotransfection of the SCIP expression construct (at DNA mass ratios as low as 1:100, expression plasmid–reporter plasmid) resulted in strong repression of the rat P_0 promoter. Repression by SCIP was specific to the extent that less than two fold differences in promoter activity (in the presence and absence of SCIP) were seen for CAT reporters driven by the mouse c-jun, SV40 early, or Rous sarcoma virus promoters. SCIP repression of the P_0 promoter required an intact DNA-binding domain–introduction of a frameshift mutation within the SCIP homeobox resulted in complete loss of repressor activity (Monuki et al., 1990). This domain is not sufficient for transcriptional repression, however, since amino terminal deletion mutants of the SCIP protein retain the ability to bind to SCIP recognition sites, but are nonetheless completely ineffective as transcriptional repressors. These studies indicate that SCP does not repress major myelin gene expression through simple competition to the binding sites of transcriptional activators. They suggest that repression instead occurs through negative interaction between SCIP and

  Molecular Mechanisms of Axonal Regeneration

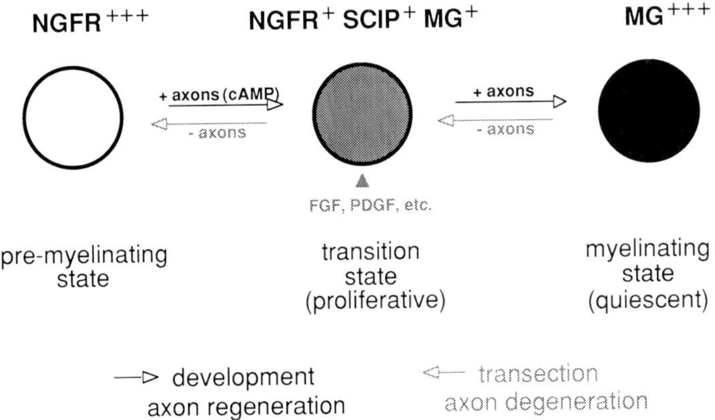

Figure 6.1 A hypothetical synopsis of axon-driven Schwann cell differentiation. In this model, Schwann cells are placed into one of three developmental states. The earliest of these corresponds to the commitment of a subpopulation of neural crest cells to a glial lineage (premyelinating state). These early cells are marked by high-level expresion of the nerve growth factor receptor (*NGFR*) p75. Upon contact with axons, these early cells progress to a proliferative blast phase (transition state) uniquely marked by high-level expression of the POU domain transcription factor SCIP. In the continued presence of axons of sufficient caliber (>1 μm), these proliferative progenitors eventually develop into quiescent myelinating cells and express high levels of myelin-specific genes (*MG*). Upon loss of axon contact (transection), this developmental progression is reversed. In cultured Schwann cells, the progression from the premyelinating state to the proliferative transition state can be mimicked by agents that elevate intracellular *cAMP* (cAMP). *FGF* and *PDGF* indicate that cell division during the proliferative transition state is thought to be driven by polypeptide growth factors such as fibroblast growth factor (FGF) and platelet-derived growth factor (PDGF). CAMP treatment of cultured Schwann cells strongly up-regulates expression of the FGF and PDGF receptors. (Adapted from Monuki et al., 1990.)

other transactivators, an interaction that may be mediated by a repressor domain at the amino terminus of the SCIP protein.

SUMMARY

Together, our studies demonstrate that high-level SCIP expression is uniquely associated with the blast phase of Schwann cell differentiation, and suggest that during this period SCIP serves to dampen transcription of genes that are properly expressed only in myelinating Schwann cells. This is an important job, since myelin-specific transcripts account for a substantial fraction of the total mRNA pool in actively myelinating Schwann cells. The P_0 mRNA alone, for example, has been estimated to account for nearly 8% of the mRNA in these cells.

Proliferative progenitor cells are characteristic not only of glial development in the PNS, but also of glial development in the CNS. One such CNS progenitor cell—the O-2A cell—gives rise to both myelinating glia (oligodendrocytes) and one form of nonmyelinating glia (type 2 astrocytes) (Raff, 1989). We have recently found that just as high-level SCIP expression marks proliferative Schwann cell progenitors, so does high-level SCIP expression mark these O-2A progenitors in the CNS. When these cells differentiate into either oligodendrocytes or type 2 astrocytes, SCIP expression is substantially reduced. Increasing evidence suggests that the presence of a transcriptional repressor of end-stage differentiation genes will prove to be a general feature of dividing blast cells. In the case of muscle development, for example, myoblasts express a helix-loop-helix repressor—Id—that blocks high-level expression of end-stage muscle-specific genes (Benezra et al., 1990). When myoblasts stop dividing and fuse to form myotubes, expression of Id is reduced and muscle-specific genes (such as the muscle creatine kinase gene) are actively transcribed. We hypothesize that SCIP plays a similar role in the differentiation of myelinating glia in the CNS and PNS, and are currently performing several experiments that test this hypothesis directly.

REFERENCES

Benezra,R., Davis, R.L. Lockshon, D. Turner, D.L., and Weintraub H. (1990). The protein Id: A negative regulator of helix-loop-helix proteins. *Cell* 61:49–59.

Bodner, M., Castrillo, J.-L., Theill, L.E., Deerinck, T., Ellisman, M., and Karin M. (1988). The pituitary-specific transcription factor GHF-I is a homeobox containing protein. *Cell* 55:505–518.

Bray, G.M., Rasminsky, M., and Aguayo, A.J. (1981). Interactions between axons and their sheath cells. *Annu. Rev. Neurosci.* 4:127–162.

Finney,M., Ruvkun, G., and Horvitz, H.R. (1988). The *C. elegans* cell lineage and differentiation gene *unc-86* encodes a protein with a homeodomain and extended similarity to transcription factors. *Cell* 55:757–769.

Herr,W., Sturm, R.A., Clerc, R.G., Corcoran, L.M., Baltimore, D., Sharp, P.A. Ingraham, H.A., Rosenfeld, M.G., Finney, M., Ruvkun, G., and H.R., Horvitz (1988). The POU domain: A large conserved region in the mammailian Pit-1, Oct-1, Oct-2, and *C. elegans unc-86* gene products. *Genes Dev.* 2:1513–1516.

Ingraham, H.A., Chen, R., Mangalam, H.J., Elsholtz, H.P., Flynn, S.E., Lin, C.R., Simmons, D.M., Swanson, L., and Rosenfeld, M.G. (1988). A tissue-specific transcription factor containing a homeodomain specifies a pituitary phenotype. *Cell* 55:519–529.

Lemke, G. (1988) Unwrapping the genes of myelin. *Neuron* 1:535–543.

Lemke, G., and Chao M. (1988). Axons regulate Schwann cell expression of the major myelin and NGF receptor genes. *Development* 102:499–504.

Lemke, G., Kuhn, R., Monuki, E.S., and Weinmaster G. (1991). Expression and activity of the transcription factor SCIP during glial differentiation and myelination. *Proc. N.Y. Acad. Sci.* 633:189–195.

Monuki, E.S., Weinmaster, G., Kuhn, R., and Lemke G. (1989). SCIP: A glial POU domain gene regulated by cyclic AMP. *Neuron* 3:783–793.

Monuki, E.S., Kuhn, R., Weinmaster, G., Trapp, B.D., and Lemke G. (1990). Expression and activity of the POU transcription factor SCIP. *Science* 249:1300–1303.

Müller, M.M., Ruppert, S., Schaffner, W., and Matthias, P. (1988). A cloned octamer transcription factor stimulates transcription from lymphoid-specific promoters in non-B cells. *Nature* 336:544–551.

Raff, M.C. (1989). Glial cell diversification in the rat optic nerve. *Science* 243:1450–1455.

     Molecular Mechanisms of Axonal Regeneration

Taniuchi, M., Clark, H.B., and Johnson, E.M. (1986). Induction of nerve growth factor receptor in Schwann cells after axotomy. *Proc. Natl. Acad. Sci. U. S. A.* 83:4094–4098.

Trapp, B.D., Hauer, P., and Lemke, G. (1988). Axonal regulation of myelin protein mRNA levels in actively myelinating Schwann cells. *J. Neurosci.* 8:3515–3521.

Yan, Q. and Johnson, E.M. (1988). An immunohistochemical study of the nerve growth factor receptor in developing rats. *J. Neurosci.* 8:3481–3498.

7 Proteases as Potential Agents for Augmenting Axon Regeneration

Randall N. Pittman, Weslia P. Hynicka, and Melissa Hunter-Ensor

Several groups have recently identified molecules associated with the surface of various cell types that inhibit axon outgrowth (for reviews, see Patterson, 1988; Schwab, 1990). A number of these molecules are present in the central nervous system (CNS) and may be in part responsible for the lack of regeneration in the CNS following injury. Characterization of these molecules indicates that they have different physicochemical properties; therefore, a number of potential inhibitors of axon regeneration are probably present in the CNS (Schwab and Caroni, 1988; Cox et al., 1990; Davies et al., 1990; Raper and Kapfhammer, 1990; Snow et al., 1990). The molecule that has been most thoroughly studied is the molecule on the surface of oligodendrocytes and myelin, recognized by the monoclonal antibody IN-1 (Caroni and Schwab, 1988a). This protein, as well as oligodendrocytes and myelin, inhibits neurite outgrowth and axon regeneration and is likely to be one of the major factors responsible for the inability of CNS neurons to regenerate axons following traumatic or pathological injuries (Caroni and Schwab, 1988b). Treatment of animals following spinal cord injury with the antibody IN-1 dramatically increases the length of regenerating axons compared to controls (Schnell and Schwab, 1990). These and other experiments support the idea that if the neurite outgrowth–inhibiting aspects of myelin could be overcome, then regeneration within the CNS would be greatly improved. There would still be a large number of other obstacles that must be overcome including acute effects of trauma, glial scarring, trophic maintenance of neurons, axonal guidance, and target recognition. Nevertheless, if the inhibitory effects of myelin on axon regeneration could be overcome, it would represent a major step toward functional recovery in the CNS following injury.

The inhibitory effects of myelin on regeneration can be overcome with antibodies such as IN-1 (Caroni and Schwab, 1988a; Schnell and Schwab, 1990). It should also be possible to overcome these inhibitory factors by selectively cleaving them with proteases. Proteases may have additional advantages of enabling axons to overcome other molecular obstacles to regeneration such as glial scars. By using genetic techniques to design proteases with very specific substrate profiles, it should be possible to create "molecular scalpels" that are capable of removing selective molecules from the surface of myelin, or "scalpels" with a broad range of substrates for penetrating scars or deposits of extracellular material.

This chapter is divided into four sections; the first section provides information on the classification and characteristics of proteases, the second section describes experiments consistent with a role for proteases in axon outgrowth in vitro, the third section presents preliminary data suggesting that proteases can effectively overcome inhibitors of axon outgrowth, and the fourth section discusses genetic manipulations for expressing proteases in regenerating neurons, and problems that are likely to be encountered.

CLASSIFICATION OF PROTEASES

Protease is a general term used to describe both endopeptidases and exopeptidases. *Proteinase* is a more selective term referring only to endopeptidases. Endopeptidases cleave peptides and proteins at internal bonds, while exopeptidases require substrates to have a free amino or C-terminus. There are four families of endopeptidases (table 7.1), named for their active sites, and several groups of exopeptidases, named primarily for their substrate specificity. Only endopeptidases or proteinases are discussed in this chapter because it is less likely that exopeptidases would be useful agents for improving regeneration.

Serine proteases have a serine at their active site and are inhibited by diisopropylfluorophosphate (DFP), phenylmethylsulfonlyl fluoride (PMSF) and *p*-nitrophenyl *p'*-guanidinobenzoate (*p*NPGB). Subfamilies of serine proteases such as trypsinlike, chymotrypsin-like, and thrombinlike proteases can be characterized by substrate preference or with more selective inhibitors such as *N*-tosyl-*l*-lys-chloromethyl ketone (for trypsinlike proteases), *N*-tosyl-*l*-phe-chloromethyl ketone (for chymotrypsin-like proteases), and D-phe-pro-arg-chloromethyl ketone (for thrombinlike proteases). Serine proteases are active at physiological pH and are most often released by cells and have extracellular functions. They are synthesized as inactive proenzymes or zymogens, and are subsequently activated by a proteolytic cleavage.

Table 7.1 Classification of Proteinases (Endopeptidases)

Serine proteases	Cysteine proteases
Proteases: trypsin, chymotrypsin	Proteases: cathepsin B, calpains
Inhibitors: DFP, PMSF	Inhibitors: iodoacetate, E64
Properties: activity at pH 7–9; synthesized as inactive zymogen; extracellular functions	Properties: activity at pH 2–7, most often pH 4–6; intracellular and lysosomal functions
Metallo proteases	Aspartic proteases
Proteases: collagenase, thermolysin	Proteases: pepsin, renin
Inhibitors: EDTA, 1,10-phenanthroline	Inhibitors: pepstatin
Properties: activity at pH 7–9; some are synthesized as zymogens; extracellular functions	Properties: activity at pH 2–7, most often pH 2–4; most are present in the stomach

DFP = diisopropyl fluorophosphate; PMSF = phenylmethylsulfonyl fluoride; EDTA = ethylenediaminetetraacetic acid.

Like serine proteases, metalloproteases are active at neutral pH and are often secreted from cells as zymogens and have extracellular functions. As their name implies, metalloproteases have a metal ion at their active site. In general, zinc is the metal present and therefore, most metalloproteases are susceptible to inhibition by the zinc chelating agent, 1,10-phenanthroline.

Aspartic and cysteine proteases are most active at acidic pH conditions found in lysosomes (generally cysteine proteases), and gastric environment (generally aspartic proteases), although exceptions do exist. Renin, an aspartic protease, is active at neutral pH and the calpains are a family of cytosolic Ca^{2+}-activated cysteine proteases active at physiological pH. Cysteine proteases are inhibited by the protease inhibitor E64, or by alkylating agents such as iodoacetate or N-ethylmaleimide, while aspartic proteases are inhibited by pepstatin.

Based on the biochemical characteristics of the four families of endopeptidases, the ones most likely to be useful as adjuvants for improving regeneration would be serine proteases or metalloproteases. Most members of both families have optimum activity at neutral pH, detailed active site structures are known for a large number of proteases in both families, and they can be genetically engineered to be released as an active protease or as an inactive zymogen requiring cleavage for activation.

Designer Proteases

Advances in the fields of protein chemistry and crystallography have made it possible to identify the amino acids involved in the interactions between proteases and substrates with considerable resolution. This not only includes interactions at the active site but also includes interactions with other parts of the protease. With this information, it is now possible to use molecular biological techniques to design proteases with very specific substrate profiles (Jallat et al., 1986; Carter and Wells, 1987; Craik et al., 1987). Once inhibitors of axon regeneration associated with myelin or glial scars have been identified and sequences determined (and some secondary structure determined), it should be possible to design proteases that cleave and inactivate these inhibitors and but few other molecules.

ROLE OF PROTEASES IN AXON OUTGROWTH IN VITRO

Axons of sympathetic and sensory neurons release a urokinase plasminogen activator (uPA) and a calcium-dependent metalloprotease (Krystosek and Seeds, 1984; Pittman, 1985). Approximately 40% of the protease activity released by neurons is from the growth cone, even though the growth cone constitutes less than 0.1% of the tissue of a developing neuron (Pittman, 1985; see also Krystosek and Seeds, 1981, 1984). Therefore, the specific activity of these proteases at the growth cone is several orders of magnitude higher than in other parts of the neuron. This suggests that uPA and the metalloprotease may be involved in growth cone functions such as neurite outgrowth. Several studies have shown that inhibitors of serine proteases increase neurite outgrowth in vitro (Monard et al., 1983; Hawkins and Seeds, 1986; Pittman and Patterson, 1987; Zurn et al., 1988; Gurwitz and Cunningham, 1988; Pittman et al., 1989). Some studies are consistent with a thrombinlike serine protease being involved in neurite outgrowth, while others are more consistent with a uPA-like serine protease being involved. Because of the different species being used as well as differences between cell lines and primary cultures, it is not clear whether multiple serine proteases are involved in neurite outgrowth or whether different proteases serve the same function in different species. What is clear, however, is that inhibition of serine protease activity in vitro increases the overall length of neurites and alters growth cone dynamics. Time lapse videomicroscopy of growth cone motility indicates that inhibition of uPA activity increases the rate of neurite outgrowth about twofold, and decreases membrane ruffling and activity around the entire circumference of the growth cone, except at the leading edge (Pittman et al., 1989). At the leading edge of the growth cone, membrane activity is unchanged or even increased following inhibition of uPA activity.

A number of endogenous inhibitors of serine proteases have been purified and shown to increase neurite outgrowth in vitro (Guenther et al., 1985; Pittman and Patterson, 1987; Zurn et al., 1988; Gurwitz and Cunningham, 1988). The most extensive studies have been carried out with glial-derived nexin (GDN; also known as protease nexin), a 43-kD inhibitor purified from C6 glioma (Monard et al., 1983; Guenther et al., 1985). GDN increases neurite outgrowth from neuroblastoma cells and primary cultures of chick sympathetic neurons (Monard et al., 1983; Zurn et al., 1988). The only area of the adult nervous system that has high levels of GDN is the olfactory bulb, which is also the only area of the nervous system in higher vertebrates that continually degenerates and regenerates throughout life. The high concentration of GDN in the olfactory system may indicate that GDN plays a key role in neurite outgrowth in this system or it may indicate that high levels of protease inhibitors are required in areas where protease activity is concentrated (the protease activity would be required for neurite outgrowth, or would be involved in the degeneration of neurons; GDN would be present to protect local cells from proteolytic activity).

It is somewhat unexpected and surprising that inhibitors of serine proteases increase neurite outgrowth. Intuitively it would seem that proteases should increase neurite outgrowth and protease inhibitors should decrease neurite outgrowth. This may in fact occur when studies are eventually performed in vivo, that is, inhibition of serine protease activity may actually decrease neurite outgrowth in vivo. It appears that the relative levels of proteases and inhibitors in a given system is very important in determining the effects of exogenously added inhibitors (see below and figure 7.1). In general, tissue culture systems that have been used to determine the effects of proteases and inhibitors on neurite outgrowth are carried out in serum-free medium containing excess protease activity.

    Molecular Mechanisms of Axonal Regeneration

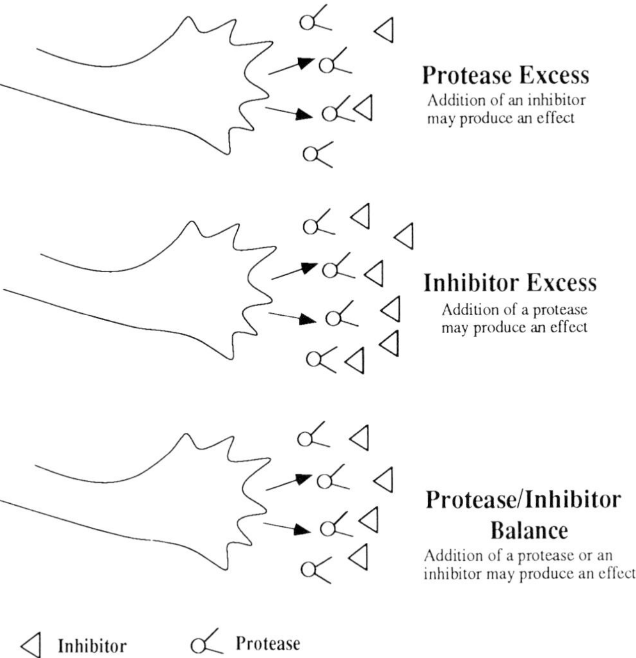

Figure 7.1 Balance between neuronal proteases and protease inhibitors. Developing and regenerating axons release proteases and a variety of cell types, including neurons, and glia release protease inhibitors. The balance between proteases and inhibitors determines the actions of endogenous or exogenous proteases or inhibitors. This balance is responsive to local hormones and growth factors and is likely to change following pathological or physiological insults to the nervous system. It will be important to measure the protease-inhibitor balance following injury to the nervous system and determine whether this balance correlates with the decreased ability of axons to regenerate within the CNS.

A question that needs to be addressed is how inhibition of protease activity increases neurite outgrowth. The most likely explanation for this observation is that inhibition of protease activity increases adhesion of the growth cone to the substrate. This results in an increase in neurite outgrowth under conditions in which neurons are typically grown in vitro. The effects of inhibitors or antibodies that block protease activity probably depend on local concentrations of proteases and inhibitors (see figure 7.1). For instance, addition of uPA to primary cultures of sympathetic neurons has no effect on neurite outgrowth, while inhibitors of uPA increase neurite outgrowth (Pittman et al., 1989). A likely explanation for this is that in the serum-free culture system being used to grow neurons, there is an excess protease activity. In other systems, where inhibitory activity is in excess of proteolytic activity (e.g., in vivo), then addition of proteases might be expected to have an effect and inhibitors may have no effect or have the opposite effect. It should be emphasized that it is the local balance between proteases and inhibitors that determines the actions of an endogenous or exogenous protease or inhibitor (see figure 7.1). Such a balance is likely to change during development and aging and as a function of hormones and growth factors. Trauma and pathophysiological insults may also alter the balance of proteases and inhibitors (Bignami et al., 1982; Monard, 1988; Salles et al., 1990; Hantai et al., 1990).

In addition to serine proteases, a metalloprotease also appears to be involved in neurite outgrowth in vitro (Pittman, 1985; Pittman and Williams, 1989). The metalloprotease is released by distal processes and growth cones of rat sympathetic and sensory neurons and degrades components of the extracellular matrix (collagen and firbronectin) through which neurites of the peripheral nervous system grow. Inhibition of this neuronal metalloprotease blocks neurite penetration into and outgrowth within three-dimensional collagen gels in vitro, but does not affect neurite outgrowth on two-dimensional collagen substrates (Pittman and Williams, 1989). This suggests that a likely function of the metalloprotease in vivo is to degrade extracellular matrix, and to create openings within three-dimensional matrices for growing axons. A combination of plasminogen activator (PA) and plasminogen could have a similar role in degrading extracellular matrix and "opening channels" for neurite outgrowth in vivo. Both UPA and tissue PA (tPA) have binding sites on the surface of neurons (Pittman et al., 1989; Verrall and Seeds, 1989) that protect them from cellular inhibitors. Therefore, the growing axon can be "armed" with proteolytically active PA (figure 7.2) which can serve as a reservoir of proteolytic activity. If plasminogen is present in the local environment of the growing axon, then it can be converted to the active trypsinlike protease, plasmin, by the cell surface–bound PA. Once formed, plasmin could degrade many components present on cells or in the extracellular environment. In fact, uPA-dependent plasmin formation appears to play a major role in the movement and metastasis of tumor cells in vitro and in vivo (for review, see Dano et al., 1985). Therefore, it would not be surprising if PA-dependent activation of plasminogen was found to be an important regulator of axon outgrowth and regeneration in vivo. A number of studies have shown that plasminogen activator activity increases dramatically following sciatic nerve crush or transection (Bignami et al., 1982; Monard, 1988; Hantai et al., 1990). This increased PA activity with subsequent plasmin formation may be an important factor in the ability of peripheral nerves to regenerate. Following transection of the optic nerve in mammals (which does not regenerate), there is little or no increase in PA activity (Bignami et al., 1982), while transection of the goldfish optic nerve (which does regenerate) results in an increase in PA activity (Salles et al., 1990). The lack of an increase in PA activity following injury in the mammalian CNS may be one of a number of factors responsible for the inability of nerves in the CNS to regenerate.

INACTIVATING INHIBITORS OF AXON OUTGROWTH WITH PROTEASES

C6 glioma cells are invasive tumor cells that migrate into both the white and gray matter of the CNS. It is surprising that migration of these cells is not inhibited by the molecules associated with myelin that inhibit axon outgrowth and regeneration. Experiments by Schwab's group suggest that C6 glioma

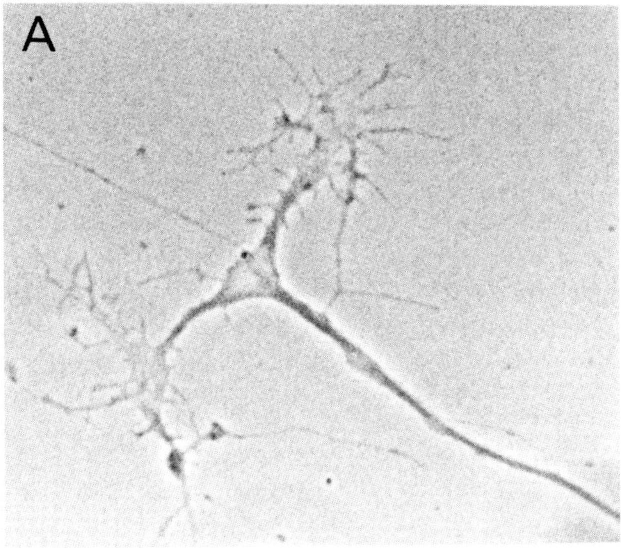

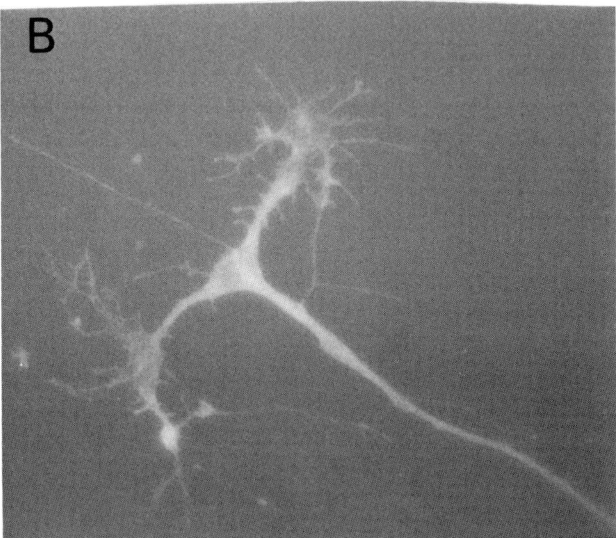

Figure 7.2 Growth cones of a living sympathetic neuron "armed" with the serine protease, tissue plasminogen activator (tPA). *A,* phase contrast micrograph of a branched axon from a rat sympathetic neuron in culture. *B,* immunohistochemical localization of cell surface–bound tPA. Note that the tPA is fairly homogeneously distributed on the axon, growth cones, and filopodia. Previous studies have shown that surface-bound plasminogen activator is proteolytically active. Surface-bound proteases probably help axons penetrate through dense extracellular material and eventually may be useful for improving regeneration in the CNS.

cells can migrate into white matter because they secrete a metalloprotease that degrades the components associated with myelin that inhibit neurite outgrowth (Paganetti et al., 1988). If this metalloprotease can be identified and characterized, it may be a useful agent for overcoming the inhibitory effects of myelin on regeneration.

Myelin is not the only component in the CNS that inhibits regeneration. It appears that glial scars, certain chondroitin sulfate proteoglycans, reactive astrocytes, and molecules associated with astrocytes such as tenascin, can all inhibit axon outgrowth or regeneration, or both (Liuzzi and Lasek, 1987; Eng et al., 1987; Verna, 1989; Snow et al., 1990; Faissner and Kruse, 1990). Fawcett has developed an interesting in vitro model system for investigating regeneration in the CNS (Fawcett et al., 1989). The system consists of three-dimensional cultures of astrocytes and incorporates a number of nonmyelin components present in the CNS that inhibit regeneration. Neither peripheral nervous system (PNS) nor CNS neonatal neurons will grow axons into the three-dimensional cultures of astrocytes; however, embryonic day 15 mouse retinal neurons and dorsal root ganglion (DRG) neurons grow axons through the astrocytes. Inhibitors of serine proteases decrease outgrowth of embryonic neurons in three-dimensional cultures of astrocytes (Fawcett and Housden, 1990) which is consistent with the idea that embryonic neurons elaborate a serine protease that can degrade molecules that inhibit axon outgrowth. Identifying and characterizing such a protease would be potentially very important because it may represent a down-regulated "genetic trait" used for growing axons in the developing CNS. Eventually, it should be possible, using genetic manipulations, to reintroduce this protease into regenerating neurons (discussed below).

For a variety of reasons it is important to identify the metalloprotease associated with C6 glioma and the serine protease associated with embryonic neurons that enable cells and axons to move in a CNS environment that is resistant to cell movement and axon outgrowth. However, even without knowing the nature of these proteases, it should still be possible to determine the susceptibility of cellular and molecular inhibitors of axon regeneration to proteases by exposing them to low concentrations of a variety of common proteases. If proteases are identified that can effectively inactivate inhibitors of axon regeneration at low concentrations, then initial studies can be performed with these proteases to determine if neurons transfected with them are able to regenerate through inhibitory environments such as myelin or three-dimensional cultures of astrocytes. Eventually it may be advantagous to genetically modify these common proteases to increase specificity, or to use the more "natural" proteases from C6 glioma or embryonic neurons.

Preliminary data from two different systems suggest that it may be possible to use low concentrations of commercially available proteases to inactivate inhibitors of neurite outgrowth. Trigeminal ganglion sensory neurons grown in co-culture with epidermal cells consisting of epithelial cells and Merkel cells actively grow onto and interact with their normal targets, the Merkel cells, while axons from sympathetic neurons are actively repelled (collapse and

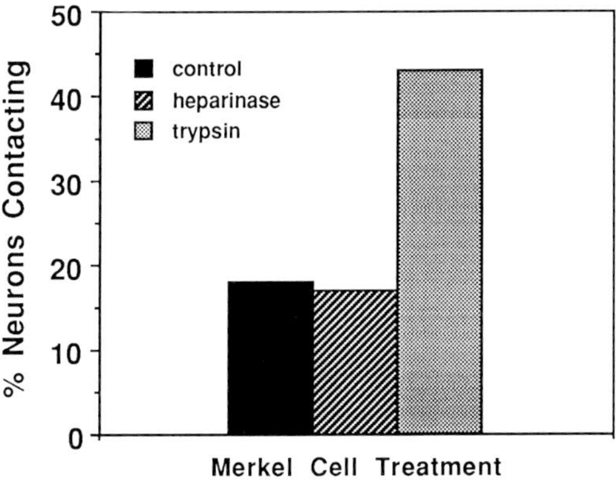

Figure 7.3 Increase in the number of sympathetic neurons contacting Merkel cells following exposure to low concentrations of trypsin. Under normal conditions in vitro, growth cones of sympathetic neurons are actively repelled when they contact living or fixed Merkel cells. Treatment of fixed (1% paraformaldehyde) Merkel cells with 2.5 μg/ml trypsin (300-fold lower concentration than that used to subculture cells), but not heparinase (200 μg/ml) increases the number of sympathetic neurons contacting Merkel cells. These and other data (see text) suggest that low concentrations of commercially available proteases may be able to inactivate inhibitors of neurite outgrowth present on myelin, astrocytes, and extracellular material. By transfecting neurons with these proteases, it may be possible to overcome a number of the molecular obstacles to regeneration in the CNS.

Table 7.2 Neurite Outgrowth in the Presence of Myelin*

	Total No. of Neurons	Neurons with Axons	Neurons Growing Axons (%)
Control	87	13	15
Plasmin-treated	114	56	49

* Myelin from rat cerebral cortex was treated with 10 μg/ml plasmin or buffer for 30 minutes at 37°C and absorbed onto polylysine-treated tissue culture dishes. Sympathetic neurons from 1-day-old neonatal rats were plated onto the dishes for 18 hours and the number of neurons with and without axons (twice the length of the cell body diameter) was determined in nine random fields from three wells in each condition.

retract) when they contact Merkel cells (Vos et al., 1991). This inhibition of neurite outgrowth of sympathetic neurons by Merkel cells is reminiscent of the inhibition of axon regeneration by myelin. Treatment of Merkel cells with 2.5 μg/ml trypsin (approximately 300-fold lower concentration than the concentration used to remove cells from a culture dish) increases the number of sympathetic axons that make stable contacts with Merkel cells by two- to threefold (figure 7.3).

Axon outgrowth in the presence of myelin is another system in which low concentrations of a commercially available protease appear to inactivate an inhibitor of neurite outgrowth. The number of neurons growing axons in the presence of myelin increases threefold when myelin is incubated with low concentrations (10 μg/ml) of plasmin (table 7.2). If myelin is not incubated

     Pittman et al.: Proteases as Potential Agents

with plasmin, but rather low concentrations of the inactive zymogen plasminogen are included in the myelin solution that is absorbed to the culture dish, there is also an increase in neurite outgrowth (preliminary observations). Presumably, in this case neurons release PA from growing axons and growth cones and this cleaves plasminogen to form plasmin, which then inactivates the neurite outgrowth inhibitors associated with myelin. If these data are substantiated by further experiments, then a next step would be to transfect neurons with plasminogen to determine whether or not they can grow axons in the presence of myelin and overcome inhibitors of axon regeneration by proteolytically inactivating them.

GENE THERAPY WITH PROTEASES

If the only molecular or cellular barriers to axon regeneration were at the site of a traumatic or pathological lesion, then local application of proteases might be a useful therapy to improve regeneration. However, molecular barriers appear to exist throughout the CNS. Therefore, it would be useful to provide the regenerating neuron with the genetic machinery required for making the protease. Although this is desirable, it creates a series of potential problems that must be overcome. Some of the problems are general ones involved with high efficiency transfer of a gene to a select population of postmitotic neurons, while other problems are more specific and deal with secondary problems associated with regulating proteolytic activity so that unwanted side effects are minimal.

Delivery of Genes into Postmitotic Neurons

Genetic information can be introduced into neurons as either complementary DNA (cDNA) or messenger RNA (mRNA), and a variety of vectors and vehicles can be used to increase the efficiency of uptake and translation. The major observations from in vitro studies using plasmid vectors to deliver cDNAs (primarily unpublished observations by a number of groups) is that uptake and translation of cDNA in plasmid vectors in neurons is not efficient ($<1\%$ of the neurons express reporter genes even when using cationic lipids such as lipofection as a vehicle) and is not stable (translation decreases after 2–3 days). Introduction of mRNA into neurons by lipofection results in efficient translation ($>20\%$ of the neurons can express reporter mRNA); however, RNA is more difficult to work with than DNA and is typically degraded within the cells during the first 12 to 24 hours after transfection. Therefore, neither mRNA nor cDNA in plasmid vectors is very effective in stably introducing genetic information into a significant fraction of neurons within a given population in vitro or in vivo. Techniques such as microinjecting mRNA or plasmid cDNA increases the fraction of neurons expressing a foreign protein; however, the number of neurons that can be injected is limited and foreign genes are still not stably expressed in postmitotic neurons using this technique.

     Molecular Mechanisms of Axonal Regeneration

At present, the only realistic means of stably transfecting postmitotic neurons appears to be with herpes simplex virus type 1 (HSV-1) as a vector (Geller and Breakefield, 1988; Dobson et al., 1990; Geller et al., 1990; Geller and Freese, 1990). In humans, HSV-1 produces "cold sores" (HSV-2 causes genital herpes) and is present in a large fraction of the US population in a latent form in neurons of the PNS. Therefore, HSV-1 is a natural vector that infects the neurons system and is an obvious choice as a vector for gene therapy of the nervous system. HSV-1 has a number of advantages for gene therapy including its ability to stably transfect postmitotic neurons, its high efficiency (most neurons in a population become infected), its ability to be transported retrograde (e.g., from the the site of an injury), and its ability to incorporate large amounts of foreign DNA into its genome (its genome is 150 kb, much of which can be replaced with genes to be expressed). The use of HSV-1 as a vector for gene transfer into the nervous system is just beginning to be explored. At present, there are two basic types of HSV-1 vectors that are being used to introduce reporter genes (*lacZ*) into neurons in vivo and in vitro. One is a plasmid vector containing HSV-1 DNA sequences that allow it to be packaged into virus particles, and an HSV-1 origin of replication. This plasmid vector has been used by Geller, Breakefield, and colleagues (Geller and Breakefield, 1988; Geller et al., 1990; Geller and Freese, 1990) to express *lacZ* in neurons of the PNS and CNS in vitro and in vivo. A next obvious step is to use this vector to introduce genes other than *lacZ* into postmitotic neurons and to determine the longitudinal stability of transfected genes.

The second type of HSV-1 vector that has been used to introduce a foreign gene (*lacZ*) into postimitotic neurons is a variant HSV-1 virus in which the genes for viral replication (ICP4) and reactivation from a latent state (LAT) have been deleted (Dobson et al., 1990). This vector is a modified form of the HSV-1 wild-type virus and appears to have many of the characteristics of the wild-type virus including neuronal tissue specificity. It is very different from the plasmid vector developed by Geller and Breakefield. Although both vectors can be used for transfecting adult neurons in vitro or in vivo, it seems that at least at the present time the best vector for attempting gene therapy studies in vivo will be the HSV-1 variant developed by Dobson et al. (1990). The reason for this is that it is clear that this variant can create a latent state in neurons in vivo with continued expression of a foreign gene. It is unlikely that the plasmid vector in its present form can create a true latent state inside neurons. Eventually, as more detailed information becomes available on the genes and the steps involved in creating a permanent latent neuronal infection, it should be possible to develop plasmid vectors with the appropriate genetic elements.

Potential Problems Associated with Transfecting Neurons with Protease

To be clinically useful, a protease transfected into neurons would not only be required to inactivate inhibitors of axon regeneration present on myelin or other structures but would also need to be safe for the transfected neurons and

Table 7.3 Potential Problems Associated with Having Neurons Containing
Transfected Proteases

Problems	Solutions
1. Uncontrolled proteolytic activity	1. Genetically engineer proteases to limit substrate profile 2. Include genetic sequences to direct proteases to the axon 3. Select proteases that are only active extracellularly 4. Limit protease distribution/diffusion with transmembrane domain 5. Select proteases having neuronal receptors 6. Up-pregulate cellular protease inhibitors
2. Transient need for proteases only during regeneration	1. Nonneuronal promoters that slowly inactivate inside neurons 2. Neuronal promoters/repressors regulated by target contact 3. Developmentally regulated or regeneration-dependent promoters

surrounding cells. There are a number of ways to limit unwanted protease
activity and to control the potential destructive effects of a protease (table
7.3). One of the most effective means of controlling unwanted proteolytic
activity is to genetically engineer proteases with very specific substrate profiles. There are many examples of naturally occurring proteases with similar
active sites but with vastly different substrates. For instance, uPA and plasmin
have similar active sites, but uPA cleaves three known proteins (plasminogen,
fibronectin, and PAI-1) whereas plasmin cleaves thousands of proteins. If
specific CNS proteins are identified that block regeneration, then it should be
possible to design proteases that fairly selectively cleave these inhibitors but
are not generally destructive. Alternatively, it may be advantagous to have a
protease with a broad substrate profile for penetrating glial scars or deposits
of extracellular material. This would require additional molecular safeguards to
protect the neuron containing the protease and cells in the local area (including the regenerating axon).

To protect the neuron from extensive intracellular proteolysis, neurons
could be transfected with proteases that only become activated in the extracellular environment. At present, there are two physiological ways in which
this is accomplished. Proteases can be released as proenzymes (known as
zymogens) that are converted by extracellular proteases to active proteases.
Most serine proteases and many metalloproteases are released as zymogens,
bind to cellular or matrix receptors, and then are activated by a second
protease. Another way of activating proteases extracellularly is to have an
extracellular molecule act as a cofactor or nonproteolytic activator. Most
metalloproteases require high concentrations (> 0.2mM) of Ca^{2+} for activity.
Therefore inside the neuron where Ca^{2+} levels are 50 to 500nM, these

     Molecular Mechanisms of Axonal Regeneration

proteases are inactive. Once they are released, metalloproteases are exposed to millimolar concentrations of Ca^{2+} and become activated.

Once activated extracellularly, a protease with a broad substrate profile may not only degrade molecules that inhibit regeneration but may also degrade molecules associated with the regenerating axon or proteins on the surface of cells in the area of protease release. Ways to limit excessive extracellular proteolysis include limiting diffusion of the protease by engineering the protease so that it has a transmembrane domain (i.e., an integral membrane protease) or to have the protease bind to a cellular receptor on the surface of the regenerating axon (PAs and plasminogen appear to have neuronal receptors that direct proteolytic activity away from the cell surface; see figure 7.2). It would also be important to direct most of the proteolytic activity into the regenerating axon rather than having it released from the neuronal cell body. Recent studies have indicated that specific sequences in the growth-associated protein GAP-43 may direct its transport into the axon (Zuber et al., 1989; Liu et al., 1991).

Another means of limiting excessive extracellular proteolysis is to increase the production of cellular protease inhibitors. Although a number of hormones and growth factors have been identified that increase the synthesis of protease inhibitors, this may not be the best means of controlling excessive proteolysis for several reasons: (1) it may not be easy to restrict protease inhibitors to areas of axon regeneration; (2) it is unknown what the effects on the organism would be of globally increasing cellular protease inhibitors for an extended period of time; and (3) hormones and growth factors that increase protease inhibitors also alter expression of many other proteins.

With essentially no information available concerning the effects of uncontrolled proteolysis following the tranfection of neurons with a protease, it is easy to speculate about the characteristics of a protease that would be desirable. Good candidates to start with might include the metalloprotease stromelysin (also known as transin), with or without a transmembrane domain or plasminogen, which appears to have a neuronal binding site (unpublished observations). Stromelysin would be activated by the high concentration of extracellular Ca^{2+} and plasminogen would be activated by local PAs or by co-transfected PA. Because stromelysin and plasminogen cleave a large number of proteins, it may be necessary to genetically engineer them to decrease the extent of their proteolytic activity.

Transient Need for Proteases only During Regeneration

In most cases of gene therapy, there is a requirement to maintain the exogenously added gene in an active state. This is unlikely to be the case for regeneration, because once an axon has regenerated to its appropriate target area and synaptogenesis has begun, a number of the factors important for active axon regeneration may no longer be required. In fact, some of the molecules important for axon outgrowth, such as proteases, may be detrimental to stablization of synapses. Therefore, it may be necessary to inacti-

     Pittman et al.: Proteases as Potential Agents

vate the transfected proteases (see table 7.3). One means of doing this is to have the protease under the control of a promoter that slowly "inactivates" in the neuronal environment. This appears to be the case with genes under control of the long terminal repeat (LTR) promoter in hypoglossal neurons (Dobson et al., 1990). Activity is robust for about 3 weeks following transfection but then precipitously decreases during the next 1 to 2 weeks. Understanding the mechanism involved in the loss of gene activity in this system will be important for designing genetic elements to control proteolytic activity. Although slowly inactivating regulatory elements may effectively limit proteolytic activity to the period of regeneration, an even better means of doing this is with endogenous neuronal elements that are active only during regeneration.

Very little is known about neuronal regulatory elements and transacting factors in neurons; however, it is an area of active interest and research. It is likely that over the next several years a variety of developmentally or axon outgrowth–regulated neuronal elements will be identified and characterized. As an example of this type of molecule, GAP-43 expression appears to be regulated by the growth status of the axon (Skene and Willard, 1981). During axon growth or regeneration, GAP-43 is synthesized in large amounts while very little is produced during periods when axons are not growing (for review, see Skene, 1989). Therefore, a protease gene being driven by GAP-43 regulatory elements would probably "turn off" its synthesis once axon regeneration was complete and synaptogenesis was initiated. It is anticipated that other proteins will also be identified that show similar regulation during axon outgrowth and regeneration. Regulatory elements of these genes will likely be important genetic elements for maintaining proteolytic activity only during regeneration.

SUMMARY AND SPECULATIONS

Proteases appear to be involved in one or more events during axon outgrowth in vitro. They can be genetically engineered to cleave a broad range of substrates or to cleave very selective substrates. It should be possible to use genetically engineered proteases (either serine proteases or metalloproteases) as "molecular scalpels" for inactivating inhibitors of axon regeneration present on myelin, glia, or extracellular material. To stably transfect postmitotic neurons at a high efficiency with a protease will probably require some form of HSV-1 as a vector. Potential problems resulting from transfecting regenerating neurons with a protease include uncontrolled proteolytic activity and the need to have proteolysis only during the period of regeneration and not during synaptogenesis. These problems can be dealt with by controlling temporal expression of the protease with regeneration or target-dependent genetic elements, by limiting the substrate profile of the protease, transfecting proteases that are only active extracellularly, and by decreasing diffusion away from the regenerating axon by selecting proteases with neuronal receptors or by adding a transmembrane domain to the protease. Given these constraints, a likely starting candidate for protease gene therapy for axon regeneration in the CNS would be a genetically engineered serine or metalloprotease under the control of regeneration-dependent genetic elements (e.g., GAP-43 regulatory elements) and packaged in a nonpathogenic variant of HSV-1.

REFERENCES

Bignami, A., Cella, G., and Chi, N.H. (1982). Plasminogen activators in rat neural tissues during development and in Wallerian degeneration. *Acta Neuropathol. (Berl.)* 58:224–228.

Caroni, P., and Schwab, M.E. (1988a). Antibody against myelin-associated inhibitor of neurite growth neutralizes nonpermissive substrate properties of CNS white matter. *Neuron* 1:85–96.

Caroni, P., and Schwab, M.E. (1988b). Two membrane protein fractions from rat central myelin with inhibitory properties for neurite growth and fibroblast spreading. *J. Cell Biol.* 106:1281–1288.

Carter, P., and Wells, J.A. (1987). Engineering enzyme specificity by substrate-assisted catalysis. *Science* 237:394–399.

Cox, E.C., Muller, B., and Bonhoeffer, F. (1990). Axonal guidance in the chick visual system: Posterior tectal membranes induce collapse of growth cones form temporal retina. *Neuron* 4:31–37.

Craik, C.S., Roczniak, S., Largman, C., and Rutter, W.J. (1987). The catalytic role of the active site aspartic acid in serine proteases. *Science* 237:909–913.

Dano, K., Andreasen, P.A., Grondahl-Hansen, J., Kristensen, B., Nielsen, L.S., and Skriver, L. (1985). Plasminogen activators, tissue degradation and cancer. *Adv. Cancer Res.* 44:146–239.

Davies, J.A., Cook, G.M.W., Stern, C.D., and Keynes, R.J. (1990). Isolation from chick somites of a glycoprotein fraction that causes collapse of dorsal root ganglion growth cones. *Neuron* 4:11–20.

Dobson, A.T., Margolis, T.P., Sedarati, F., Stevens, J.G., and Feldman, L.T. (1990). A latent, nonpathogenic HSV-1–derived vector stably expresses β-galactosidase in mouse neurons. *Neuron* 5:353–360.

Eng, L.R., Reier, P.J., and Houle, J.D. (1987). Astrocyte activation and fibrous gliosis: Glial fibrillary acidic protein CNS tissue. *Prog. Brain Res.* 71:439–455.

Faissner, A., and Kruse, J. (1990). J1/Tenascin is a repulsive substrate for central nervous system neurons. *Neuron* 5:627–637.

Fawcett, J.W., and Housden, E. (1990) The effects of protease inhibitors on axon growth through astrocytes. *Development* 109:59–66.

Fawcett, J.W., Housden, E., Smith-Thomas, L., and Meyer, R. (1989). The growth of axons in three-dimensional astrocyte cultures. *Dev. Biol.* 135:449–458.

Geller, A.I., and Breakefield, X.O. (1988). A defective HSV-1 vector expresses *Escherichia coli* β-galactosidase in cultured peripheral neurons. *Science* 241:1667–1669.

Geller, A.I., and Freese, A. (1990). Infection of cultured central nervous system neurons with a defective herpes simplex virus 1 vector results in stable expression of *Escherichia coli* β-galactosidase. *Proc. Natl. Acad. Sci. U.S.A.* 87:1149–1153.

Geller, A.I., Keyomarsi, K., Bryan, J., and Pardee, A.B. (1990). An efficient deletion mutant packaging system for defective herpes simplex virus vectors: Potential applications to human gene therapy and neuronal physiology. *Proc. Natl. Acad. Sci. U.S.A.* 87:8950–8954.

    Pittman et al.: Proteases as Potential Agents

Guenther, J., Hanspeter, N., and Monard, D. (1985). A glia-derived neurite promoting factor with protease inhibitory activity. *EMBO J.* 4:1963–1966.

Gurwitz, D., and Cunningham, D.D. (1988). Thrombin modulates and reverses neuroblastoma neurite outgrowth. *Proc. Natl. Acad. Sci. U.S.A.* 85:3440–3444.

Hantai, D., Rao, J.S., and Festoff, B.W. (1990). Rapid neural regulation of muscle urokinase-like plasminogen activator as defined by nerve crush. *Proc. Natl. Acad. Sci. U.S.A.* 87:2926–2930.

Hawkins, R.L., and Seeds, N.W. (1986). Effect of proteases and their inhibitors on neurite outgrowth from neonatal mouse sensory ganglia in culture. *Brain Res.* 398:63–70.

Jallat, S. Carvallo, D., Tessier, L.H., Roecklin, D., Roitsch, C., Ogushi, F., Crystal, R.G., and Courtnay, M. (1986). Altered specificities of genetically engineered alpha-1 antitrypsin variants. *Protein Eng.* 1:29–35.

Krystosek, A., and Seeds, N.W. (1981). Plasminogen activator release at the neuronal growth cone. *Science* 213:1532–1534.

Krystosek, A., and Seeds, N.W. (1984) Peripheral neurons and Schwann cells secrete plasminogen activator. *J. Cell Biol.* 98:773–776.

Liu, Y., Chapman, E.R., and Storm, D.R. (1991). Targeting of neuromodulin (GAP-43) fusion proteins to growth cones of cultured rat embryonic neurons. *Neuron* 6:411–420.

Liuzzi, F.J., and Lasek, R.J. (1987). Astrocytes block axonal regeneration in mammals by activating the physiological stop pathway. *Science* 237:642–645.

Monard, D. (1988). Cell-derived proteases and protease inhibitors as regulators of neurite outgrowth. *Trends Neurosci.* 11:541–544.

Monard, D., Miday, E., Limat, A., and Solomon, R. (1983). Inhibition of protease activity can lead to neurite extension in neuroblastoma cells. *Prog. Brain Res.* 58:359–364.

Paganetti, PA., Caroni, P., and Schwab, M.E. (1988). Glioblastoma infiltration into central nervous system tissue in vitro: Involvement of a metalloprotease. *J. Cell Biol.* 107:2281–2291.

Patterson, P.H. (1988). On the importance of being inhibited, or saying no to growth cones. *Neuron* 1:263–267.

Pittman, R.N. (1985). Release of plasminogen activator and a calcium-dependent metalloprotease from cultured sympathetic and sensory neurons. *Dev. Biol.* 110:91–101.

Pittman, R.N., and Patterson, P.H. (1987). Characterization of an inhibitor of neuronal plasminogen activator released from heart cells. *J. Neurosci.* 7:2664–2673.

Pittman, R.N., and Williams, A.G. (1989). Neurite penetration into collagen gels requires calcium-dependent metalloproteinase activity. *Dev. Neurosci.* 11:41–51.

Pittman, R.N., Ivins, J.K., and Buettner, H.M. (1989). Neuronal plasminogen activators; Cell surface binding sites and involvement in neurite outgrowth. *J. Neurosci.* 9:4269–4286.

Raper, J.A., and Kapfhammer, J.P. (1990). The enrichment of a neuronal growth cone collapsing activity from embryonic chick brain. *Neuron* 4:21–29.

Salles, F.J., Schechter, N., and Strickland, S. (1990). A plasminogen activator is induced during goldfish optic nerve regeneration. *EMBO J.* 9:2471–2477.

Schnell, L., and Schwab, M.E. (1990). Axonal regeneration in the rat spinal cord produced by an antibody against myelin-associated neurite growth inhibitors. *Nature* 343:269–272.

Schwab, M.E. (1990). Myelin-associated inhibitors of neurite growth. *Exp. Neurol.* 102:2–5.

Schwab. M.E., and Caroni. P. (1988) Oligodendrocytes and CNS myelin are nonpermissive substrates for neurite growth and fibroblast spreading in vitro. *J. Neurosci.* 8:2381–2393.

Skene, J.H.P. (1989). Axonal growth-associated proteins. *Annu. Rev. Neurosci.* 12:127–156.

Skene, J.H.P., and Willard, M. (1981). Axonally transported proteins associated with axon growth in rabbit central and peripheral nervous systems. *J. Cell Biol.* 89:96–103.

Snow, D.M., Steindler, D.A., and Silver, J. (1990). Molecular and cellular characterization of the glial roof plate of the spinal cord and optic tectum: A possible role for a proteoglycan in the development of an axon barrier. *Dev. Biol.* 138:359–376.

Verna, J.-M. (1989). Influence of glycosaminoglycans on neurite morphology and outgrowth patterns in vitro. *Int. J. Dev. Neurosci.* 7:389–399.

Verrall, S., and Seeds, N.W. (1989). Characterization of [125]-I-tissue plasminogen activator binding to cerebellar granule neurons. *J. Cell Biol.* 109:265–272.

Vos, P., Stark, F., and Pittman, R.N. (1991). Merkel cells in vitro: Production of nerve growth factor and selective interactions with sensory neurons. *Dev. Biol.* 144:281–300.

Zuber, M.X., Strittmatter, S.M., and Fishman, M.C. (1989). A membrane-targeting signal in the amino terminus of the neuronal protein GAP-43. *Nature* 341:345–348.

Zurn, A.D., Nick, H., and Monard, D. (1988). A glia-derived nexin promotes neurite outgrowth in cultured chick sympathetic neurons. *Dev. Neurosci.* 10:17–24.

8 GAP-43 and Regrowth of Retinal Ganglion Cell Axons

Susan Spencer and Mark B. Willard

To extend an axon, developing and regenerating neurons elaborate growth cones, organelles specialized for directed locomotion. The behavior of such growth cones can be influenced by a multitude of extrinsic elements, such as growth factors and the molecular constituents of the substrate, which convey signals to the motile machinery via specific receptors on the growth cone surface; these signals can modify the speed and direction of the growth cone's movement. The intrinsic metabolism of the neuron may also influence the behavior of the growth cone. For example, alterations in protein synthesis that would optimize the concentration of proteins composing the machinery for directed locomotion could be important in establishing the potential of the neuron for axon growth. If so, the nature of these changes, and the signals that regulate them would be of interest in understanding the requirements for a neuron to recover from an injury to its axon. We consider here certain properties of the growth-associated protein, GAP-43, whose increased synthesis may reflect metabolic changes that augment the potential of a neuron for axon growth.

ASSOCIATION OF GAP-43 WITH AXON GROWTH

Our laboratory first encountered GAP-43 in experiments investigating whether axon regeneration is accompanied by changes in the composition of proteins that are transported down axons. GAP-43 was among the small number of rapidly transported proteins whose labeling with ^{35}S-methionine, provided to the cell bodies of amphibian retinal ganglion cells, increased dramatically (as much as 100 fold) after the axons of the retinal ganglion cells were crushed to initiate regeneration (Skene and Willard, 1981a). Increased synthesis and transport of GAP-43 has also been observed during regeneration of fish retinal ganglion cell axons (Benowitz and Lewis, 1983; Perry et al., 1987), and mammalian peripheral nerve (Skene and Willard, 1981b). Furthermore, the expression of GAP-43 in mammalian retinal ganglion cells (Skene and Willard, 1981b) and certain other central nervous system (CNS) neurons (Kalil and Skene, 1986) declines during postnatal development. Injury to the distal regions of the axons of adult mammalian retinal ganglion cells (Skene and

Willard, 1981b) and pyramidal track neurons (Kalil and Skene, 1986; Reh et al., 1987) that do not spontaneously regenerate did not trigger increases in GAP-43. (However, the response of GAP-43 expression to injury in mammalian retinal ganglion cells depends upon the location of the injury, as discussed below). This widespread correlation with both developmental and regenerative axon growth suggested that such changes in GAP-43 may reflect metabolic changes that favor axon growth.

The location of GAP-43 in cultured neurons is consistent with this notion; antibodies against GAP-43 bind preferentially to the growth cones (DeGraan et al., 1985; Meiri et al., 1986; Skene et al., 1986). Moreover, the growth cones of rapidly extending neurites from superior cervical ganglion cell neurons cultured from embryonic rats are more intensely labeled by antibodies against GAP-43 than the growth cones of more slowly extending neurites from postnatal rat superior cervical ganglia (Johnson, Meiri, and Willard, in preparation), suggesting a relationship between the rate of axon extension and the amount of GAP-43 in the growth cone. In the case of cultures of hippocampal neurons, the neurites that correspond to axons are more reactive with anti–GAP-43 than neurites that correspond to dendrites, suggesting that this protein may be a marker for the differentiation of these neurites (Goslin et al., 1990). In this case also, GAP-43 content correlates with the rate of neurite extension, because axonal neurites generally extend more rapidly than dendritic neurites. The abundance of GAP-43 in growth cones is consistent with the idea that its function is important for the operation of these organelles, and that its increased synthesis and transport during periods of axon elongation serve to optimize this function.

A more direct evaluation of the potential importance of GAP-43 for axon growth has been provided by recent experiments designed to alter the amounts of GAP-43 in neurons. Transient transfection of cultured hippocampal neurons with antisense GAP-43 RNA, expected to reduce specifically the synthesis of this protein, inhibited the extension of neurites (Fidel et. al., 1990). In the case of PC12 cells, a pheochromocytoma cell line that can be induced to differentiate into neuronlike cells by exposure to nerve growth factor (NGF), transfection with antisense GAP-43 has been reported to inhibit neurite extension (Schotman et al., 1990), whereas transfection with the coding strand (to increase GAP-43 synthesis) facilitated neurite extension and rendered it less dependent upon exposure to NGF (Fidel et al., 1990). It has also been reported that non-neuronal (fibroblastic) cells generate longer and more numerous processes after they have been induced to express GAP-43 by transfection (Zuber et al., 1989). On the other hand, a particular line of PC12 that is deficient in the synthesis of GAP-43 extended the neuritic process normally in response to NGF, suggesting that a high concentration of GAP-43 is not an absolute requirement for the extension of such processes (Baetge and Hammang, 1991). However, the relationship of these PC12 processes to authentic axons or dendrites is not clear. With this exception, these observations provide direct support for a role for GAP-43 in axon growth.

     Molecular Mechanisms of Axonal Regeneration

MOLECULAR PROPERTIES, PHOSPHORYLATION, AND POSSIBLE FUNCTIONS OF GAP-43

The precise function of GAP-43 within the growth cone is not yet known, but certain properties that it exhibits in vitro provide clues suggesting that it has the potential to interact with several second messenger systems. These clues have been supplied by the discovery of GAP-43 in different contexts, each providing this protein with a new module of characteristics, and often with an additional name. Hence, the homonym protein B-50 was initially identified as a brain-specific phosphoprotein whose phosphorylation was inhibited by adrenocorticotrophic hormone (ACTH), a peptide hormone that induces grooming behavior in rats (Zwiers et al., 1976). Subsequent studies of this protein have shown that it is a substrate for protein kinase C (Aloyo et al., 1983), and that antibodies against it can inhibit transmitter release from synaptic vesicles (Dekker et al., 1989). In addition, in its phosphorylated form, B-50 has been reported to inhibit the enzyme that produces phosphatidylinositol diphosphate, the precursor of the second messengers that can stimulate the activity of protein kinase C (Gispen et al., 1985). A second homonym protein, F1, was identified by virtue of its increased phosphorylation by protein kinase C in tissue slices of the hippocampus after induction of long-term potentiation, a process by which synaptic efficacy is increased following high-frequency stimulation of certain presynaptic neurons (Nelson and Routtenberg, 1985). Thus, studies of F1 and B-50 have shown that, in addition to a function within growth cones, this protein also performs a function that may influence synaptic plasticity and transmitter release in the presynaptic terminals of certain mature neurons. This raises the question of whether the presence of GAP-43 in both growth cones and certain presynaptic terminals reflects a common function shared by both. The discovery that B-50 and F1 are substrates for protein kinase C, an enzyme that can be activated indirectly by the interaction between receptors on the cell surface and certain external ligands, suggests that GAP-43 phosphorylation may be an element in the transformation of information from the environment into the appropriate response of the growth cone's motility.

A potential function for the phosphorylation of GAP-43 by protein kinase C has been suggested by the properties of a third homonym, neuromodulin, formerly designated P57 (Andreasen et al., 1983). This protein was identified by virtue of its binding to calmodulin. Unlike most calmodulin-binding proteins, whose enzymatic activities are altered by binding a complex of Ca^{2+} and calmodulin, the affinity of neuromodulin for calmodulin is lower in the presence of Ca^{2+} than in its absence under certain conditions. In addition, the affinity for calmodulin decreased when neuromodulin was phosphorylated by protein kinase C, and conversely, the phosphorylation by protein kinase C was inhibited by the binding of calmodulin to neuromodulin (Cimler et al., 1987). This mutually inhibitory effect is explicable in terms of the proximity of the single site (serine 41) that is phosphorylated by protein kinase C (Apel et al., 1990; Coggins and Zwiers, 1989; Schuh et al., 1989), and the region of

MLCCMRRTKQVEKNDEDQKIEQDGVKPEDKAHKAATKIQA**SFRGHITRKKL**

KGDEKKGDAPAAEAEAKEKDDAPVADGVEKKEGDGSATTDAAPATS̲PKEPS

KAGDAPSEEKKGEGDAAPSEEKAGSAETESAAKATTDNSPSSKAEDGPAKE

EPKQADVPAAVTDAAATT̲PAAEDAAKAAQPPTETAESSQAEEEKDAVDEAK

PKESARQDEGKEDPEADQEHA

Figure 8.1 The amino acid sequence of GAP-43 showing the sites (*arrows*) that are phosphorylated by protein kinase C, or unidentified protein kinases. The region that binds to calmodulin (Alexander et al., 1988) is shown in outline.

the protein that has been identified (Alexander et al., 1988) as the calmodulin-binding domain (figure 8.1). These observations have led to the hypothesis that a function of this protein is to sequester calmodulin at appropriate sites beneath the plasma membrane; the release of calmodulin, triggered either by an increase in the concentration of Ca^{2+}, or by the phosphorylation of GAP-43 with protein kinase C, might then influence Ca^{2+}-calmodulin–sensitive processes that would in turn influence the behavior of the growth cone (Estep et al., 1990). We have considered that these same properties could be employed to increase the velocity of axonal tranport of calmodulin in neurons with growing axons (Spencer and Willard, 1992); according to this hypothesis, the increased amounts of rapidly transported GAP-43 would serve as a carrier to deliver calmodulin (transported slowly in mature neurons) rapidly to the distal portions of the growing axon, where its release would be regulated by the phosphorylation of GAP-43 by protein kinase C.

The physiological significance of phosphorylation of GAP-43 by protein kinase C at serine 41 is supported by the observation that this site is phosphorylated in living superior cervical ganglion cells and neuroblastoma cells (Schuh et al., 1989). Furthermore, an antibody that reacts specifically with GAP-43 phosphorylated at this site has been used to locate the phosphorylated form in nervous tissue by means of immunohistochemistry (Meiri et al., 1991). During development, this antibody labels growing axons only after they have extended for some distance from the cell body, and then it only reacts with the distal portion of the axons. This indicates that the phosphorylation of GAP-43 by protein kinase C is subject to positional and temporal constraints during development.

In addition to protein kinase C, GAP-43 is a substrate for phosphorylation by other protein kinases. When superior cervical ganglion cells growing in culture were incubated with ^{32}P-orthophosphate, five tryptic peptides of GAP-43 were phosphorylated; the labeling of only one of these peptides, which proved to contain serine 41, was stimulated when the cultures were incubated with phorbol ester, a specific stimulator of protein kinase C (Schuh et al., 1989). Analysis of the sequence and phosphoamino acids of the other labeled peptides indicates that their labeling can be accounted for by two additional sites: serine 96 and threonine 172 (Spencer et al., in preparation). The sequence around these sites is similar, suggesting that both sites may be phosphorylated by the same protein kinase. These sites are located in a region of the GAP-43 sequence that is less conserved among species than the amino terminal region containing the protein kinase C phosphorylation site and the calmodulin-binding domain (see figure 8.1). However, these sites are labeled with $^{32}PO_4$ as actively as the protein kinase C site in cultured rat superior cervical ganglion cell neurons (Spencer et al., in preparation).

In vitro, purified GAP-43 is a substrate for casein kinase II (Pisano et al., 1988), which phosphorylates it predominantly at a single site, serine 192 (Spencer et al., in preparation). However, this site was not among the major sites that were phosphorylated by living superior cervical ganglion cells in culture, suggesting that either phosphorylation by casein kinase II is not important in vivo, or that it occurs only under circumstances different from those that prevail in these cultures.

A final clue to the function of GAP-43 is the observation that, in vitro, it stimulates the binding of guanosine nucleotide to the G protein G_0 (Strittmatter et al., 1990), a reaction that would be anticipated to modulate the G_0-dependent process in vivo. It has been considered that GAP-43 might serve as a substitute for, or a competitor of, the receptor-ligand interactions that typically activate G_0 (Strittmatter et al., 1990). Thus, GAP-43 may interact with three second messenger systems: the Ca^{2+}-calmodulin system, the Ca^{2+}-phospholipid system, and G_0 systems.

REGULATION OF SYNTHESIS OF GAP-43

Insofar as the synthesis of GAP-43 responds to signals that regulate the entry of a neuron into a state that is advantageous for axon growth, its induction may serve as an assay for such signals. Several observations suggest that in certain mature neurons, GAP-43 synthesis may be subject to repression by factors arriving from the periphery via retrograde transport. For example, the application of cholchicine to rat peripheral nerve, which is expected to block retrograde axonal transport, has been reported to induce the synthesis of GAP-43 in dorsal root ganglion cells (Woolf et al., 1990). The acquisition of such hypothetical repressors may be sensitive to the state of the synaptic terminal; when regenerating retinal ganglion cells of goldfish were prevented from making synapses by removal of the optic tectum (Perry et al., 1990), the level of radiolabeling of axonally transported GAP-43 remained elevated long after the level had returned to normal in control axons that were permitted to make synapses. Potential sources of such synapse-dependent repressive elements would include the postsynaptic neurons, other cells close to the synapse, or intrinsic neuronal molecules that become repressors only after interacting with an intact presynaptic terminal (Willard and Skene, 1982).

During neonatal development, GAP-43 in mammalian retinal ganglion may also be subject to repression by synapse-specific elements. The amount of GAP-43 declines approximately 20-fold between early neonatal life and adulthood: this reduction is evident both in the labeling of axonally transported GAP-43 (Skene and Willard, 1981b; Freeman et al., 1986) with ^{35}S-methionine and in the staining of retinal whole mounts with an anti–GAP-43 antibody (Doster et al., 1991). It has been noted that synapse-dependent inhibition might be useful for linking the repression of synthesis of proteins that facilitate axon growth to the requirement for axon growth (Willard and Skene, 1982).

An additional mechanism for the regulation of GAP-43 in mature retinal ganglion cells is suggested by its response to injury. In adult rats, axotomy of the optic nerve is not followed by spontaneous regeneration. However, injured retinal ganglion cell axons can regenerate into a graft of peripheral nerve (So and Aguayo, 1985; reviewed in Aguayo, 1985; Aguayo et al., 1990), provided that the graft and injury are close to the eye (Richardson et al., 1982). In recently reported experiments, injury to rat retinal ganglion cells led to an accumulation of GAP-43 that was detected by the staining of retinal whole mounts with anti–GAP-43; as in the case of regeneration into a graft, this response was only observed when the injury was close to the eye (Doster et al., 1991). A speculative explanation for the positional dependence of this response is that axotomy close to the eye removes a larger source of repression for GAP-43 than does axotomy far from the eye. For example, this situation would prevail if repressive elements were generated by non-neuronal cells of the optic nerve, and required intact axons to exert their repressive effects in the cell body. Indeed, factors originating in non-neuronal cells of the optic nerve (e.g. oligodendrocytes) have been observed to elicit negative affects upon axon growth (Caroni and Schwab, 1988; Schwab, 1990; Carbonetto et al., 1987); perhaps these or other factors also serve to alter the metabolism of the injured neuron, repressing growth-related functions. If such a mechanism is indeed responsible for the regulation of growth-related functions in the mature mammalian visual system, it is apparently differentially effective within the CNS, because GAP-43 is differentially regulated during development of different CNS systems (Neve et al., 1988; Benowitz et al., 1988). Moreover, in some cases such a mechanism must be secondary to other means of regulation. For example, GAP-43 can be induced in the cell bodies of dorsal root ganglion cells by axotomy of the peripheral nerve (Woolf et al., 1990) despite the maintenance of an intact axonal branch that enters the spinal cord; this might have been expected to provide a conduit for repressive elements generated by non-neuronal cells of the CNS.

This position-dependent induction of GAP-43 accumulation in injured mammalian retinal ganglion cells indicates that GAP-43 accumulation can occur without concomitant axon growth, and that axotomy provides a sufficient signal to induce this accumulation. However, both GAP-43 induction and growth into a peripheral nerve graft appear to be favored by proximal,

    Molecular Mechanisms of Axonal Regeneration

but not distal, axotomy, consistent with the notion that the induction of GAP-43 may reflect metabolic changes that are related to an increased potential for axon growth: this potential is not realized unless the appropriate substrate for axon growth—i.e., the peripheral nerve graft—is supplied (Doster et al., 1991). This notion is also compatible with the observation that the efficiency of regeneration of the central branches of dorsal root ganglion cell axons into a graft of peripheral nerve is greatly enhanced when the peripheral branch of these axons is also injured (Richardson and Issa, 1984), a process that augments transport of GAP-43 into both branches of these neurons (Woolf et al., 1990; Schreyer and Skene, 1988).

Acknowledgments

This work was supported by NIH grant EYO 2682. We thank Jim Lagasse and Arlene Loewy for discussion and technical assistance.

REFERENCES

Aguayo, A.J. (1985). Axonal regeneration from injured neurons in the adult mammalian central nervous system. In *Synaptic Plasticity*, ed. W. Cotman, 457–484, New York: Guilford Press.

Aguayo, A.J., Carter, D.A., Zwimpfer, T.J., Vidal-Sanz, M., and Bray, G.M. (1990). Axonal regeneration and synapse formation in the injured CNS of adult mammals. In *Brain Repair*, ed. A. Björklund, A. Aguayo, and D. Ottoson, 251, New York: Stockton Press.

Alexander, K.A., Wakim, B.T., Doyle, G.S., Walsh, K.A., and Storm, D.R. (1988). Identification and characterization of the calmodulin binding domain of neuromodulin, a neurospecific calmodulin binding protein. *J. Biol. Chem.* 263:7544–7549.

Aloyo, V.J., Zwiers, H., and Gispen, W.H. (1983). Phosphorylation of B-50 protein by calcium-activated, phospholipid-dependent protein kinase and B-50 protein kinase. *J. Neurochem.* 41:649–653.

Andreason, T.J., Luetje, C.W., Heidman, W., and Storm, D.R. (1983). Purification of a novel calmodulin binding protein from bovine cerebral cortex. *Biochemistry* 22:4615–4618.

Apel, E.D., Byford, M.F., Au, D., Walsh, K.A., and Storm, D.R. (1990). Identification of the protein kinase C phosphorylation site in neuromodulin. *Biochemistry* 29:2330–2335.

Baetge, E.E., and Hammang, J.P. (1991). Neurite outgrowth in PC12 cells deficient in GAP-43. *Neuron* 6:21–30.

Benowitz, L.I., Apostolides, P.J., Perrone-Biozzozero, N., Finklestein, S., and Zwiers, H. (1988). Anatomical distribution of the growth-associated protein GAP-43–B-50 in the adult brain. *J. Neurosci.* 8:339–352.

Benowitz, L.I., and Lewis, E.R. (1983). Increased transport of 44,000 to 49,000-dalton acidic proteins during regeneration of the goldfish optic nerve: a two-dimensional gel analysis. *J. Neurosci.* 3:2153–2163.

Carbonetto, S., Evans, D., and Cochard, P. (1987). Nerve fiber growth in culture on tissue substrata from central and peripheral nervous systems. *J. Neurosci.* 7:610–620.

Caroni, P., and Schwab, M.E. (1988). Two membrane protein fractions from rat central myelin with inhibitory properties for neurite growth and fibroblast spreading. *J. Cell. Biol.* 106:1281–1288.

Cimler, B.M., Giebelhaus, D.H., Wakim, B.T., Storm, D.R., and Moon, R.T. (1987). Characterization of murine cDNAs encoding P-57 a neural-specific calmodulin-binding protein. *J. Biol. Chem.* 262:12158–12163.

Coggins, P.J., and Zwiers, H. (1989). Evidence for a single protein kinase C–mediated phosphorylation site in rat brain protein B-50. *J. Neurochem.* 53:1895–1901.

DeGraan, P.N.E., Van Hoof, C.O.M., Tilly, B.C., Oestricher, A.B., Schotman, P., and Gispen W.H. (1985). Phosphoprotein B-50 in nerve growth cones from fetal rat brain. *Neurosci. Lett.* 61:235–241.

Dekker, L.V., DeGraan, P.N.E., Pijnappel, P., Oestreicher, A.B., and Gispen, W.H. (1991). Noradrenaline release from streptolysin O–permeated rat cortical synaptosomes: Effects of calcium, phorbol esters, protein-kinase inhibitors, and antibodies to the neuron-specific protein-kinase-C substrate B-50 (GAP-43). *J. Neurochem.* 56:1146–1153.

Dekker, L.V., DeGraan, P.N.E., Versteeg, D.H.G., Oestreicher, A.B., and Gispen, W.H. (1989). Phosphorylation of B-50 (GAP-43) is correlated with neurotransmitter release in rat hippocampal slices. *J. Neurochem.* 52:24–30.

Doster, S.K., Lozano, A.M., Aguayo, A.J., and Willard, M.B. (1991). Expression of the growth-associated protein GAP-43 in adult rat retinal ganglion cells following axon injury. *Neuron* 6:635–647.

Estep, R.P., Alexander, K.A., and Storm, D.R. (1990). Regulation of free calmodulin levels in neurons by neuromodulin: Relationship to neuronal growth and regeneration. *Curr. Top. Cell Regul.* 31:161–180.

Fidel, S.A., Dawes, L.R., Neve, K.A., and Neve, R.L. (1990). Effects of manipulation of GAP-43 expression on morphology in PC12 cells and cultured hippocampal neurons. *Soc. Neursci. Abstr.* 16:339.

Freeman, J.A., Bock, S., Deaton, M., McGuire, B., Norden, J.J., and Snipes, G.J. (1986). Axonal and glial proteins associated with development and response to injury in the rat and goldfish optic nerve. *Exp. Brain Res.* 13(suppl.):34–47.

Gispen, W.H., Van Dongen, C.J., De Graan, P.N.E., Oestreicher, A.B., and Zwiers, H. (1985). The role of phosphoprotein B-50 in phosphoionsitide metabolism in synaptic plasma membranes. In *Inositol and Phosphoinositides*, (ed. J.E. Blaesdale, G. Hauser, and J. Eichberg). 399–413. Clifton, N.J.: Humana Press.

Goslin, K., Schreyer, D.J., Skene, J.H., and Banker, G. (1990). Changes in the distribution of GAP-43 during the development of neuronal polarity. *J. Neurosci.* 10:588–602.

Kalil, K., and Skene, J.H.P. (1986). Elevated synthesis of an axonally transported protein correlates with axon outgrowth in nomal and injured pyramidal tracts. *J. Neurosci.* 6:2563–2570.

Meiri, K.F., Bicherstaff, L.E., and Schwob, J.E. (1991). Monoconal antibodies show that kinase C phosphorylation of GAP-43 during axonogenesis is both spatially and temporally restricted in vivo. *J. Cell Biol.* 112:991–1005.

Meiri, K.F., Pfenninger, K.H., and Willard, M.B. (1986). Growth-associated protein, GAP-43, a polypeptide that is induced when neurons extend axons, is a component of growth cones and corresponds to pp46, a major polypeptide of a subcellular fraction enriched in growth cones. *Proc. Natl. Acad. Sci. U. S. A.* 83:3537–3541.

Nelson, R., and Routtenberg, A. (1985). Characterization of protein F1 (47 kDa, 4.5 pI): A kinase C substrate directly related to neural plasticity. *Exp. Neurol.* 89:213–244.

Neve, R.L., Finch, E.A., Bird, E.D., and Benowitz, L.I. (1988). Growth-associated protein GAP-43 is expressed selectively in associative regions of the adult human brain. *Proc. Natl. Acad. Sci. U. S. A.* 85:3638–3642.

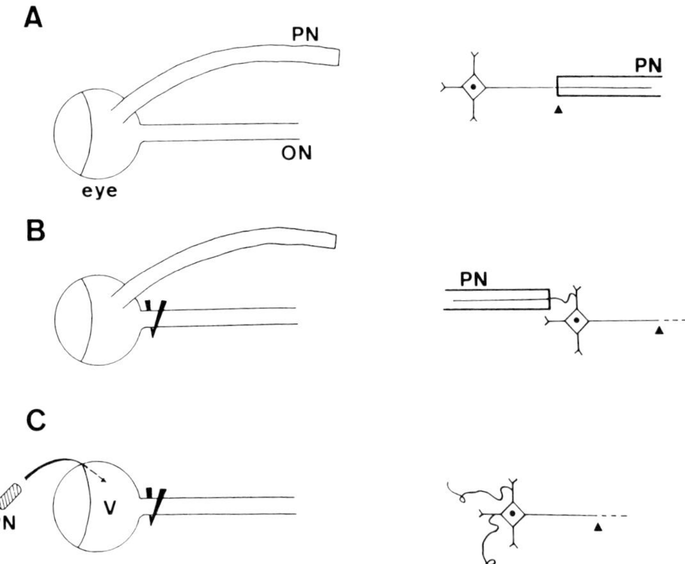

Figure 9.1 Schematic diagrams illustrating the experimental protocols (*left-hand column*) used to study the responses of retinal ganglion cells after axotomy (*right-hand column*). *(A) Left*: transplantation of an autologous peripheral nerve *(PN)* segment to the retina of the eye. *ON* = optic nerve. *Right*: extensive axonal regeneration in the graft is induced when the tip of the damaged axon is in contact with the PN. *Arrowhead* denotes site of axotomy. *(B) Left*: grafting of a PN to the retina together with intraorbital crushing of the ON. *Right*: axotomized ganglion cells located close and central to the graft elicit axonlike processes which undergo long-distance growth in the PN when their damaged axons reside in the ON and cannot regenerate. *(C) Left*: implantation of a short PN into the vitreous body *(V)* of an eye which had the ON crushed intraorbitally. There is no direct physical contact of the PN with the retina. *Right*: ganglion cells are induced to sprout axonlike processes from the somatodendritic compartment and intraretinal axon. The sprouts in this case elongate randomly in the various retinal laminae since the PN was inaccessible for innervation.

FACTORS INFLUENCING ALP FORMATION FROM RGCs

The Role of the Axon

Axotomy of RGCs is a prerequisite in inducing ALPs. This is indicated by the fact that when PN grafting to the retina is performed in the absence of ON crush, the central population of sprouting RGCs (which emit ALPs) do not appear. Thus, intact RGCs or those which suffer damage to the dendritic tree alone do not elaborate ALPs even in the presence of a PN.

The idea that axonal damage provides a specific signal for sprouting is further suggested by the finding that the distance of axotomy from the soma dictates whether ALPs could be elicited. If a PN is grafted to the retina and concurrently the optic pathway is lesioned at distances from the eye greater than that of the intraorbital ON crush, the central population of sprouting RGCs becomes greatly diminished (Cho and So, 1991). This decrease of the sprouting stimulus as a result of the distant axotomy stands in contrast to the

    So et al.: Peripheral Nerve Transplantation

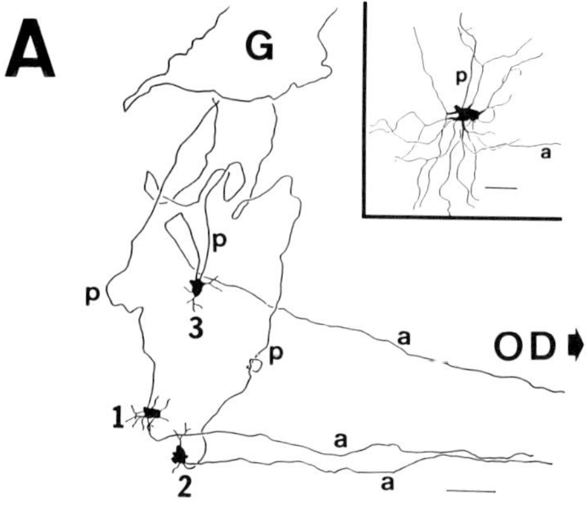

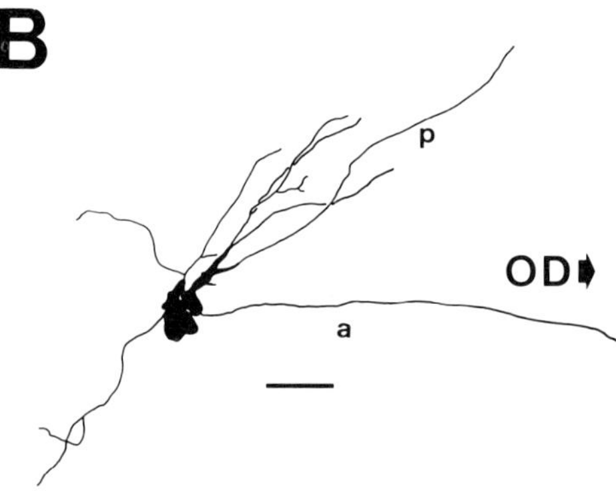

Figure 9.2 Camera lucida tracings of axotomized retinal ganglion cells from silver-stained retinal whole mounts of animals in which a peripheral nerve was grafted to the retina concurrent with intraorbital optic nerve crush. *A*, three silver-stained ganglion cells located central to the graft exhibit sprouting of an axonlike process from the cell body growing toward the graft. The processes have the characteristics of axons in that they are long and sparsely branched, and they tend to maintain a constant thickness without tapering. In their course of elongation toward the graft, they can exhibit either a relatively undeviated trajectory (e.g., cell *1*) or form loops and turns (cells *2* and *3*). In each cell, the original axon (which had the damaged stump residing in the optic nerve) can still be traced toward the optic disc. *G*, grafting site; *OD*, optic disc; *p*, axonlike process: *a*, axon. Scale bar: 100 μm. The inset shows the detailed morphology of cell *1*. Scale bar: 50 μm. *B*, an axotomized ganglion cell with an axonlike process (*p*) emerging from the dendrite. The process heads toward the graft (located beyond the upper right corner) while the axon (*a*) runs in the direction of the optic disc (*OD*). Scale bar: 50 μm.

     Retinal Responses to Injury and Transplantation

less severe neuronal cell death seen after similar axonal injury (Lieberman, 1974; Villegas-Pérez et al., 1989). Further studies with our model may shed light on the nature of the axotomy signal and how it regulates neuronal sprouting and survival differentially.

The growth status of the damaged axon dictates whether ALPs can be produced. When the proximal stump of the injured axon is in contact with the PN graft, only extensive axonal regeneration into the graft occurs. In contrast, RGCs of the central population whose damaged axons reside in the ON and cannot regenerate because of the unfavorable CNS environment will elaborate ALPs to innervate the graft.

The Role of the PN Graft

Sprouting of processes which resemble axons have been described in some vertebrate CNS neurons after axotomy (lamprey anterior bulbar neurons: Hall and Cohen, 1988; cat α-motoneurons: Lindå et al., 1985; Havton and Kellerth, 1987), but they do not seem to require any favorable extrinsic stimulus to support their formation. However, the presence of a PN graft placed close to the axotomized RGCs is necessary to stimulate the formation of ALPs in the retina. In the above-described PN grafting and concurrent ON crush paradigm, the central population of sprouting RGCs is confined at most only to a distance 1.5 mm from the graft, with most cells situated less than 500 μm from it. This suggests that the trophic stimulus arising from the PN takes the form of a diffusible factor(s) and exerts its action on the RGCs with a diffusion gradient effect.

Further evidence supporting a role of the active influence of the graft on the growth of ALPs comes from examining the trajectories of ALPs. When the initial trajectory of each ALP (defined as the first 100 μm of length after initiation from the cell) was measured relative to the grafting site, it was found that greater than 60% of them have very small orientation angles (30 degrees or less) with respect to the PN graft, suggesting that at least during its early phase of formation and growth, the ALP is actively guided by the PN (Cho, 1990).

INTRAVITREAL IMPLANTATION OF PN STIMULATES SPROUTING OF AXOTOMIZED RGCs

In order to gain further insights into how the PN influences ALP formation and to study the pattern of ALP growth, a new experimental paradigm was developed: the ON was crushed intraorbitally and concurrently a small piece of autologous PN (2 mm long) was implanted into the vitreous body (figure 9.1,C) of the ON-crushed eye (Cho and So, 1989b, 1992). This resulted in the PN being located in the vitreous and separated physically from the retina by a small distance. Thus, any influence arising from the PN is likely to operate only via a diffusion mode. Silver staining was used to examine the morphology of RGCs at 2 weeks to 2 months post axotomy.

The presence of an intravitreous PN stimulates on average 323 axotomized RGCs per retina to sprout ALPs at 2 weeks post ON crush, this value dropping to 116 and 52 cells at 1 and 2 months post ON crush respectively. A maximum of 16, 20, and 10 sprouts per cell could be observed at 2 weeks, and 1 and 2 months post ON crush, respectively. The sprouts wander randomly in the various retinal laminae since the PN in this case was inaccessible for innervation. When ON crush was performed *without* intravitreous PN implantation, no RGCs were observed to sprout. These results suggest that diffusible factors emanating from the intravitreal PN alone are sufficient to induce sprouting of ALPs and that innervation of the PN graft is not necessary, at least for the short term development of ALPs.

The ALPs arising from the axotomized RGCs could originate from three sites of the cell: the dendritic tree, soma, and intraretinal axon (figure 9.3). However, a distinct preference for certain sprout initiation loci was observed: ALPs tend to arise most commonly from the dendrites, while only 6% to 16% of the cells sampled from 2 weeks to 2 months post ON crush possessed ALPs coming directly from the soma. The frequency of sprouting from the intraretinal axon lay in between, with 26% to 40% of the sampled cells bearing axonal sprouts. These observations suggest the existence of a hierarchical order of sprouting within an axotomized RGC, with the injured axonal stump being the most favored sprouting site. Only when the damaged axon cannot regrow will ALPs be sprouted from other parts of the cell, and in this case dendrites are more attractive than the intraretinal axon and soma. Determining the mechanisms which govern the intracellular distribution of sprouting loci could provide insights on how a developing neuron achieves its highly specific morphology.

In addition to ALP formation, the somata of the sprouting RGCs also exhibited changes in parallel with the sprouting response. For example, a drastic increase in the cross-sectional area of the soma occurred which at the peak could be more than four times the area of normal RGCs. Sprouting RGCs also displayed irregular somatic profiles such as surface foldings and filamentous protrusions. The temporal pattern of variation of these somatic changes can be correlated with the intensity of sprouting of ALPs from the

Figure 9.3 Photomicrographs of silver-stained retinal ganglion cells which exhibit sprouting of axonlike processes from various cellular compartments after axotomy. *A*, sprouting from the dendritic tree. Three sprouts (labeled by an *asterisk, arrow*, and *arrowhead*) are seen originating from a single primary dendrite. Sprout elongation occurred in various retinal laminae and was extremely random as suggested by the complex looping behavior. Scale bar: 50 μm. *B*, sprouting from the soma. The axonlike sprout (*asterisk*) arises at a point (*arrowhead*) on the cell almost directly opposite to the axon initiation site (*arrow*). The two processes are distinguished by the trajectory and location: the original axon (*a*) resides in the nerve fiber layer and projects toward the optic disc (*OD*), whereas the sprout displays loops and is not confined to a specific lamina. Scale bar: 25 μm. *C*, sprouting from the intraretinal axon. Three sprouts (initiation sites denoted by *arrows*) can be identified arising from the parent axon (*a*) but one sprout per axon is a more common feature. The sprouts are not directed toward the optic disc (*OD*), as is the parent axon, but instead exhibit random growth. Scale bar: 50 μm.

     Retinal Responses to Injury and Transplantation

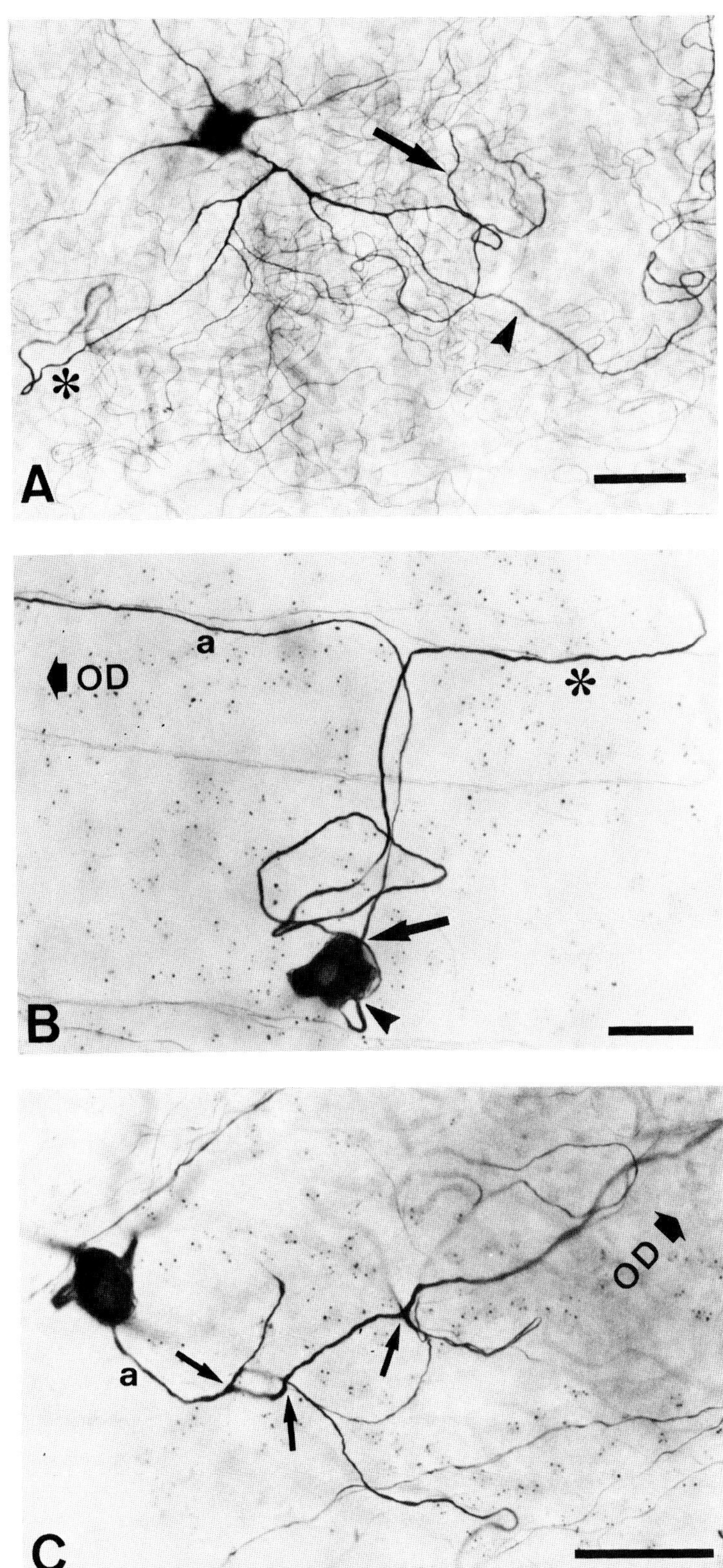

    So et al.: Peripheral Nerve Transplantation

dendritic tree, suggesting that the morphological changes of the soma are another manifestation of the growth behavior exhibited by the sprouting RGCs. Interestingly, these somatic changes are more vigorous when compared with those of RGCs undergoing axonal regeneration in a PN graft, an indication that RGCs sprouting ALPs are in a more active growth state than RGCs regenerating their axons.

The above results highlight the exceptional ability of a mature mammalian CNS neuron to reorganize its neuronal geometry after injury. Sprouting of ALPs can be viewed as an attempt of the injured neuron to replace its damaged axon under circumstances in which axonal regeneration becomes impossible. In this regard, the feasibility of utilizing ALPs as a means of reconstructing interrupted neural pathways should be examined. However, the structural and functional properties of ALPs must first be characterized and compared with those of axons. In addition, the factors governing the initiation, growth, stabilization, and elimination of ALPs have to be elucidated in order to avoid the formation of aberrant and misdirected target connections. Studies of the ultrastructure and biochemical features of ALPs can also shed light on how a neuron maintains the identity of its processes.

Exhibition of Spinelike Processes on Dendrites of RGCs Regenerating Axons Along the PN Graft or Sprouting Axonlike Processes Within the Retina

During normal development of RGCs, transient SLPs have been observed on dendrites of RGCs (Ramoa et al., 1987; Dann et al., 1987; Wong, 1990; Lau et al., 1992). Since there is a temporal correlation of the formation and elimination of these transient SLPs with the synaptogenesis within the inner plexiform layer of the retina, it has been speculated that these transient SLPs are potential sites for making synaptic connections by "catching" bipolar and amacrine cell processes (Wässle, 1988). These transient SLPs disappear when the RGCs attain their adult morphology.

It is well known that afferent synaptic inputs to neurons may fall off and reorganize following axotomy (Kerns and Hinsman, 1973; Purves, 1975; Mendell et al., 1976). Thus, in order for an axotomized RGC to regenerate and regain function, reestablishment of the appropriate synaptic connections between the regenerating RGC with the bipolar and amacrine cells is required in addition to the reconnection of the RGC axon with its target neurons. Recently, we have been using the intracellular injection of Lucifer Yellow to reveal the detailed morphology of RGCs undergoing axonal regeneration along a PN graft (Lau et al., 1991a) or ectopic sprouting of ALPs within the retina (authors' unpublished observation). SLPs similar to those observed on dendrites of developing RGCs were also found on dendrites of these RGCs undergoing axonal regeneration (figure 9.4 and 9.5), while the dendrites of these regenerating RGCs continue to retract or deteriorate as postaxotomy time increases (see below). SLPs were also observed on dendrites of ALP-sprouting cells. It is reasonable to speculate that those SLPs observed on the

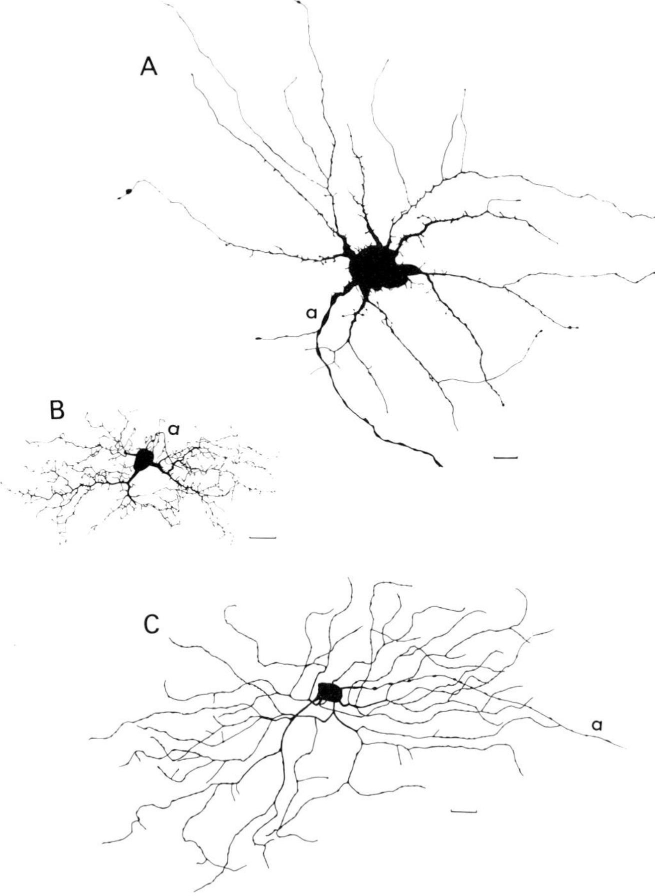

Figure 9.4 Reconstructed drawings of three Lucifer yellow–injected retinal ganglion cells. *A*, a regenerating cell at 5 to 6 weeks post grafting. This cell is the same cell shown in figure 9.5. *B*, a developing type I retinal ganglion cell at postnatal day 10. *C*, a normal adult type I retinal ganglion cell. Note the presence of the spinelike processes (SPLs) on dendrites of the regenerating and developing cells but not on the dendrites of the normal adult type I cell. SPLs can also be observed on the soma of the regenerating cell. *a*, axon. Scale bars: 20 μm.

regenerating or ALP-sprouting RGCs may be sites for making synaptic connections with afferent elements as has been speculated to occur during development (Wässle, 1988). Thus, these results suggest that the damaged adult mammalian RGCs, when challenged by a favorable stimulus, may be able to reattract and reestablish their afferent inputs by producing SLPs on their dendrites. However, unlike the developing RGCs, SLPs were found to persist on some of the regenerating or sprouting RGCs for a long period of time.

FACTORS INFLUENCING THE FORMATION AND ELIMINATION OF SLPs

The formation of SLPs requires that RGCs be in an active growing state following axotomy and presentation of a PN: they have to be regenerating an

    So et al.: Peripheral Nerve Transplantation

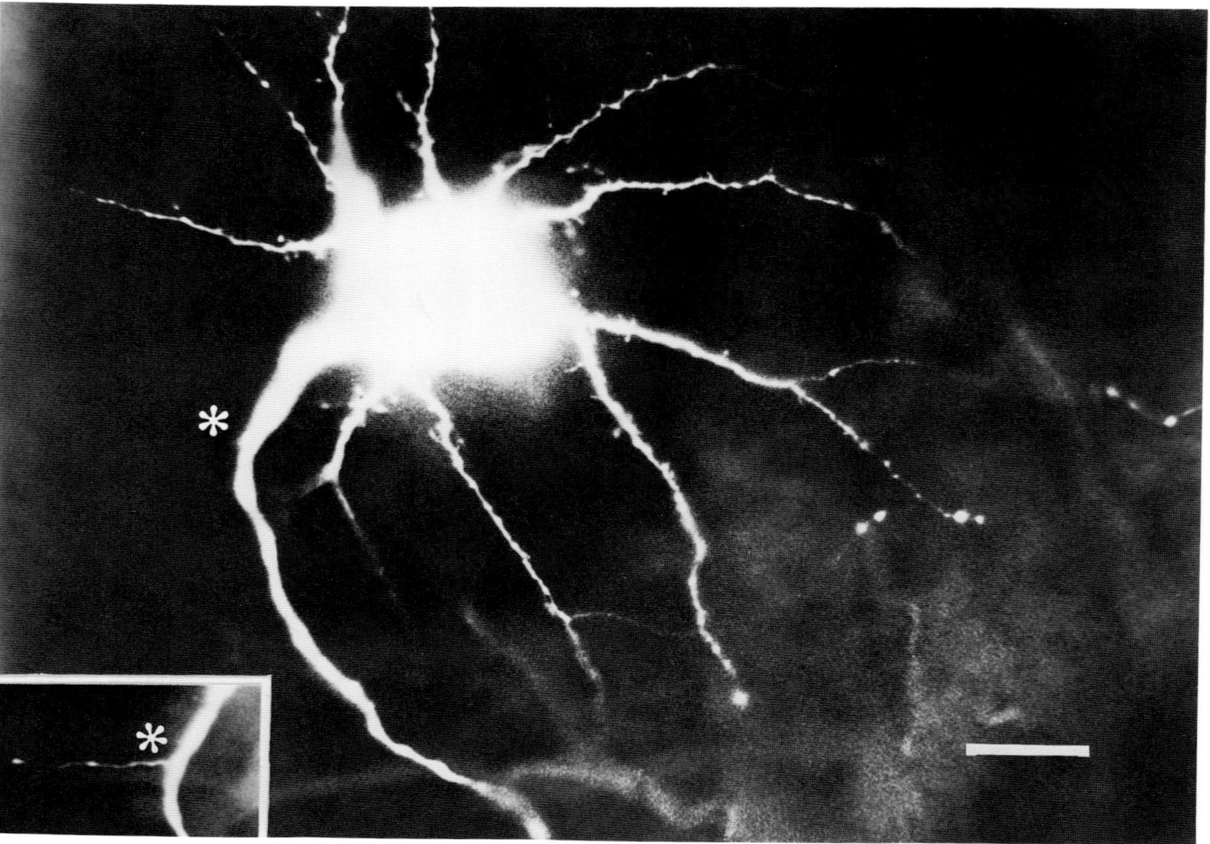

Figure 9.5 Photograph of a Lucifer yellow–injected regenerating cell at 5 to 6 weeks post grafting. Note the spinelike processes on dendrites. Because of the difference in the focal plane of the dendrites and the axon, an axon collateral arising from the axon at the position indicated by the *asterisk* cannot be seen when most of the dendrites are in focus. Inset shows the the axon collateral. A reconstructed drawing of this cell is shown in figure 9.4A. Scale bar: 40 μm.

axon or sprouting ALPs. Axotomy alone, however, is not adequate to cause the formation of the SLPs. We examined RGCs in adult hamsters at 2 and 4 weeks after axotomy using Lucifer Yellow injection technique and did not observe any SLPs on these cells (Lau et al., 1991a).

Normal light stimulation and visual experience do not seem to be important in underlying the elimination of the SLPs in the regenerating RGCs because the animals are reared in normal conditions and the SLPs on some of the regenerating RGCs can persist for up to 9 months after transplantation (Lau et al., 1991a). Although we have not conducted light deprivation experiments in the transplanted animals, the results obtained from similar experiments carried out in developing hamsters support the above point. Thus, rearing hamsters in the dark or suturing their eyelids during development (therefore depriving them of light or visual experience) does not prevent the SLPs from being eliminated, as would normally occur (Lau et al., 1990).

Connection with target might be important for the elimination of the SLPs. Similar SLPs have also been observed on regenerating RGCs in goldfish, and these SLPs disappeared when the RGCs reestablished functional connections with their targets (Becker and Cook, 1990). In both our models for studying the morphology of regenerating and sprouting RGCs, the RGCs were deprived of their targets once they had been axotomized. The persistence of SLPs on these regenerating or sprouting RGCs suggests that the elimination of SLPs is target-dependent. However, the results of our recent study on the morphology of the ipsilaterally projecting RGCs in rats with neonatal unilateral thalamotomy suggest that the process of elimination or retraction of transient SLPs on dendrites of RGCs occurs during development regardless of whether they make connections with correct or incorrect loci in the visual targets (Lau et al., 1991b). Therefore, topographic specificity within an appropriate target may not be essential for the elimination of the SLPs on dendrites.

The results of the above studies indicate that even mature mammalian RGCs may have the potential to reestablish connections with their afferents after damage once they are provided with a proper stimulus and environment to regenerate. Future studies on the mechanism underlying the formation and elimination of the SLPs on RGCs during development and regeneration may provide us with information on how to enhance the reestablishment of synaptic connections between the regenerating RGCs and their afferents.

Dendritic Morphology of Retinal RGCs Regenerating an Axon Along a Peripheral Nerve Graft

Using the Lucifer Yellow intracellular injection and reduced silver staining methods, we have also examined the dendritic morphology of the RGCs with their axons regenerating along a peripheral nerve graft at different postgrafting periods. The branching patterns of the dendrites were analyzed using the concentric circles method of Sholl (Sholl, 1953) and were compared with those obtained from normal RGCs.

    So et al.: Peripheral Nerve Transplantation

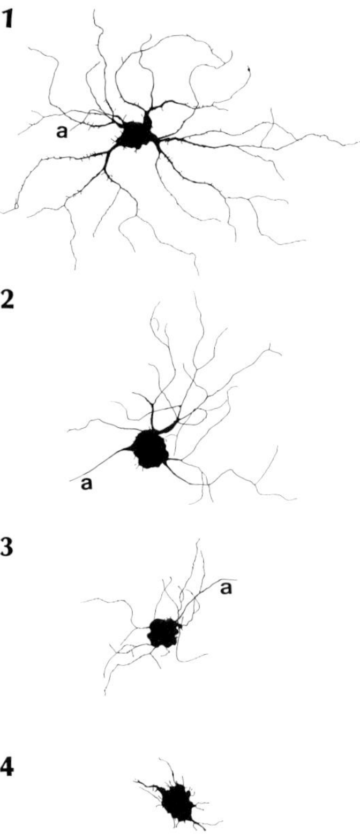

Figure 9.6 Four Lucifer yellow–injected regenerating cells with different dendritic complexity at 5 to 6 weeks post grafting. Note that spinelike processes on the dendrites and soma can be observed on some of the cells. *a*, axon. Scale bar: 50 μm.

Our results from both methods demonstrated that the complexity of the dendrites of RGCs decreases markedly after axotomy and PN transplantation, as has been described recently (Thanos, 1988; Thanos and Aguayo, 1988). However, regenerating RGCs with different degrees of dendritic complexity could be observed in all postgrafting periods studied (figure 9.6) and the dendritic complexity seems to decrease continuously with the increase in the postgrafting time (figure 9.7).

The variations in the complexity of the dendrites of the regenerating RGCs suggests that either the dendrites of the same population of RGCs are reacting differently in response to the PN graft, or the differential dendritic responses are associated with different types or subtypes of RGCs. It would be useful to have an independent cellular marker for specific types of RGCs (e.g., substance P–containing RGCs: Brecha et al., 1987) so that the dendritic responses could be better compared under different experimental situations.

When the regenerating RGCs are considered as a group at each postgrafting period, there is a gradual decrease in the complexity and total length of the dendrites as the postgrafting period increases. Although retraction of the dendrites of the RGCs is expected following axotomy, as has been ob-

     Retinal Responses to Injury and Transplantation

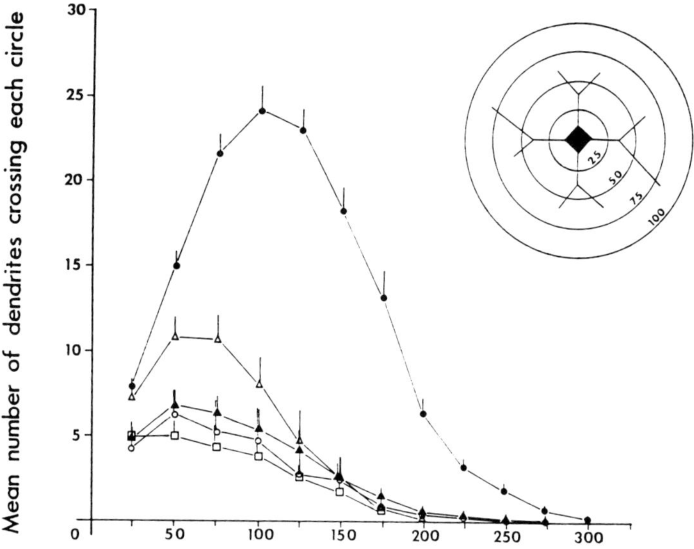

Distance from the center of the soma (μm)

Figure 9.7 Branching pattern analysis of the dendrites of the normal type I cells and regenerating cells from different postgrafting periods studied by the Lucifer yellow injection method. A schematic diagram illustrating the concentric circles method for analysis of the branching pattern of dendrites is shown at upper right. Concentric circles were drawn on top of the cell with the soma as the center. The results of the branching pattern of the dendrites of the cells are presented by plotting the mean number of dendrites intersecting each circle against the distance from the soma. (*Solid circles*, normal type I cells; *open triangles*, 2 to 3 weeks post grafting; *solid triangles*, 5 to 6 weeks post grafting; *open circles*, 10 to 12 weeks post grafting; *open squares*, 20 to 26 weeks post grafting. Note that the dendritic complexity of the regenerating cells decreased with the increase in the postgrafting time. Error bars: SEM.

served in nerve cells that regenerate readily (Sumner and Watson, 1971; Yawo, 1987), our results suggest that the trophic influence provided by the PN graft cannot prevent the continuous deterioration and retraction of the dendrites of the RGCs. Since reexpansion of the dendrites of axotomized hypoglossal and superior cervical ganglion neurons has been observed in mammals once the regenerating axons have reconnected with the appropriate targets (Sumner and Watson, 1971; Yawo, 1987), it offers the hope that this might also be achieved in the regenerating RGCs were a similar reconnection carried out. In fact, successful bridging of the axotomized optic axons in adult rodents with the denervated superior colliculus (Vidal-Sanz et al., 1987; Carter et al., 1989) or with transplanted fetal superior colliculi (Tan et al., 1990; Thanos and Vanselow, 1990) using a PN graft have been reported for the regenerating RGCs. However, since the number of RGCs that have reconnected with the target is still very low, an enhancement of target reconnection is necessary before one can confidently assess the influence of the target on RGCs following reconnection.

     So et al.: Peripheral Nerve Transplantation

CONCLUSION

Past studies of the response of CNS neurons after axonal injury have concentrated mainly on the axonal compartment, such as the pattern of degeneration and regeneration, whereas other cell sites have been relatively neglected. Our results have shown that many reorganizations are in fact taking place on the somatodendritic compartment and many of them may be events which aim at restoring the neuron to its normal state of function. Future work designed to elucidate the mechanisms behind these cellular events may allow the manipulation of injured CNS neurons to promote their functional recovery.

Acknowledgments

We thank the Croucher Foundation of Hong Kong for its support of the research carried out in our laboratory.

REFERENCES

Aguayo, A.J., Bray, G.M., Rasminsky, M., Zwimpfer, T., Carter, D., and Vidal-Sanz, M., (1990). Synaptic connections made by axons regenerating in the central nervous system of adult mammals. *J. Exp. Biol.* 153:199–224.

Becker, D.L., and Cook, J.E. (1990). Changes in goldfish retinal ganglion cells during axonal regeneration. *Proc. R. Soc. Lond. [Biol.]* 241:73–77.

Berry, M., Rees, L., and Sievers, J. (1986). Unequivocal regeneration of rat optic nerve axons into sciatic nerve isografts. In *Neural Tissue Transplantation Research*, ed. R. Wallace and G. Das, 63–79. New York: Springer-Verlag.

Brecha, N., Johnson, D., Bolz, J., Sharma, S., Parnavelas, J.G., and Lieberman, A.R. (1987). Substance P–immunoreactive retinal ganglion cells and their central axon terminals in the rabbit. *Nature* 327:155–158.

Carter, D.A., Bray, G.M., and Aguayo, A.J. (1989). Regenerated retinal ganglion cell axons can form well-differentiated synapses in the superior colliculus of adult hamsters. *J. Neurosci.* 9:4042–4050.

Cho, E.Y.P. (1990). *Axonal Regrowth and Morphological Plasticity of Retinal Ganglion Cells in the Adult Hamster.* (Thesis, University of Hong Kong)

Cho, E.Y.P., and So, K.-F. (1989a). De novo formation of axon-like processes from axotomized retinal ganglion cells which exhibit long distance growth in a peripheral nerve graft in adult hamsters. *Brain Res.* 484:371–377.

Cho, E.Y.P., and So, K.-F. (1989b). Trophic factors from peripheral nerve can stimulate sprouting of neurites from dendrites and soma of axotomized retinal ganglion cells. *J. Neurotrauma.* 6:221–222.

Cho, E.Y.P., and So, K.-F. (1991). Induction of axon-like processes from axotomized retinal ganglion cells by a peripheral nerve graft is influenced by the distance of axotomy from the cell body. *J. Anat.* 176:229.

Cho, E.Y.P., and So, K.-F. (1992). Characterization of the sprouting response of axon-like processes from retinal ganglion cells after axotomy in adult hamsters: A model using intravitreal implantation of a peripheral nerve. *J. Neurocytol.* (in press).

  Retinal Responses to Injury and Transplantation

Dann, J.F., Buhl, E.H., and Peichl, L. (1987). Dendritic maturation in cat retinal ganglion cells: a Lucifer yellow study. *Neurosci. Lett.* 80:21−26.

Hall, G.F., and Cohen, M.J. (1988). The pattern of dendritic sprouting and retraction induced by axotomy of lamprey central neurons. *J. Neurosci.* 8:3584−3597.

Havton, L., and Kellerth, J.-O. (1987). Regeneration by supernumerary axons with synaptic terminals in spinal motoneurons of cats. *Nature* 325:711−714.

Keirstead, S.A., Rasminsky, M., Fukuda, Y., Carter, D.A., Aguayo, A.J., and Vidal-Sanz, M. (1989). Electrophysiologic responses in hamster superior colliculus evoked by regenerating retinal axons. *Science* 246:255−257.

Kerns, J.M., and Hinsman, E.J. (1973). Neuroglial response to sciatic neurectomy. II. Electron microscopy. *J. Comp. Neurol.* 151:255−280.

Kiernan, J.A. (1985). Axonal and vascular changes following injury to the rat's optic nerve. *J. Anat.* 141:139−154.

Lau, K.C., So., K.-F., and Tay, D. (1990). Effects of visual or light deprivation on the morphology, and the elimination of the transient features during development, of type I retinal ganglion cells in hamsters. *J. Comp. Neurol.* 300:583−592.

Lau, K. C., So, K.-F., and Cho, E.Y.P. (1991a). Morphological changes of retinal ganglion cells regenerating axons along peripheral nerve grafts: A Lucifer yellow and silver staining study. *Restorative Neurol. Neurosci.* 3:235−246.

Lau, K.C., So, K.-F., Tay, D., and Jen, L.S. (1991b). Elimination of transient dendritic spines in ipsilaterally projecting retinal ganglion cells in rats with neonatal unilateral thalamotomy. *Neurosci. Lett.* 121:255−258.

Lau, K. C., So, K.-F., and Tay, D. (1992). Postnatal development of type I retinal ganglion cells in hamsters: A Lucifer yellow study. *J. Comp. Neurol.* 315:375−381.

Leicester, J., and Stone, J. (1967). Ganglion, amacrine and horizontal cells of the cat's retina. *Vision Res.* 7:695−705.

Lieberman, A.R. (1974). Some factors affecting retrograde neuronal responses to axonal lesions. In *Essays on the Nervous System*, ed. R. Bellairs and E. G. Gray, 71−105, Oxford, England: Clarendon Press.

Lindå, H., Risling, M., and Cullheim S. (1985). "Dendraxons" in regenerating motoneurons in the cat: do dendrites generate new axons after central axotomy? *Brain Res.* 358:329−333.

McConnell, P., and Berry, M. (1982). Regeneration of ganglion cell axons in the adult mouse retina. *Brain Res.* 241:362−365.

Mendell, L.M., Munson, J.B., and Scott, J.G. (1976). Alterations of synapses on axotomized motoneurones. *J. Physiol. (Land.)* 255:67−79.

Politis, M.J., and Spencer, P.S. (1986). Regeneration of rat optic axons into peripheral nerve grafts. *Exp. Neurol.* 91:52−59.

Purves, D. (1975). Functional and structural changes in mammalian sympathetic neurones following interruption of their axons. *J. Physiol. (Land.)* 252:429−463.

Ramoa, A.S., Campbell, G., and Shatz, C.J. (1987). Transient morphological features of identified ganglion cells in living fetal and neonatal retina. *Science* 237:522−525.

Ramón y Cajal, S. (1928). *Degeneration and Regeneration of the Nervous System*, trans. R.M. May. New York: Hafner.

Sholl, D.A. (1953). Dendritic organization in the neurons of the visual and motor cortices of the cat. *J. Anat.* 87:387−407.

    So et al.: Peripheral Nerve Transplantation

So, K.-F., and Aguayo, A.J. (1985). Lengthy regrowth of cut axons from ganglion cells after peripheral nerve transplantation into the retina of adult rat. *Brain Res.* 328:349–354.

So, K.-F., Xiao, Y.M., and Diao, Y.C. (1986). Effects on the growth of damaged ganglion cell axons after peripheral nerve transplantation in adult hamster. *Brain Res.* 377:168–172.

Sumner, B.E.H., and Watson, W.E. (1971). Retraction and expansion of the dendritic tree of motor neurones of adult rats induced in vivo. *Nature* 233:273–275.

Tan, M.M.L., Harvey, A.R., and So, K.-F. (1990). Regeneration of retinal axons in grafts of peripheral and central nervous tissue in the adult rat. *Neurosci. Lett.* 117:14–19.

Thanos, S. (1988). Alterations in the morphology of ganglion cell dendrites in the adult rat retina after optic nerve transection and grafting of peripheral nerve segments. *Cell Tissue Res.* 254:599–609.

Thanos, S., and Aguayo, A.J. (1988). Changes in dendrites of adult rat ganglion cells regenerating axons into peripheral grafts. In *Post-Lesion Neural Plasticity*, ed. H. Flohr, 129–138, Heidelberg: Springer-Verlag.

Thanos, S., and Vanselow, J. (1990). Fetal tectal transplants in the cortex of adult rats become innervated both by retinal ganglion cell axons regenerating through peripheral nerve grafts and by cortical neurons. *Restor. Neurol. Neurosci.* 2:63–75.

Vidal-Sanz, M., Bray, G.M., Villegas-Pérez, M.P., Thanos, S., and Aguayo, A.J. (1987). Axonal regeneration and synapse formation in the superior colliculus by retinal ganglion cells in the adult rat. *J. Neurosci.* 7:2894–2909.

Villegas-Pérez, M., Vidal-Sanz, M., Bray, G.M., and Aguayo, A.J. (1989). The distance of axotomy from the neuronal cell body influences rate of retrograde degeneration but not long term survival of retinal ganglion cells. *Soc. Neurosci. Abstr.* 15:457.

Wässle, H. (1988). Dendritic maturation of retinal ganglion cells. *Trends Neurosci.* 11:87–89.

Wong, R.O.L. (1990). Differential growth and remodelling of ganglion cell dendrites in the postnatal rabbit retina. *J. Comp. Neurol.* 294:109–132.

Yawo, H. (1987). Changes in the dendritic geometry of mouse superior cervical ganglion cells following postganglionic axotomy. *J. Neurosci.* 7:3703–3711.

10 Intracerebral Retinal Transplants

Raymond D. Lund, Jeffrey D. Radel, Mark H. Hankin, Kathleen T. Yee, Ranjita Banerjee, Peter J. Coffey, and Gwynn M. Horsburgh

The use of transplant technology for studying development and regeneration has been a standard approach in nonmammalian vertebrates for many years (see Harris, 1984). Major application of intracerebral transplantation to problems of mammalian neurobiology developed in the 1970s largely as a result of morphological studies by Das (Das, 1974), regeneration experiments by Björklund (Björklund et al., 1976), and our own studies on development (Lund and Hauschka, 1976). The field has expanded greatly and has provided insight into a variety of issues ranging from immunological consequences of transplantation (Mason et al., 1986; Lawrence et al., 1990) to the use of transplants in correcting deficient neuroendocrine functions (Krieger et al., 1982). The use of transplanted non-neuronal tissue to provide regenerative or trophic support to neurons is another and important application of this technique.

Overall, transplantation research falls into three main categories. The first category comprises those studies in which the transplanted cells may function as neuromodulators, as support for the growth and survival of host neurons, and as relays of specific information. Examples of this group include nigral transplants to the striatum (Björklund and Stenevi, 1979), septal grafts to hippocampus (Gage and Björklund, 1986), and basal forebrain grafts to cortex (Fine et al., 1985). These studies serve as an important experimental model for correcting deficits encountered in Parkinson's disease, Alzheimer's disease, and other forms of memory loss.

In the second category, the role for grafts in providing trophic support has been shown to advantage in the series of studies by Aguayo and his colleagues (see David and Aguayo, 1981; Vidal-Sanz et al., 1987; and chapters 3 and 16 of this book) where in a sciatic nerve graft can act as a conduit for regeneration of the damaged axons of host neurons. Other studies have shown that genetically modified cells, capable of producing nerve growth factor, can sustain axotomized basal forebrain cells (Breakefield and Gage, 1988).

The third type of transplant involves the formation of neural circuits that integrate with host neural pathways. A growing number of situations in which this is possible have been identified, some of which are clearly capable of relaying functional information (Harvey et al., 1982; Neafsey et al., 1989; Sotelo et al., 1990; Wictorin et al., 1990; Silverman et al., 1991). In our early studies, we were interested in how transplanted tectum and cortex integrated with host neural pathways during development (Lund and Hauschka, 1976; Jaeger and Lund, 1980; Lund and Harvey, 1981; Harvey and Lund, 1981; Harvey et al., 1982). Subsequent work demonstrated that embryonic retinas placed over the midbrain of newborn or adult rats form specific connections with visual centers of the host brain, and that these connections are capable of relaying light intensity information to host brain circuits to elicit appropriate functional responses. This work is summarized in this chapter.

EXPERIMENTAL PREPARATION

Donor tissue is taken from rats or mice between 12 and 14 days of gestation. The neural retinas are dissected free of investing tissues (including the pigment epithelium) and are transferred to the host brain using a small pipette attached by polyethylene tubing to a $50\mu l$ syringe. Grafts to newborn rats can be introduced by making a small cut in the skull and releasing the graft directly over the midbrain (Lund and Yee, 1991). In adult mice and rats, while the graft can be introduced over the midbrain using a caudal approach, it is also possible to remove overlying cortex and place the graft directly on the surface of the brain or in a lesion cavity. While even xenografts can frequently survive transplantation to neonatal rat hosts (Lund et al., 1988) in the absence of immunosuppression, they are generally rejected within a week of transplantation to adult hosts (Klassen and Lund, 1988). Under certain conditions, allografts are also subject to immune destruction (Mason et al., 1986; Lawrence et al., 1990; Rao et al., 1989).

OBSERVATIONS

Transplant Organization

Light microscopic studies have shown that retinas placed in neonatal brains develop much of the organization of a normal retina, with all the normal layers present, including photoreceptor outer segments (figure 10.1). There is a diversity of ganglion cells similar to that seen normally (Perry et al., 1985). If the retinas are transplanted with minimal disruption and maintained with a lens intact, they generally retain the sheetlike organization of a normal retina: if they are damaged or disrupted during transplantation (the most extreme disruption being dissociation), they still show a recognizable lamination, but the layers are configured into rosette formations around a central lumen lined by receptor cells. In general, retinal transplants to adult animals show more rosette formations with fewer sheetlike regions (McLoon and Lund, 1983; Klassen and Lund, 1988).

Transplants placed in neonates show all the synaptic features of normal retina when examined electron microscopically (Matthews et al., 1982; Radel et al., 1992). Embryonic retinal transplants develop over a time course similar to that for normal retinas, but lag behind the developmental state of the

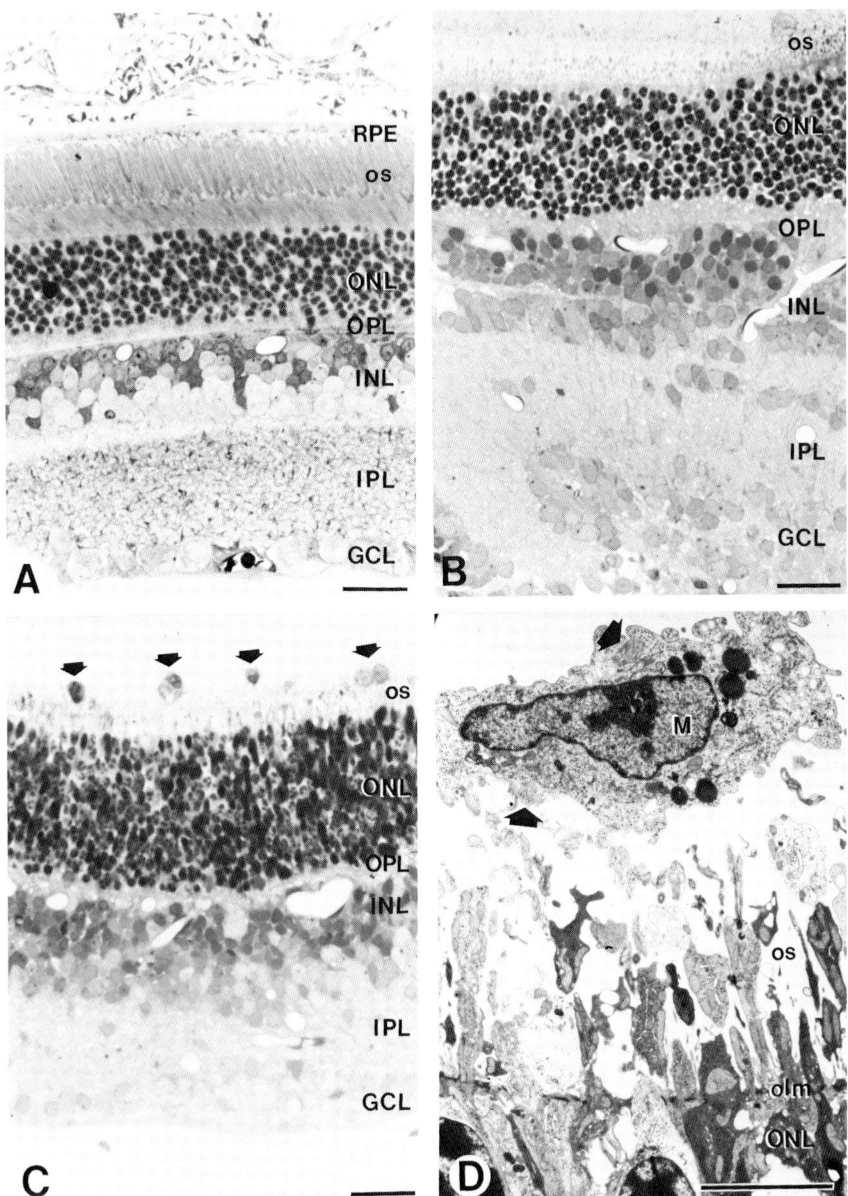

Figure 10.1 Normal and transplanted retinas possess similar patterns of laminar organization. *A*, retina taken from the eye of an adult Long-Evans rat exhibits normal lamination. Transplanted albino retinas have laminar patterns characteristic of normal retinas, but lack pigment epithelium. *B*, mature transplant 30 days after transplantation. *C*, a transplanted retina 22 days after transplantation, at an age equivalent to that of a normal retina when a rat's eyes first open. Note the presence of macrophages adjacent to photoreceptor outer segments (*arrows*). *A–C* are sections 1 μm thick stained with toluidine blue. *D*, electron microscopic view of the transplant shown in *C* illustrating a macrophage (*M*) in close proximity to outer segments, containing undigested fragments of heavily folded membrane (*arrows*). *RPE*, retinal pigment epithelium; *os*, outer segments; *ONL*, outer nuclear layer; *OPL*, outer plexiform layer; *INL*, inner nuclear layer; *IPL*, inner plexiform layer; *GCL*, ganglion cell layer; *olm*, outer limiting membrane. Calibration bars: 25 μm *(A–C)* and 5 μm *(D)*.

     Lund et al.: Intracerebral Retinal Transplants

surrounding host brain by 1 week (Hankin and Lund, 1987; Radel et al., 1992). Outer segments are clearly evident, but they are usually less well aligned than in normal retinas. One point of significance is that during the dissection process, the neural retina is separated from the pigment epithelial layer and it is clear that there are very few, if any, pigment epithelial cells associated with a mature transplant. The absence of these cells might be expected to compromise normal visual function in the light of studies on pigment epithelium and receptor cell interrelations in the intact eye (Bok and Hall, 1971; LaVail, 1981). However, it appears that cells showing morphological and antigenic features of microglia may substitute, at least in part, for the absent pigment epithelial cells. These microglia-like cells line the outer border of the transplant, as do pigment epithelial cells in a normal eye, and engulf outer segment membranes in a manner similar to pigment epithelial cells (Perry and Lund, 1989; Sharma and Lund, 1990; Banerjee and Lund, 1992).

Transplants show substantial projections to the host brain which can be first identified within a few days of transplantation (Hankin and Lund, 1990a). The cells of origin show all the characteristics of ganglion cells with cell bodies located mainly in the ganglion cell layer and sometimes on the inner border of the inner nuclear layer, as would normally be expected of "displaced" ganglion cells (Perry et al., 1985).

DEVELOPMENT OF TRANSPLANT CONNECTIONS

The results from an extended series of studies indicate that the formation of specific connections between transplanted retinas and visual nuclei in the brainstem may depend upon, at the least, the following conditions. First, appropriate substrates that promote the outgrowth of retinal axons must be present in the region of implantation. Related to this must be a consideration of the host brain's reaction to implantation, especially where it influences neurite outgrowth (either positively or negatively). Second, in lieu of random outgrowth, cues must be present which not only promote axonal growth in general, but which are sufficient to direct the retinal fibers to the appropriate target regions. Third, the target must support innervation by optic axons.

We have approached these issues by studying the early events following intracerebral transplantation of neural retina. Immediately after implantation of a retina into the brain of a newborn host, there is an injury site associated with the damage caused by the injection pipette (M.H.H. unpublished observation). During the first 2 to 3 days, there is a gradual condensation of vimentin-positive cells, presumably developing glia, upon the edges of the lesion. A glial scar is not seen in newborn animals, although the extent of the astrocytic reaction may depend upon several factors, including the type and location of the lesion (Sumi and Hager, 1968; Bignami and Dahl, 1974; Suard et al., 1989; Trimmer and Wunderlich, 1990), and the age of the animal (Berry et al., 1983; Krüger et al., 1986). When the implantation is into the midbrain, occasional hypertrophied astroctytes are observed with elevated glial fibrillary acidic protein (GFAP) levels. The implantation cavity progressively diminishes in size and within 1 to 2 weeks the only indication of the injection tract is a line of GAP-positive cells that may persist into maturity.

The first outgrowth from retinal grafts placed either in the region of the midbrain or cerebral cortex can be detected within 24 hours of transplantation (Hankin and Lund, 1990a). For grafts with adjacent lesion damage, there is a transient axonal growth along the borders of the lesion that persists for 3 to 5 days (Sefton et al., 1991). If placed on the surface of the cortex, transplant-derived fibers may grow along layer 1 (unrelated to the direct surgical damage), frequently extending as much as 1 mm and persisting for approximately 5 days after implantation. Axons emanating from a retina grafted to the cortex can survive for longer periods, however, if a natural target (e.g., superior colliculus) is also transplanted to the cortex (Sefton and Lund, 1987; Sefton et al., 1991).

Transplants placed on the brainstem surface extend axons for considerable distances close to the surface, much as do normal optic tract axons. Grafts located within approximately 200 μm of the brainstem surface show substantial outgrowth along the surface, extending several hundred micrometers from the graft within 2 days of transplantation (Hankin and Lund, 1990a). Eventually, transplant axons grow toward the tectum even over distances that may exceed 5 mm (Hankin and Lund, 1990a; Radel et al., 1990), well beyond the range over which diffusible substances are thought to be effective. By contrast, retinas embedded in the brainstem show directed outgrowth toward the tectum only if located within a distance of 1 mm (Hankin and Lund, 1987; Hankin and Lund, 1990a). It is suggested therefore that the oriented growth along the surface of the brainstem may depend more on substrate cues than on target-derived events. Studies in developing *Xenopus*, in accordance with this idea, indicate the presence of polarity cues associated with the brainstem surface which define the direction of growth of optic axons (Harris, 1989). Growth through the parenchyma may be dependent on a target-derived diffusible factor.

It is proposed that the differential outgrowth patterns of superficially located and embedded grafts may reflect two aspects of normal optic axon growth (Hankin and Lund, 1991). Axons may extend toward the tectum guided by substrate molecules that may be encoded for polarity at the surface of the brainstem. Once in the vicinity of the tectum, a target-derived factor may serve to focus more axons upon the tectum and perhaps provide a signal that the growing axons should change their developmental program and ramify terminal arbors, form synapses, and become dependent on the target for the continued survival of the parent cell. The transplant paradigm may have artificially separated the two events.

PATTERNS OF CONNECTIVITY

The superior colliculus is invariably innervated by the transplants but substantial projections are frequently also seen to other visual centers including pretectum (olivary pretectal nucleus and nucleus of the optic tract), and accessory optic nuclei (McLoon and Lund, 1980; Radel et al., 1990). There is also a lesser projection to the dorsal lateral geniculate nucleus which generally shows a restricted or preferential distribution to the superficial aspect of the nucleus. No projection has been shown to the suprachiasmatic nucleus and projections were not seen in earlier studies to the ventral lateral geniculate nucleus or to the intergeniculate leaflet. More recently, by modifying fixation conditions, we have on occasion been able to demonstrate a network of graft-derived axons to the intergeniculate leaflet and sometimes to the ventral lateral geniculate nucleus. All projections are heaviest when the host optic innervation to these various regions is removed at the time of transplantation, but they can still be seen if the eyes are intact (figure 10.2; McLoon and Lund, 1980; Radel et al., 1991a). The density of the projection is enhanced but does not change its regional specificity significantly if the graft is introduced before birth (Yee and Lund, 1991). The possibility that the projections may be guided by intact optic axons or by the effects of removing optic inputs was studied by examining the projections of retinas transplanted to anophthalmic mice in which the eye cup fails to develop properly and no axons ever leave the eye (Silver and Robb, 1979). Transplants in these animals (figure 10.3) project with an equal or greater density to most of the nuclei innervated in eye-enucleated genetically normal hosts (see figure 10.3; Hankin and Lund, 1990b; Horsburgh et al., 1990; Horsburgh et al., 1991).

Anatomical studies using two retrogradely transported labels showed that the transplant projection to the superior colliculus does not appear to be topographically ordered: adjacent ganglion cells in the transplant are as likely to project to the opposite pole of the tectum as they are to project to the same area (Galli et al., 1989).

The terminal fields of optic axons from the two eyes segregate from one another during normal development, often into laminae or stripes in those regions where they converge (Hayhow, 1958; Harting and Guillery, 1976; Hubel and Wiesel, 1969, 1972). Such segregation does not seem to occur between inputs from transplanted rodent retinas and host optic projections, despite the fact that in frogs transplanted retinas do form segregated stripes with the normal host input in the tectum (Constantine-Paton and Law, 1978). Even when two embryonic retinas are transplanted into a newborn rat, the projections from the two retinas appear to overlap substantially (Yee and Lund, 1991).

Fine structural studies have so far examined transplant terminals only in the superior colliculus and olivary pretectal nucleus, where transplant axons exhibit characteristics of normal optic terminals and form similar synaptic arrays (Horsburgh et al., 1990).

PHYSIOLOGICAL STUDIES

Physiological studies have demonstrated that gross potential responses, the amplitude of which is intensity-dependent, can be recorded from light-stimulated transplants and that unit responses can be recorded from the

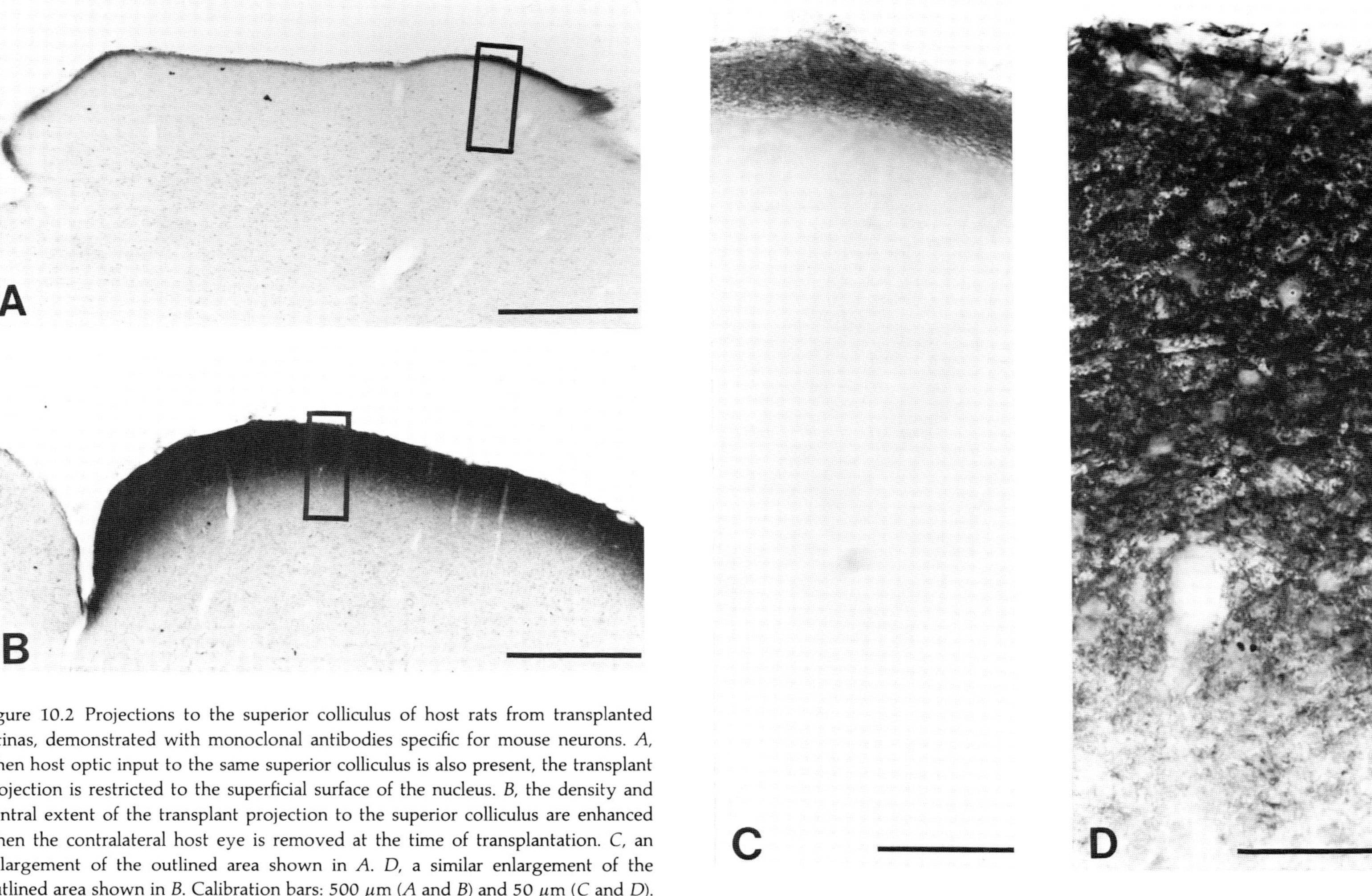

Figure 10.2 Projections to the superior colliculus of host rats from transplanted retinas, demonstrated with monoclonal antibodies specific for mouse neurons. *A,* when host optic input to the same superior colliculus is also present, the transplant projection is restricted to the superficial surface of the nucleus. *B,* the density and ventral extent of the transplant projection to the superior colliculus are enhanced when the contralateral host eye is removed at the time of transplantation. *C,* an enlargement of the outlined area shown in *A. D,* a similar enlargement of the outlined area shown in *B.* Calibration bars: 500 µm (*A* and *B*) and 50 µm (*C* and *D*).

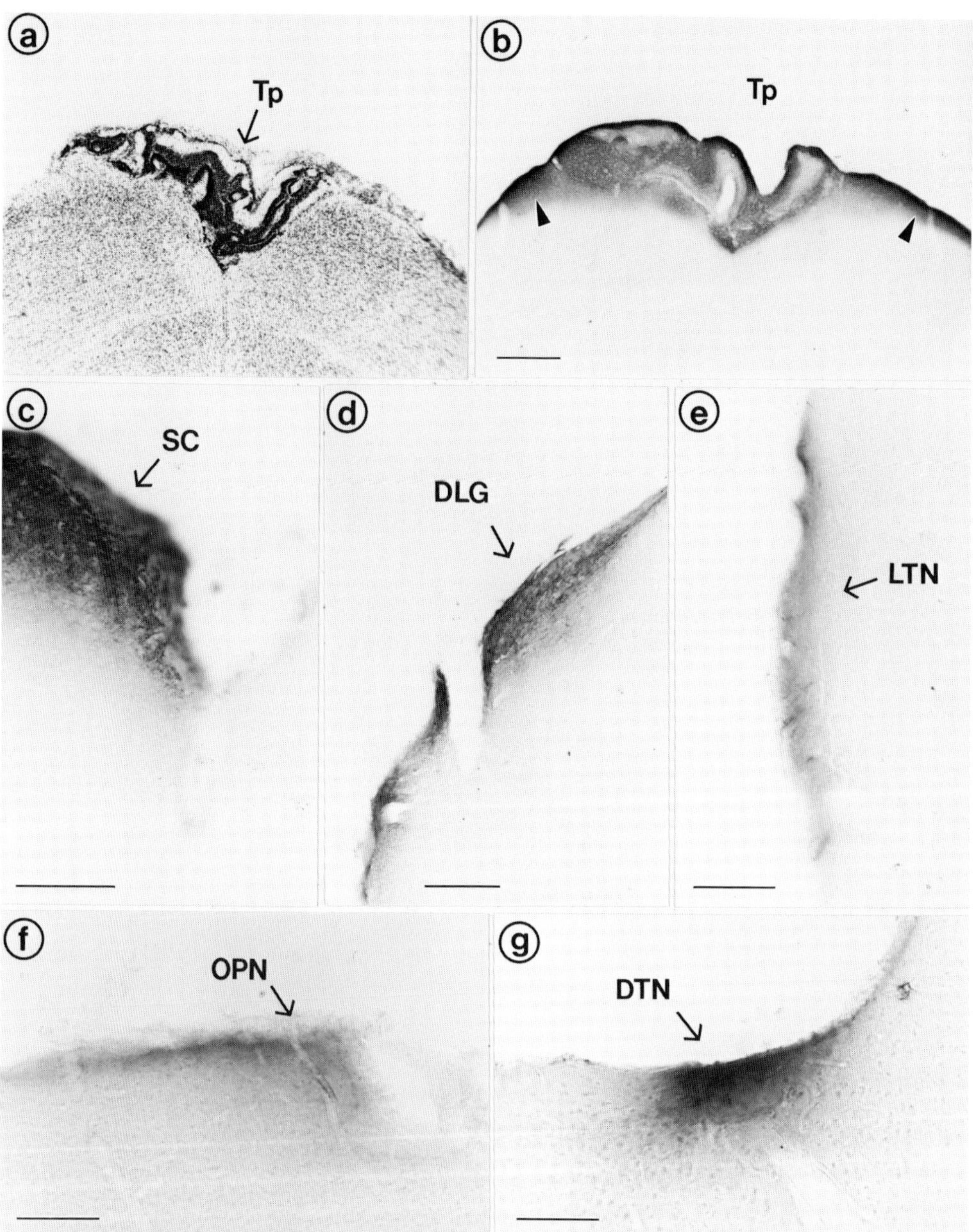

Figure 10.3 Example of a mouse retina (*Tp*), 5 weeks after transplantation to the dorsal surface of the midbrain of a newborn congenitally anophthalmic mouse. The retina was taken from an E12 AKR donor. Such retinas (*a*, cresyl violet; *b*, immunohistochemistry with anti-Thy-1.1 antibodies) show histological features typical of retinas transplanted to genetically normal animals. Anti-Thy-1 immunostaining (*b–g*) also shows transplant-derived projections to retino-recipient nuclei in the host brainstem: *b* (*arrowheads*) and *c*, superior colliculus (*SC*); *d*, dorsal lateral geniculate nucleus (*DLG*); *e*, lateral terminal nucleus (*LTN*); *f*, olivary pretectal nucleus (*OPN*); *g*, dorsal terminal nucleus (*DTN*). Transplant-derived labeling was not apparent in the medial geniculate nuclei (in contrast to the situation in normal hosts) or suprachiasmatic nuclei. Calibration bars: 500 μm (*a* and *b*), 100 μm (*c*, *e–g*), and 200 μm (*d*).

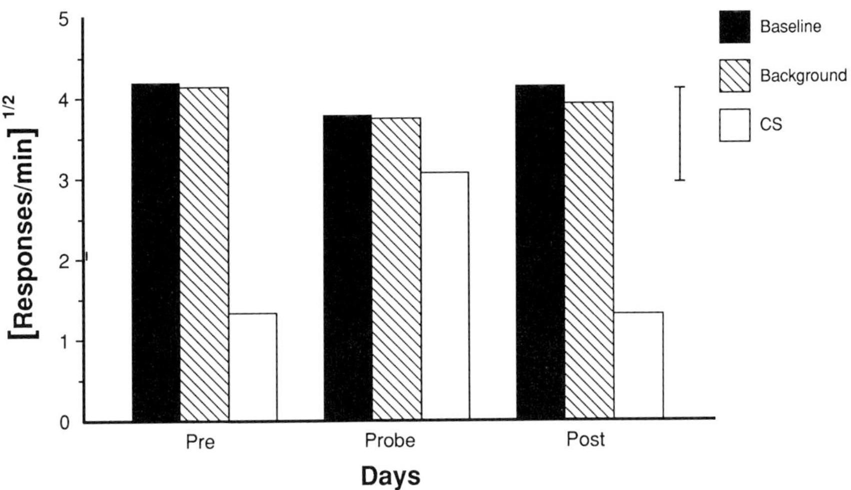

Figure 10.4 Conditioned suppression (*CS*) of lever pressing in rats with a transparent window over the transplanted retina and the host eye covered with a patch. Baseline (*solid*), background (*hatched*), and CS (open) bars represent rate of bar pressing with the window uncovered (*Pre*), covered (*Probe*), and uncovered again (*Post*) on 3 successive test days. Bar to the right indicates 2 SE from significant "stimulus × days" interaction by ANOVA (analysis of variance). (Reproduced with permission from Coffey et al., 1990.)

superior colliculus that are specific to light-on, light-off, and to ambient light levels (Simons and Lund, 1985). Examination of cortical responsiveness has defined a subdivision of area 18a that is activated by illumination of transplants. The pathway by which this input reaches the cortex is likely to be by way of the superior colliculus and lateral posterior nucleus of the thalamus (Craner et al., 1989).

Light not only elicits transient electrical responses of the kind described above but it has also been shown to effect changes that occur over a longer time course: changes in protein synthesis can be demonstrated using antibodies for Fos protein. Photic stimulation of transplants induces c-Fos expression in regions such as the superior colliculus and pretectum, most notably the olivary pretectal nucleus (Craner et al., 1990; 1992).

BEHAVIORAL OBSERVATIONS

A series of studies has shown that stimulation of transplants by light flashes can elicit a variety of behaviors. These include a conditioned suppression response, light avoidance behavior in an open field, a startle response, and pupilloconstriction of the host eye.

The conditioned suppression response requires host animals to learn that light delivered to the transplanted retina is an accurate predictor of mild foot shock, in contrast to a tone that serves as a less precise predictor of the shock. Having learned the association between light and foot shock, conditioned animals show a reduced rate of ongoing bar pressing for food when the light stimulus is presented but not when the stimulus is a tone burst (figure 10.4;

  Lund et al.: Intracerebral Retinal Transplants

Coffey et al., 1989). Subsequent work has shown that the learned behavior fails to generalize when rats are trained using transplant stimulation alone and then tested with normal vision only, and vice versa (Coffey et al., 1991).

The light avoidance response depends on the fact that rats, when placed in a brightly lighted environment, in this case an open field with a shadowed region, will tend to spend more time within the dark region. Host rats exhibit this photophobic behavior when using their remaining eye when initially tested prior to conditioned suppression training, but not when using the transplant alone. After conditioning, however, they continue to exhibit photophobia when surveying the open field through their remaining eye, and also when surveying it through only the transplant (figure 10.5; Coffey et al., 1990). This implies that the animals have in some way learned to use transplant-mediated information to direct their behavior in an open field test.

The startle response was assessed in free-moving animals with a fiberoptic light guide attached over the transplant. When illuminated, the animals initially show a freezing response followed by a period of random exploration (Coffey et al., 1991). This suggests that light-activated startle responses, which are normally mediated through the superior colliculus (Mitchell et al.,

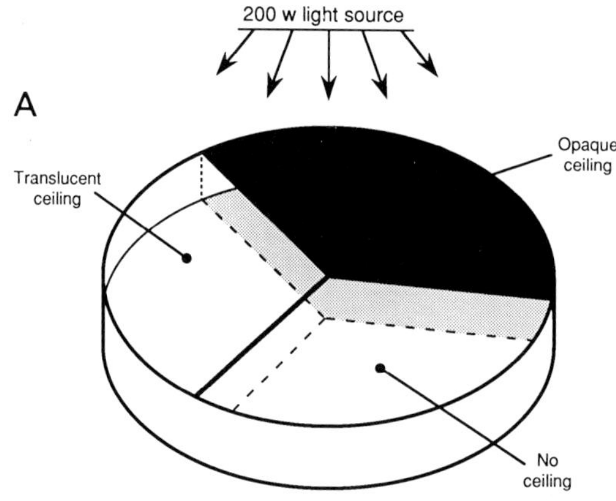

B	View of the Open Field		
	Host eye	Transplant	No input
Before conditioning	65%	30%	36%
After conditioning	60%	62%	36%

Figure 10.5 Open field assessment of light avoidance in transplant recipient rats before and after conditioned suppression training. A, the test apparatus. B, percent of time spent in the dark region of the area before and after conditioning, for rats viewing the arena through the host eye alone (transplant patched), the transplant alone (host eye patched), or with both the transplant and host eye patched (no input). (Reproduced with permission from Coffey et al., 1990.)

     Retinal Responses to Injury and Transplantation

1988; Dean et al., 1989), can also be activated by transplant stimulation, presumably through the same neural circuit.

The pupilloconstrictor response requires that information concerning the level of illumination entering the transplant be relayed to the host circuit that effects constriction of the iris musculature (figure 10.6). The first synapse in this pathway is in the olivary pretectal nucleus, which functions as a pupilloconstrictor center. From there luminance information is relayed to the Edinger-Westphal nucleus, which projects in turn to the ciliary ganglion that contains cells which innervate the pupilloconstrictor muscles of the iris. The studies conducted so far show that illumination of a transplant does indeed drive pupilloconstriction of the host eye, and that transplant-mediated responses are lost if either the transplant or the olivary pretectal nucleus is damaged (Klassen and Lund, 1987, 1988, 1990a). Furthermore, while the amplitude of the response varies among animals, it is highly consistent for a single animal from one testing session to another, provided the intensity of illumination is held constant. The pupil diameter does, however, vary inversely with the intensity of transplant illumination. The density of innervation of the olivary pretectal nucleus by the transplant also varies across animals and correlates directly with the amplitude and briskness of the pupillary response (Klassen and Lund, 1990b). It was also found that if host and transplant are illuminated simultaneously at submaximal intensity levels, the amplitude of pupilloconstriction is greater than that due to illumination of either alone (Lund et al., 1989). A further aspect of the interaction of host and transplant inputs was shown in a study in which the pupilloconstrictor response was measured across a range of intensities while the host eye being

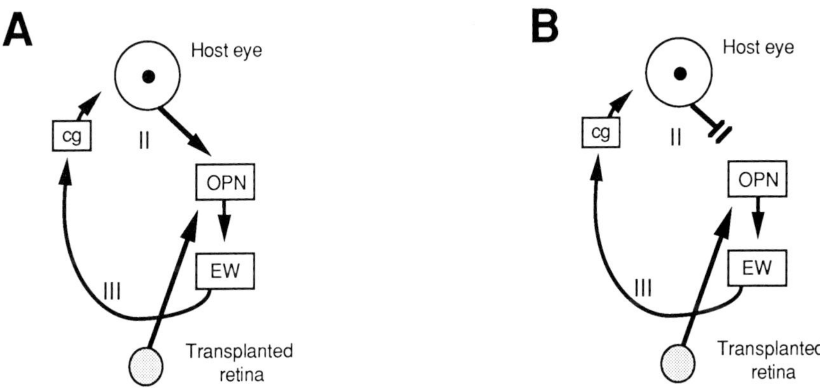

Figure 10.6 Schematic representation of the transplant procedure. *A*, the host eye is maintained in darkness while the pupillary response of that eye to transplant illumination is recorded. Information about luminance levels passes from the transplant to the host olivary pretectal nucleus (*OPN*), and is relayed from there to the Edinger-Westphal nucleus (*EW*) along the oculomotor nerve (*III*) to the ciliary ganglion (*cg*) and finally to the iris musculature. *B*, after testing animals as illustrated in *A*, the host optic nerve (*II*) is sectioned intracranially to eliminate all optic input from the host while preserving the transplant input and the output pathway for the pupillomotor response, and the testing is repeated. (Reproduced with permission from Radel et al., 1991b.)

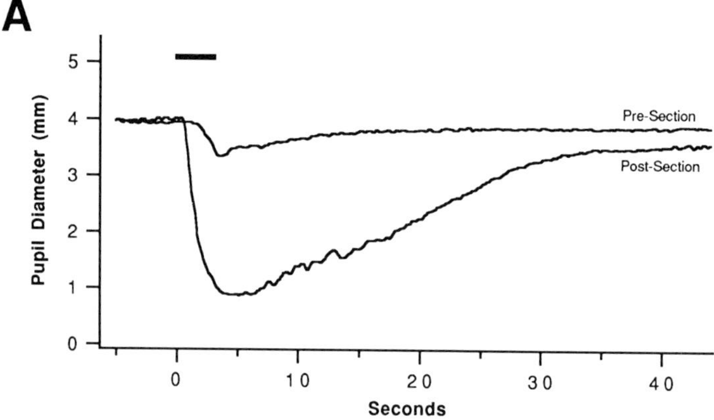

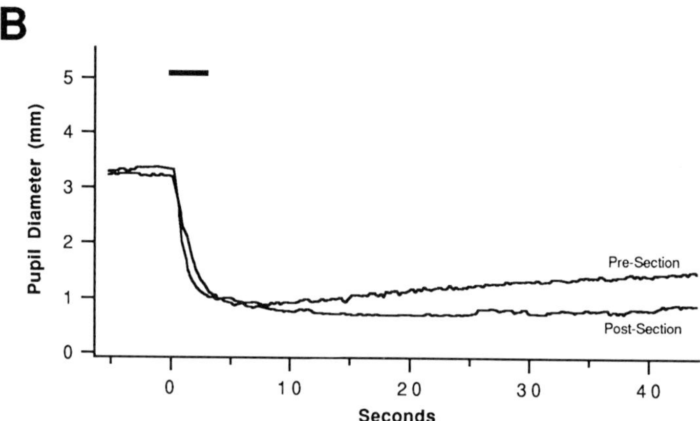

Figure 10.7 Changes in pupil diameter elicited by a light flash of the same intensity, delivered before and after optic nerve section. *A*, illumination of an intracranial retinal transplant produces pupilloconstriction in the eye of a host rat. The transplant-mediated response to the same stimulus is enhanced after elimination of all host optic input by intracranial sectioning of the optic nerve. *B*, the pupillary response of the left eye after stimulation of the right eye in a normal rate is shown for comparison. Stimuli were 3 seconds in duration (indicated by the *solid bar* above each graph). (Reproduced with permission from Radel et al., 1991b.)

tested was maintained in darkness. The optic nerve serving that eye was then cut and the transplant-driven response tested 1 and 2 days later under similar conditions (figure 10.7; Radel et al., 1991b). The amplitude, rate, and latency of response were all significantly enhanced after host optic nerve section (figure 10.8). This suggests an immediate enhancement of transplant effectiveness which would occur before there was time for significant axonal sprouting. This improvement may be due to a better signal-noise ratio caused by eliminating input from spontaneous activity in the host nerve or to receptor up-regulation in response to deafferentation.

The value of the pupilloconstrictor response in relation to other behaviors is that it is mediated by a relatively circumscribed pathway and that several

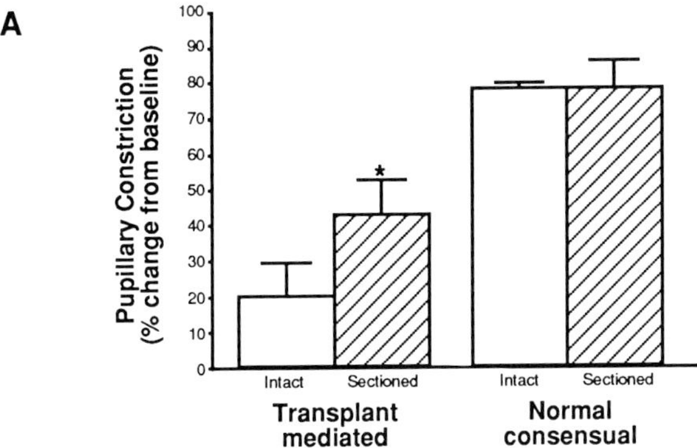

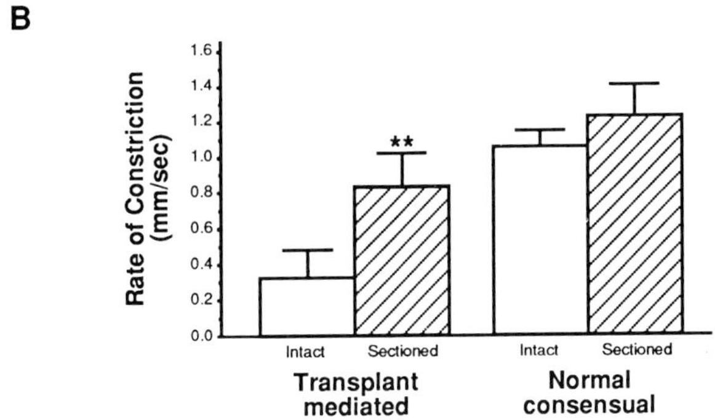

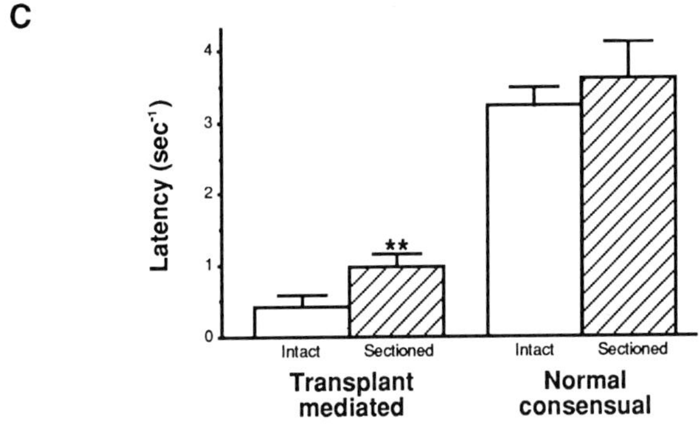

Figure 10.8 Comparison of changes in the response parameters of the transplant-mediated and normal consensual pupillary response, before and after intracranial sectioning of the optic nerve. Columns represent mean values from eight experimental rats and seven normal rats for each parameter, with the standard error of the mean indicated by bars. Changes in each parameter were compared statistically before and after intracranial optic nerve section for individual rats; statistically significant changes are indicated (* $p < .05$; **, $p < .01$). A, maximum pupillary constriction. B, maximum rate of constriction. C, latency of the pupil to respond, expressed as an inverse value for presentation purposes. (Reproduced with permission from Radel et al., 1991b.)

parameters of the response can be precisely quantified. This permits an in-depth examination of events that may influence the relay function of such a transplant, providing its use as a valuable model for studying factors that may improve transplant functioning where defined circuitry serves as the substrate. This preparation also serves as a useful system for examining how convergent input systems are processed and interact to provide an output function.

ADULT HOSTS

Much of the work so far has described the consequences of transplantation to neonatal hosts. Under these conditions, the transplant becomes integrated into a developing system, albeit at a somewhat more advanced stage of development. It is likely that many of the local environmental cues that support growth of the developing axons are still present and that certain inhibitory factors have yet to develop.

Transplantation to the adult nervous system presents a somewhat more complex situation. In general, the transplants do not differentiate quite as well: there are many more rosettes and less of the transplant appears as a sheet of retinal tissue: the long-distance projections seen after transplantation to neonates are not evident (McLoon and Lund, 1983; Rao et al., 1988). However, if the transplant is placed close to a region normally receiving optic innervation, axons from the transplant will ramify within that region and at least in the case of grafts placed over the pretectum, these axons will form the connections necessary to elicit a pupilloconstrictor response (Klassen and Lund, 1990a).

DISCUSSION

Developmental Consequences

Evidence from studies of retinal transplant development suggest that the initial outgrowth from retinas is highly directed and that the patterns seen at maturity are not simply the product of retraction of an initial random outgrowth process.

To achieve the specific connectivity underlying the behavioral responses elicited after transplantation to neonatal animals, the transplant cells must respond to a set of cues that serve to guide their axons in a highly targeted fashion. This occurs despite the fact that the transplants are placed in an anomalous location and in a host brain that is developmentally more mature. One point of note is that developing axons do not appear to make anomalous connections with inappropriate brain regions, even when embedded in structures such as cerebral cortex and cerebellum (McLoon et al., 1985; Sefton et al., 1991). This is in marked contrast to the patterns exhibited by optic axons regenerating through sciatic nerve guides, which are capable of innervating nonretinal targets such as the cerebellum, inferior colliculus, and cerebral cortex (Zwimpfer et al., 1990). The specificity of innervation by intracranially transplanted retinas is clearly not due to prior optic innervation, since it is also achieved in anophthalmic mutants. The experiments in intact hosts and in mutants also emphasize that degeneration associated with host optic deafferentation is not a necessary factor in guiding transplant axons to visual targets in the brain. It is suggested that a combination of surface-associated substrate cues and target-derived factors guide the axons to the appropriate regions (Hankin and Lund, 1991). The factors that organize the elaborate synaptic neuropil within these regions remain to be determined.

Transplants clearly interact differently when placed in adult hosts. Failure of long-distance growth by transplants placed in mature brains may be explained by the down-regulation of growth-promoting factors (Cohen et al., 1986; Cohen et al., 1989) and the added presence of growth-inhibiting molecules (Schwab, 1990) as the brain matures. Further investigation is clearly required in this area. However, it is apparent that the local circuitry necessary to subserve at least one specific response (the pupilloconstrictor response) can still be assembled.

RELAY FUNCTIONS

It is clear that transplants are capable of analyzing luminance information sufficiently for cells in the superior colliculus to respond in a highly stereotypic fashion to transplant activity and relay the information through several synapses to the cerebral cortex. Similarly, transplant input to the olivary pretectal nucleus drives host cells to generate a response to light which is transmitted through several nuclei to effect a clearly defined pupillomotor response. Evidence from normal animals indicates that the startle response is likely to be generated in the superior colliculus (Mitchell et al., 1988; Dean et al., 1989), a region that also receives a massive input from retinal transplants. It is not clear what the pathway for the conditioned response may be; suggested routes include the superior colliculus and the central gray matter of the midbrain and the amygdala, but other routes may involve cortical circuitry (Le Doux et al., 1990; Davis, 1991).

Each of these situations illustrates that (1) the analysis of photic information normally manifest in the retina still occurs, despite the fact that the retina undergoes most of its differentiation in an anomalous location; (2) the connections made with the host nervous system are sufficiently precise to elicit specific responses rather than random activity; (3) once the transplant has accessed the host circuitry, it is able to affect host functions in much the same way as normal optic input; and (4) while the complete repertoire of transplant-mediated functions has yet to be catalogued, evidence collected so far suggests that the axons from retinal transplants are as likely to drive parallel visual functions as is the normal visual input.

An interesting point raised by the light avoidance test in the open field is that it may be necessary for the input from transplants to be given "significance" before that input can drive a behavior. The fact that the pupilloconstrictor response to transplant illumination is immediately effective suggests that the early failure in the open field was not due to some limiting factor of the transplant or its primary connections, but rather reflected the ability of the host systems to recognize that the transplant input contained information. It is yet to be determined whether the conditioned suppression training simply alerted the animal to the fact that transplant inputs were functionally significant and should be attended to, or that the training provoked a light-avoidance response that was generalized from one task to another. There are a number of previous studies showing that behaviors can be primed pharmacologically (Segal and Mandell, 1974; Robinson and Becker, 1986) and similar priming is also effective in eliciting a transplant-mediated response (Snyder-Keller and Lund, 1990). The general principle that new circuits recruited to subserve a behavior may need to be primed in order to function is a fundamental tenet of much of the work examining recovery of function after injury. Indeed, the strategies of physiotherapy are in part concerned with giving "significance" to new pathways that may replace damaged circuits. The relatively simple system provided by the present transplant paradigm provides an opportunity to examine what is involved in the process of making a circuit accessible to new information.

INTERACTIONS BETWEEN TRANSPLANT AND HOST OPTIC INPUTS

The interrelation between transplant and host optic afferents is complex and depends on the particular function under investigation. In those situations in which transplant and host axons terminate in the same regions, there is usually substantial overlap in terminal distribution. This is heaviest when the transplant is at a competitive advantage, as in rats enucleated at birth or when placed in fetal hosts. Behavioral responses attributable to a region receiving convergent inputs, such as the olivary pretectal nucleus, encode inputs coming from host and transplant as comparable: the size of the constriction is larger when both the transplant and eye are stimulated with submaximal stimuli than when either is stimulated alone.

The host-transplant interactions in pupilloconstriction contrast with conditioned suppression studies where the response learned through the host eye does not transfer to the transplant, and vice versa. The failure of transfer could reflect the possibility that different pathways are involved, the transplant having a restricted projection to the lateral geniculate nucleus in contrast to the normal optic input. The lack of transfer may also reflect differences in the characteristics or quality of the perceived stimuli. The better optics of the host eye are likely to ensure that the host retina will be illuminated at a higher intensity and more focally than the transplant. Furthermore, the absence of topographic order in the transplant projection to the superior colliculus stands in marked contrast to the host input. Thus, the failure could also be one of stimulus generalization rather than of central connectivity. This deserves further examination.

   Retinal Responses to Injury and Transplantation

TRANSPLANTED RETINAS AS SURROGATE VISUAL SYSTEMS?

The observations presented here demonstrate that retinal transplants can mature to mediate specific visual response patterns in host rodents despite the absence of many normal developmental contextual cues. The question then arises: Might a transplanted retina eventually serve to replace a damaged primary optic pathway in a human? At present, this is a somewhat ambitious goal and more work is clearly needed before it can be realized. Certainly, an eye implanted in the back of the head is not optimally located for visual function. Recent work has shown, however, that axons from transplanted embryonic retinas can grow along sciatic nerve tubes providing a means whereby a replacement eye grafted to the orbit can establish connections with the brain (Hallas et al., 1991). There are many other issues yet to be addressed. These include the difficulties of stabilizing an eye with proper optics in the orbit, the establishment of a topographic order in the primary visual projection, and the extrapolation of results from experiments in small mammals to adult human systems. While this line of investigation does not presently offer a cure for blindness, it has proved to be an invaluable preparation for addressing questions significant in the field of developmental neurobiology and information processing in a sensory system.

References

Banerjee, R., and Lund, R.D. (1992). A role for microglia in the maintenance of photoreceptors in retinal transplants lacking pigment epithelium. *J. Neurocytol.* 21:235–243.

Berry, M., Maxwell, W.L., Logan, A., Mathewson, A., McConnell, P., Ashhurst, D.E., and Thomas, G.H. (1983). Deposition of scar tissue in the central nervous system. *Acta Neurochir. Suppl. (Wien)* 32:31–53.

Bignami, A., and Dahl, D. (1974). Astrocyte-specific protein and radial glia in the cerebral cortex of the newborn rat. *Nature* 252:55–56.

Björklund, A., and Stenevi, U. (1979). Reconstruction of the nigrostriatal dopamine pathway by intracerebral nigral transplants. *Brain Res.* 117:555–560.

Björklund, A., Stenevi, U., and Svendgaard, N.-A. (1976). Growth of transplanted monoaminergic neurons into the adult hippocampus along the perforant path. *Nature* 262:787–790.

Bok, D., and Hall, M.O. (1971). The role of the pigment epithelium in the etiology of inherited retinal dystrophy in the rat. *J. Cell Biol.* 49:664–682.

Breakefield, X.O., and Gage, F.H. (1988). Grafting genetically-modified cells to the damaged brain: Restorative effects of NGF expression. *Science* 242:1575–1578.

Coffey, P.J., Lund, R.D., and Rawlins, J.N.P. (1989). Retinal transplant-mediated learning in a conditioned suppression task in rats. *Proc. Natl. Acad. Sci. U. S. A.* 86:7248–7249.

Coffey, P.J., Lund, R.D., and Rawlins, J.N.P. (1990). Detecting the world through a retinal implant. *Proc. Brain Res.* 82:269–276.

Coffey, P.J., Lund, R.D., Rawlins, J.N.P. (1991). Transfer of information between retinal transplants and host visual systems in a conditioned suppression task in rats. *Eur. J. Neurosci. [Suppl.]* 4:249.

Cohen, J., Burne, J.F., Winter, J., and Bartlett, P. (1986). Retinal ganglion cells lose response to laminin with maturation. *Nature* 322:465–467.

Cohen, J., Nurcombe, V., Jeffrey, P., and Edgar, D. (1989). Developmental loss of functional laminin receptors on retinal ganglion cells is regulated by their target tissue, the optic tectum. *Development* 107:381–387.

Constantine-Paton, M., and Law, M.I. (1978). Eye-specific termination bands in tecta of three-eye frogs. *Science* 202:639–641.

Craner, S.L., Radel, J.D., Jen, L.S., and Lund, R.D. (1989). Light-evoked cortical activity produced by illumination of intracranial retinal transplants: Experimental studies in rats. *Exp. Neurol.* 104:93–100.

Craner, S.L., Hoffman, G.E., Lund, J.S., and Lund, R.D. (1990). Use of c-Fos to determine the neural pathway activated by intracranial retinal transplants in rats. *Soc. Neurosci. Abstr.* 16:656.

Craner, S.L., Hoffman, G.E., Lund, J.S., Humphrey, A.L., and Lund, R.D. (1992). c-Fos labelling in the superior colliculus: Activation by normal retinal pathways and pathways from intracranial retinal transplants. *Exp. Neurol.* (in press).

Das, G.D. (1974). Transplantation of embryonic neural tissue in the mammalian brain. I. Growth and differentiation of neuroblasts from various regions of the embryonic brain in the cerebellum of neonate rats. *Tower Int. Technomed. Inst. J. Life Sci.* 4:93–124.

David, S., and Aguayo, A.J. (1981). Axonal elongation into peripheral nervous system "bridges" after central nervous system injury in adult rats. *Science* 214:931–933.

Davis, M. (1991). The role of the amygdala in conditioned fear. In *The Amygdala*, ed. J. Aggleton, New York: John Wiley & Sons, (in press).

Dean, P., Redgrave, P., and Westby, G.W.M. (1989). Event or emergency? Two response systems in the mammalian superior colliculus. *Trends Neurosci* 12:137–146.

Fine, A., Dunnett, S.B., Björklund, A., and Iversen, S.D. (1985). Cholinergic Ventral forebrain grafts into the neocortex improve passive avoidance memory in a rat model of Alzheimer disease. *Proc. Natl. Acad. Sci. U. S. A.* 82:5227–5230.

Gage, F.H., and Björklund, A. (1986). Cholinergic septal grafts into the hippocampal formation improve spatial learning and memory in aged rats by an atropine sensitive mechanism. *J. Neurosci.* 6:2837–2847.

Galli, L., Rao, K., and Lund, R.D. (1989). Transplanted rat retinae do not project in a topographical fashion on the host tectum. *Exp. Brain Res.* 74:427–430.

Hallas, B.H., Guarino, L., Wells, M., and Zanakis, M.F. (1991). Peripheral nerve bridges between embryonic eyes and superior colliculus: Long-term connections. *Invest. Ophthalmol. Vis. Sci.* 32:1133.

Hankin, M.H., and Lund, R.D. (1987). Role of the target in directing the outgrowth of retinal axons: Transplants reveal surface-related and surface-independent cues. *J. Comp. Neurol.* 263:455–466.

Hankin, M.H., and Lund, R.D. (1990a). Directed early axonal outgrowth from retinal transplants into host rat brain. *J. Neurobiol.* 21:1202–1218.

Hankin, M.H., and Lund, R.D. (1990b). Induction of target-directed optic axon outgrowth: Effects of retinae transplanted to anophthalmic mice. *Dev. Biol.* 138:136–146.

Hankin, M.H., and Lund, R.D. (1991). How do retinal axons find their targets in the developing brain? Interactions with substrates cells and target-derived factors may be critical. *Trends Neurosci.* 14:224–228.

Harris, W.A. (1984). Neural transplants in lower vertebrates. In *Neural Transplants: Development and Function*, ed. J.R. Sladek and D.M. Gash, 43–97. New York: Plenum Press.

     Retinal Responses to Injury and Transplantation

Harris, W.A. (1989). Local positional cues in the neuroepithelium guide retinal axons in embryonic *Xenopus* brain. *Nature* 339:218–221.

Harting, J.K., and Guillery, R.W. (1976). Organization of retinocollicular pathways in the cat. *J. Comp. Neurol.* 166:133–144.

Harvey, A.R., and Lund, R.D. (1981). Transplantation of tectal tissue in rats. II. Distribution of host neurons which project to transplants. *J. Comp. Neurol.* 202:505–520.

Harvey, A.R., Golden, G.T., and Lund, R.D. (1982). Transplantation of tectal tissue in rats. III. Functional innervation of transplants by host afferents. *Exp. Brain Res.* 47:437–445.

Hayhow, W.R. (1958). The cytoarchitecture of the lateral geniculate body in relation to the distribution of crossed and uncrossed fibers. *J. Comp. Neurol.* 110:1–51.

Horsburgh, G.M., Hankin, M.H., and Lund, R.D. (1990). Retinal transplant-derived synapses in the superior colliculus of anophthalmic mutant (or ^{J}) mice. *Soc. Neurosci. Abstr.* 16:487.

Horsburgh, G.M., Lund, R.D., and Hankin, M.H. (1991). Morphology of the terminal arbors of retinal transplant-derived projections in eyeless mutant and normal mice. *Soc. Neurosci. Abstr.* 17:558.

Hubel, D.H., and Wiesel, T.N. (1969). Anatomical demonstration of columns in the monkey striate cortes. *Nature* 221:747–750.

Hubel, D.H., and Wiesel, T.N. (1972). Laminar and columnar distribution of geniculocortical fibers in the Macaque monkey. *J. Comp. Neurol.* 146:421–450.

Jaeger, C.B., and Lund, R.D. (1980). Transplantation of embryonic occipital cortex to the tectal region of newborn rats. A light microscopic study of organization and connectivity of the transplants. *J. Comp. Neurol.* 194:571–597.

Klassen, H., and Lund, R.D. (1987). Retinal transplants can drive a pupillary reflex in host rat brains. *Proc. Natl. Acad. Sci. U. S. A.* 84:6958–6960.

Klassen, H., and Lund, R.D. (1988). Anatomical and behavioral correlates of xenograft-mediated pupillary reflex. *Exp. Neurol.* 102:102–108.

Klassen, H., and Lund, R.D. (1990a). Retinal graft-mediated pupillary responses in rats: Restoration of a reflex function in the mature mammalian brain. *J. Neurosci.* 10:578–587.

Klassen, H., and Lund, R.D. (1990b). Parameters of retinal graft-mediated responses are related to underlying target innervation. *Brain Res.* 533:181–191.

Krieger, D.T., Perlow, M.J., Gibson, M.J., Davies, T.F., Ferin, M., Zimmerman, E.A., and Charlton, H.M. (1982). Brain grafts reverse hypogonadism of gonadotropin releasing hormone deficiency. *Nature* 298:468–472.

Krüger, S., Sievers, J., Hansen, C., Sadler M., and Berry M. (1986). Three morphologically distinct types of interface develop between adult host and fetal brain transplants: Implications for scar formation in the adult central nervous system. *J. Comp. Neurol.* 249:103–116.

LaVail, M.M. (1981). Analysis of neurological mutants with inherited retinal degeneration. *Invest. Ophthalmol. Vis. Sci.* 21:638–657.

Lawrence, J.M., Morris, R.J., Wilson, D.J., and Raisman, G. (1990). Mechanisms of allograft rejection in the rat brain. *Neuroscience* 37:431–462.

Le Doux, J.E., Ciochetti, P., Xagorais, A., and Romanski, L.M. (1990). The lateral amygdaloid nucleus: Sensory interface of the amygdala in fear conditioning. *J. Neurosci.* 10:1062–1064.

Lund, R.D., and Harvey, A.R. (1981). Transplantation of tectal tissue in rats. I. Organization of transplants and pattern of distribution of host afferents within them. *J. Comp. Neurol.* 201:191–209.

Lund, R.D., and Hauschka, S.D. (1976). Transplanted neural tissue develops connections with host rat brain. *Science* 193:582–584.

Lund, R.D., and Yee, K.T. (1992). Intracerebral transplantation to immature rats. In *Neural Transplantation: A Practical Approach,* ed. Björklund and S. Dunnett, 79–91. Oxford, Oxford University Press.

Lund, R.D., Rao, K., Kunz, H.W., and Gill, T.J., III (1988). Instability of neural xenografts placed in neonatal rat brains. *Transplantation* 46:216–223.

Lund, R.D., Radel, J.D., Hankin, M.H., Klassen, H., Coffey, P.J., and Rawlins, J.N.P. (1989). Developmental and functional integration of retinal transplants with host rat brains. In *Brain Repair Symposium, Wenner-Gren Center International Conference,* Stockholm, 327–340.

Mason, D.W., Charlton, H.M., Jones, A.J., Lavy, C.B., Puklavec, M., Simmonds, S.J. (1986). The fate of allogeneic and xenogeneic neuronal tissue transplanted into the third ventricle of rodents. *Neuroscience* 19:685–694.

Matthews, M.A., West, L.C., and Riccio, R.V. (1982). An ultrastructural analysis of the development of foetal rat retina transplanted to the occipital cortex, a site lacking appropriate target neurones for optic fibres. *J. Neurocytol.* 11:533–557.

McLoon, S.C., and Lund, R.D. (1980). Specific projections of retina transplanted to rat brain. *Exp. Brain Res.* 40:273–282.

McLoon, S.C., and Lund, R.D. (1983). Development of fetal retina, tectum, and cortex transplanted to the superior colliculus of adult rats. *J. Comp. Neurol.* 217:376–389.

McLoon, L.K., McLoon, S.C., Chang, F.-L.F., Steedman, J.G., and Lund, R.D. (1985). Visual system transplanted to the brain of rats. In *Neural Grafting in the Mammalian CNS,* ed. A. Björklund and U. Stenevi, 267–283. Amsterdam, Elsevier Science Publishers.

Mitchell, I.J., Dean, P., and Redgrave, P. (1988). The projection from the superior colliculus to the cuneiform area in the rat. II. Defense-like responses to stimulation with glutamate in cuneiform nucleus and surrounding structures. *Exp. Brain Res.* 72:611–625.

Neafsey, E.J., Sørensen, J.C., Tønder, N., and Castro, A.J. (1989). Fetal cortical transplants into neonatal rats respond to thalamic and peripheral stimulation in the adult. An electrophysiological study of single-unit activity. *Brain Res.* 493:33-40.

Perry, V.H., and Lund, R.D. (1989). Microglia in retinae transplanted to the central nervous system. *Neuroscience* 31:453–462.

Perry. V.H., Lund, R.D., and McLoon, S.C. (1985). Ganglion cells in retinae transplanted to newborn rats. *J. Comp. Neurol.* 231:353–365.

Radel, J.D., Hankin, M.H., Lund, R.D. (1990). Proximity as a factor in the innervation of host brain regions by retinal transplants. *J. Comp. Neurol.* 300:211–229.

Radel, J.D., Galli-Resta, L., and Lund, R.D. (1991a). Plasticity in innervation of the rat superior colliculus by transplanted retinae as a result of eye removal at maturity. *Exp. Neurol.* 12:252–263.

Radel, J.D., Kustra, D.J., and Lund, R.D. (1991b). Rapid enhancement of transplant-mediated pupilloconstriction after elimination of competing host optic input. *Dev. Brain Res.* 60:275–278.

Radel, J.D., Das, S., and Lund, R.D. (1992). Development of the light-activated pupillary response in rats as mediated by normal and transplanted retinae. *Eur. J. Neurosci.* (in press).

Rao, K., Kunz, H.W., Gill, T.J., III, and Lund, R.D. (1988). MHC-dependent neural allograft rejection. *Ann. N.Y. Acad. Sci.* 540:493–494.

Rao, K., Lund, R.D., Kunz, H.W., and Gill, T.J., III (1989). The role of MHC and non-MHC antigens in the rejection of intracerebral allogeneic neural grafts. *Transplantation* 48:1018–1021.

Robinson, T.E., and Becker, J.B. (1986). Enduring changes in brain and behavior produced by chronic amphetamine administration: A review and evaluation of animal models of amphetamine psychosis. *Brain Res. Rev.* 11:157–198.

Schwab, M.E. (1990). Myelin-associated inhibitors of neurite growth. *Exp. Neurol.* 109:2–5.

Sefton, A.J., and Lund, R.D. (1987). Co-transplantation of embryonic mouse retina with tectum, diencephalon or cortex to neonatal rat cortex. *J. Comp. Neurol.* 269:548–564.

Sefton, A.J., Rao, K., Hankin, M.H., and Lund, R.D. (1991). Outgrowth of transplant-derived retinal axons in cerebral cortex of neonatal rats. *Soc. Neurosci. Abstr.* 17:40.

Segal, D.S., and Mandell, A.J. (1974). Long-term administration of *d*-amphetamine: Progressive augmentation of motor activity and stereotypy. *Pharmacol. Biochem. Behav.* 2:249–255.

Sharma, R., and Lund, R.D. (1990). The role of microglia in transplanted retinae. *Soc. Neurosci. Abstr.* 16:36.

Silver, J., and Robb, R.M. (1979). Studies on the development of the eye cup and optic nerve in normal mice and mutants with congenital optic nerve aplasia *Dev. Biol.* 68:175–190.

Silverman, M.S., Hughes, S.E., and Valentine, T.L. (1991). Restoration of the pupillary reflex by photoreceptor transplantation. *Invest. Ophthalmol. Vis. Sci.* 32:983.

Simons, D.J., and Lund, R.D. (1985). Fetal retinae transplanted over tecta of neonatal rats respond to light and evoke patterned neuronal discharges in the host superior colliculus. *Dev. Brain Res.* 21:156–159.

Snyder-Keller, A., and Lund, R.D. (1990). Amphetamine sensitization of stess-induced turning in animals given unilateral dopamine transplants in infancy. *Brain Res.* 514:143–146.

Sotelo, C., Alvarado-Mallart, R.M., Gardette, R., and Crepel, F. (1990). Fate of grafted embryonic Purkinje cells in the cerebellum of the adult "Purkinje cell degeneration" mutant mouse. I. Development of reciprocal graft host interactions. *J. Comp. Neurol.* 295:165–187.

Suard, I.M., Collins, V.P., Ignacio, V., and Jacque, C.M. (1989). Implantation of rabbit embryo brain fragments into newborn mice: Integration and survival of xenogeneic astrocytes. *J. Neurosci. Res.* 23:172–179.

Sumi, S.M., and Hager, H. (1968). Electron microscopic study of the reaction of the newborn rat brain injury. *Acad. Neuropathol.* 10:324–335.

Trimmer, P.A., and Wunderlich, R.E. (1990). Changes in astroglial scar formation in rat optic nerve as a function of development. *J. Comp. Neurol.* 296:359–378.

Vidal-Sanz, M., Bray, G.M., Villegas-Pérez, M.P., Thanos, S., and Aguayo, A.J. (1987). Axonal regeneration and synapse formation in the superior colliculus by retinal ganglion cells in the adult rat. *J. Neurosci.* 1:2899–2909.

Wictorin, K., Clarke, D.J., Bolam, J.P., and Björklund, A. (1990). Fetal striatal neurons grafted into the ibotenate lesioned adult striatum: Efferent projections and synaptic contacts in the host globus pallidus. *Neuroscience* 37:301–315.

Yee, K.T., and Lund, R.D. (1991). Do retinal transplant axons form segregated stripes in the rat tectum? *Invest. Ophthamol. Vis. Sci.* 32:1262.

Zwimpfer, T.J., Inoue, H., Aguayo, A.J., and Bray, G.M. (1990). Regenerating retinal ganglion cell axons can form synapses with neurons in four different non-retinal targets in the adult hamster. *Soc. Neurosc. Abstr.* 16:41.

11 Photoreceptor Cell Rescue in the Dystrophic and Aging Retina by Retinal Pigment Epithelial Cell Transplantation

Harold J. Sheedlo, Vinod Gaur, Linxi Li, Anthony D. Seaton, Suzanne V. Stovall, Keiko Yamaguchi, and James E. Turner

Degeneration of photoreceptor cells (PRCs) in retinas of Royal College of Surgeons (RCS) dystrophic rats begins in the third postnatal week (Bourne et al., 1938; LaVail, 1981; Dowling and Sidman, 1962). A debris zone accumulates in the subretinal space concomitant with PRC loss. By 6 months, few PRCs remain, while the remaining debris material is restricted to the peripheral retina (Li et al., 1990). In these inherited dystrophic retinas, retinal pigment epithelial (RPE) cells are defective in phagocytosis of shed rod outer segments (Bok and Hall, 1971; Chaitin and Hall, 1983), a primary function of this cell, which directly or indirectly leads to PRC degeneration. Some of these cells also detach from Bruch's membrane by 2 months and ultimately degenerate (Caldwell et al., 1984). In addition to PRC degeneration, a decrease in the density of deep retinal vessel beds in RCS dystrophic rats begins at about 3 months (Gerstein and Dantzker, 1969). By 4 months, retinal vessels are seen invading the retinal pigment epithelium (Caldwell, 1989). Consequently, at this time, neovascularization profiles begin to appear. More specifically, at 4 to 6 months, this new retinal vessel growth progresses from the deep vessel bed into the epithelium and even into the vitreous (Weber et al., 1989; El-Hifnawi, 1987).

Knowing that RPE cells are defective in retinas of RCS dystrophic rats raised the question of whether replacement of these cells by their normal counterparts would rescue the degenerating retina, especially PRCs. In fact, we reported that transplantation of normal RPE cells into retinas of young RCS dystrophic rats caused significant cessation of PRC degeneration, which essentially arrested the disease process under the transplant (Li and Turner, 1988b). Similar RPE cell transplant-mediated PRC rescue in retinas of RCS dystrophic rats were subsequently reported by Lopez and co-workers (1989). In these studies, the transplanted normal RPE cells developed a normal structural relationship with the rescued PRC outer segments and contained phagocytized membrane debris and outer segments (Li and Turner, 1988b; Lopez et al., 1989; Sheedlo et al., 1989a).

In humans and other animals, retinal degeneration, in particular PRCs, naturally occurs with aging (Cano et al., 1986). Age-related degeneration appears to be affected, to a large degree, by an RPE cell dysfunction that may result from gradual failure of cell function due to elevated cellular activity, exposure to toxic factors, or to lipofuscin accumulation, individually or severally (Gartner and Kenkind, 1981; Marshall et al., 1979; Lai et al., 1978; Dorey et al., 1989; Katz and Robison, 1984). In the Fischer 344 rat, a progressive loss of PRCs, most prominently in the peripheral retina, occurs with aging, even with controlled dietary and lighting conditions (Shinowara et al., 1982).

These studies were undertaken to determine the effects of normal RPE cell transplants on PRC survival and retinal vasculature in retinas of RCS dystrophic rats. Also, RPE cells isolated from neonatal normal rats were transplanted into retinas of an aging rat model, the Fischer 344 rat, to attempt to affect PRC rescue and delay the retinal aging process. Furthermore, studies were undertaken to determine the mechanism(s) by which RPE transplants rescued PRCs in retinas of RCS dystrophic rats.

CELL ISOLATION, CULTURE AND TRANSPLANTATION, IMMUNOCYTOCHEMISTRY, NORTHERN BLOTTING, AND RETINAL VESSEL ANALYSIS

RPE Cell Isolation

RPE cells were isolated from retinas of 6- to 8-day-old normal pigmented Long Evans and nonpigmented Sprague-Dawley rats, following a previously described procedure (Mayerson et al., 1985; Li and Turner, 1988a). Briefly, whole eyes were first incubated in collagenase-hyaluronidase, and then in trypsin. After removal of the sclera and choroid, the neural retinas with attached RPE cells were incubated in growth medium (MEM/F12, 20% fetal bovine serum, gentamicin, and kanamycin). During this incubation, the RPE cells detach as a sheet. The sheets were collected, treated with trypsin, dissociated, and concentrated to 60,000 cells per microliter in Ca^{2+}, Mg^{2+}-free Hanks' balanced salt solution (CMF-HBSS) for transplantation or 100,000 cells per milliliter for culture.

In addition, RPE cells were isolated from adult Long Evans and RCS dystrophic rats using an eyecup method (Timmers et al., 1984). Briefly, after removing the cornea, the neural retina was carefully removed, leaving RPE cells attached to Bruch's membrane. The eyecups were incubated in 0.1% trypsin in CMF-HBSS for 20 to 30 minutes at 37°C in 5% CO_2. The enzyme-treated eyecups were then placed in growth medium and the RPE cells were gently dislodged, then collected using a Pasteur pipette. The cells were concentrated to 60,000 cells per microliter in CMF-HBSS.

Macrophage Isolation

Cells were harvested from 26-day-old RCS dystrophic rats injected with 11.6% sucrose in 0.01M sodium phosphate–buffered saline (PBS), pH 7.4, into the peritoneum (Chang and Chang, 1982). Macrophages were isolated from the peritoneal cells by differential substrate adherence to plastic. After incubation for 90 minutes in a growth medium, the culture plate was shaken and the floating cells were discarded. This procedure was repeated three times. The remaining cells, which were greater than 98% macrophages, as shown by immunocytochemistry for a macrophage-specific antibody, were rinsed several times. These cells were dislodged by treatment with 30mM lidocaine in PBS for 15 minutes, collected, rinsed, then concentrated to 60,000 cells per microliter for transplantation.

RPE Cell Culture

For conditioned medium, RPE cells were cultured in 35-mm wells (Falcon, 3046) to confluence (about 1 week) in growth medium. The cultures were then rinsed several times with CMF-HBSS, then grown in a defined medium consisting of 1% ITS (Collaborative Research), 99% MEM/F12, and antibiotics for 4 days. The cells were returned to growth medium for at least 1 week, then replaced with defined medium. This procedure was repeated several times.

Transplantation and Injection Techniques

RPE cells were transplanted into the interphotoreceptor space of RCS dystrophic and Fischer 344 rats using a superior lesion approach (Li and Turner, 1988a; Sheedlo et al., 1989a). Briefly, the superior surface of the eye was exposed and a small lesion (< 1 mm) was made between the vorticose veins. At the lateral edge of the lesion, a 30-gauge needle, attached to a 10-μl Hamilton syringe, was used to inject a 1-μl cell suspension into the interphotoreceptor space. Macrophages were similarly transplanted into dystrophic retinas. For transplantation into retinas of Fischer 344 rats, an incision was made close to the limbus to target the interphotoreceptor space of the peripheral retina. For sham controls, 1 μl of vehicle (CMF-HBSS) was injected into this space as described for RPE cells.

RPE-CM and basic fibroblast growth factor (bFGF) were also, injected into the vitreous of young RCS dystrophic rats. In this injection procedure, a very small lesion was made through the sclera and choroid slightly posterior of the ora serrata, to limit retinal damage, and a 32-gauge needle was used to inject 1 to 10 μl of RPE-CM and 166 ng of bFGF.

Immunocytochemistry

Opsin and Na^+, K^+-adenosine triphosphatase (ATPase) were detected in paraffin sections of RPE cell–transplanted and control retinas of RCS dystrophic rats and retinas of control Long Evans rats following a previously described technique (Sheedlo et al., 1989a,b; Sheedlo and Siegel, 1987). Briefly, retinal sections were deparaffinized and rehydrated. Following incubation with normal serum, sections were incubated with 1:1,000 sheep antibovine opsin or rabbit antibovine Na^+, K^+-ATPase antisera. The next day, the sections were incubated with the appropriate secondary antibody conjugated to horseradish peroxidase. Finally, sections were treated with 0.025% diaminobenzidine plus 0.01% hydrogen peroxide in 0.05M Tris buffer, then dehydrated and mounted in Permount. The immunostained sections were examined and photographed with Nomarski optics.

RNA Extraction and Northern Blotting

Eyes of RCS dystrophic rats, RPE cell–transplanted, sham-injected and control, and control Long Evans rats were enucleated and frozen in liquid nitrogen. Total RNA was isolated from frozen retinas by extraction with guanidine isothiocyanate (Chirgwin et al., 1979). Purified RNA after electrophoresis in a 1.1% agarose-formaldehyde gel was blotted onto a Nytrannylon membrane. The blots were hybridized with a 1.64-kb bovine complementary DNA (cDNA) probe using the procedure of Nathans and Hogness (1983).

Retinal Vessel Preparation

Control Sprague-Dawley and RCS dystrophic rats, RPE cell–transplanted, and sham-injected and control rats were injected with horseradish peroxidase and 15 minutes later the rats were sacrificed. The eyes were fixed in 2.5% glutaraldehyde and the retinas were removed from the sclera and choroid. The retinas were subsequently treated with 0.05% diaminobenzidine (DAB) for 24 hours and the next day with 0.05% DAB plus 0.05% hydrogen peroxide. The retinal tissue was flat-mounted and placed under a coverslip for analysis (Raviola and Freddo, 1980). The blood vessel length and density were measured in areas beneath and lateral to RPE cell transplants and in respective areas of sham-injected dystrophic and Sprague-Dawley retinas.

EFFECTS OF RPE CELL TRANSPLANTATION IN RETINAS OF RCS DYSTROPHIC RATS

Long-Term Effects of RPE Cell Transplants

Transplantation of normal pigmented RPE cells into retinas of young (10–26 days old) RCS dystrophic rats affected significant PRC survival for up to 1 year. The outer nuclear layer (ONL) thicknesses in retinas transplanted at 17 days and examined at 1 year was 20.8 $\pm$ 1.9 μm, while the ONL in retinas of age-matched control normal Sprague-Dawley rats was 25.7 $\pm$ 1.2 μm in thickness. Nontreated dystrophic retinas had few surviving PRCs, which were confined to the peripheral retina. A decline in ONL thickness was observed from 6 to 12 months in transplanted retinas. However, this phenomenon was also observed in retinas of normal Sprague-Dawley rats during this same time period, which appeared to be due to the aging process (Li and Turner, 1991). The surviving PRCs in transplanted retinas of 1-year-old RCS dystrophic rats maintained both inner and outer segments, both of which immunostained for the photopigment opsin (figure 11.1).

Rescued PRCs were not only detected directly beneath but also lateral to RPE cell transplants (Sheedlo et al., 1989a; 1990). In a chimera study by Mullen and LaVail (1976), surviving PRCs were also observed beneath dystrophic RPE cells when these cells were positioned close to normal RPE cells. Taken together, these results suggest that RPE cells provide trophic support for PRCs.

These results clearly show that transplantation of RPE cells from neonatal normal rats into young RCS dystrophic rats will affect PRCs survival for extended time periods, up to 1 year. This is extremely important when considering that a similar transplantation method may ultimately be applied to human eyes exhibiting PRC degeneration, such as retinitis pigmentosa and macular degeneration.

Transplantation Age of RCS Dystrophic Rats

The most beneficial effect on PRC survival was observed when retinas of RCS dystrophic rats were transplanted at 17 days, although transplantation at 10 and 26 days also promoted significant PRC rescue (Li and Turner, 1991; Sheedlo et al., 1990). However, RPE cell transplants in retinas at 38 days and older affected little survival, even at 3 weeks post transplantation. The ONL thicknesses of retinas of 4-month-old RCS dystrophic rats transplanted at 10, 17, 26, and 38 days were 28.0 ± 0.99 μm, 32.5 ± 2.4 μm, 29.2 ± 2.0 μm, and 3.77 ± 0.16 μm, respectively, while retinas of age-matched Sprague-Dawley rats had an ONL thickness of 35.8 ± 1.7 μm (Li and Turner, 1991).

These results suggest that normal RPE cell transplants will not affect PRC rescue in retinas of RCS dystrophic rats when degeneration has progressed beyond 2 weeks, beginning in the third postnatal week. Maximum PRC rescue was seen in retinas transplanted at 17 days. The lessened effect of RPE cell transplantation at 10 days may be a result of the decreased size of the eye in which retinal damage may have resulted from the needle insertion and RPE cell injection. Also, at 26 days, PRC degeneration is already underway in dystrophic retinas, which may account for the reduced effect of RPE cell transplantation at this time period.

RPE Cells of Normal and Dystrophic Rats: Young and Old

Transplantation of RPE cells of neonatal RCS dystrophic rats affected PRC survival equivalent to that seen in neonatal normal RPE cells 1 month post surgery. However, the PRC layer in neonatal dystrophic RPE cell–transplanted retinas was reduced to that observed in sham control retinas 2 months later (90 days) (Li and Turner, 1991).

RPE cells of adult Long Evans rats transplanted into retinas of young RCS dystrophic rats promoted significant PRC survival for up to 3 months post transplantation; however, there was less rescue than that seen in neonatal RPE Cell–transplanted retinas (ONL thicknesses of 29.2 ± 2.0 μm and

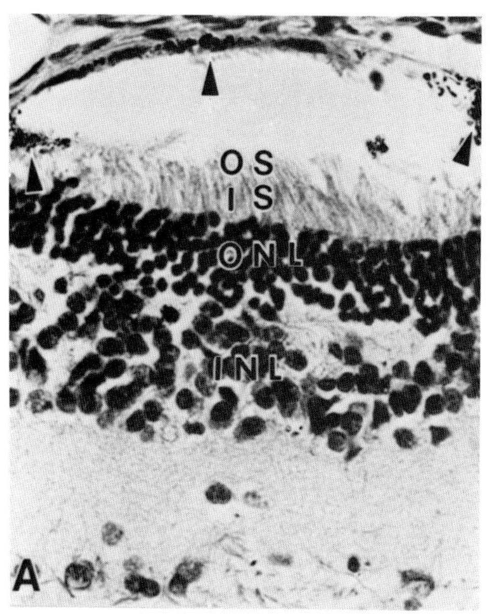

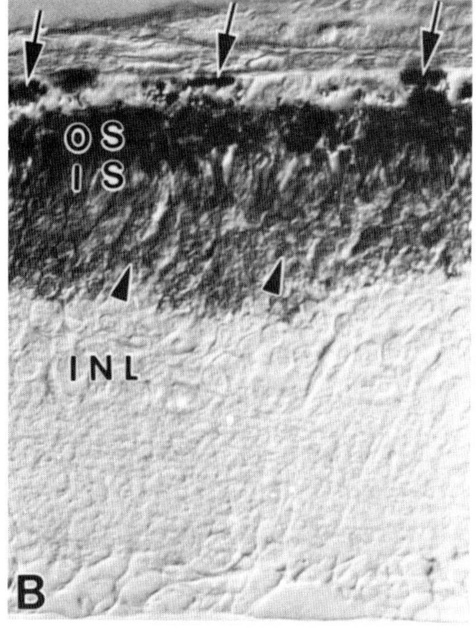

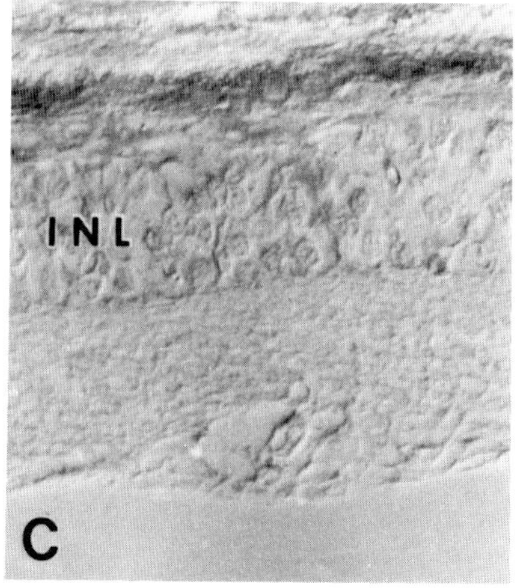

  Retinal Responses to Injury and Transplantation

16.0 ± 5.5 μm, respectively) at any time period studied (Li and Turner, 1991). Adult RCS dystrophic rat RPE cells did not affect PRC survival above that of sham control dystrophic retinas, even 1 month post transplantation. As shown at the light microscopic level, dystrophic retinas transplanted with neonatal normal RPE cells exhibited greater PRC rescue than that seen in normal adult RPE transplanted retinas (figure 11.2).

Similar results were observed in an in vitro study which showed that conditioned medium of neonatal RPE cells of Long Evans and RCS dystrophic rats affected significant PRC survival, as shown by opsin immunoreactivity, after 3 days. However, those cultures which were supplemented with RPE-CM of adult Long Evans and RCS dystrophic rats showed only about 46% and 22% surviving PRCs, respectively, when compared with neonatal normal RPE-CM supplemented cultures.

Thus, as shown both in vivo and in vitro, RPE cells from neonatal normal rats will affect greater PRC survival than RPE cells from adult rats. The decreased ability of aged RPE cells to support PRCs may involve the phagocytosis or structural relationship, but more likely represents a diminished trophic effect.

Immunocytochemical and Gene Expression Analyses of RPE Cell–Transplanted Retinas

Rescued PRCs in RPE cell–transplanted retinas of RCS dystrophic rats expressed the photopigment opsin at all time periods studied, up to 1 year of age. This protein was distributed on outer and inner segment membranes and PRC bodies (figure 11.3). In nontreated retinas of 6-month-old RCS dystrophic rats, opsin-immunostained debris was restricted to the peripheral retina (Li and Turner, 1991). At 1 year in nontreated dystrophic retinas, opsin-immunostained cell bodies were only observed adjacent to the ora serrata (Sheedlo et al., 1989b). The ubiquitous enzyme Na^+, K^+-ATPase was detected most prominently on inner segment and ganglion cell membranes, in the plexiform layers and inner nuclear layer in RPE cell–transplanted retinas of RCS dystrophic rats 3 months post transplantation, especially in areas immediately beneath the transplant. In retinas of 1-year old RCS dystrophic rats, the remaining inner retina—inner nuclear layer (INL), inner plexiform layer

Figure 11.1 Retinal pigment epithelial (RPE) cell–transplanted and nontreated retinas of 1-year-old RCS dystrophic rats. *A*, an outer nuclear layer (*ONL*) five to six cells in thickness is observed beneath transplanted pigmented RPE cells (*arrowheads*). Note that many of the rescued photoreceptor cells (RPCs) have both inner (*IS*) and outer (*OS*) segments. The separation between the OS and RPE cells is a tissue-processing artifact. In this study, normal neonatal RPE cells were transplanted at 26 days. Hematoxylin-eosin–stained paraffin section. *B*, in RPE cell–transplanted retinas, rescued PRCs (*arrowheads*) and their IS and OS immunostain for the photopigment opsin. The *arrows* indicate the transplanted RPE cells. *C*, nontreated retinas of 1-year-old RCS dystrophic rats do not show opsin-immunostained cells or debris material. *INL*, inner nuclear layer Magnification x375.

     Sheedlo et al.: RPE Cell Transplantation

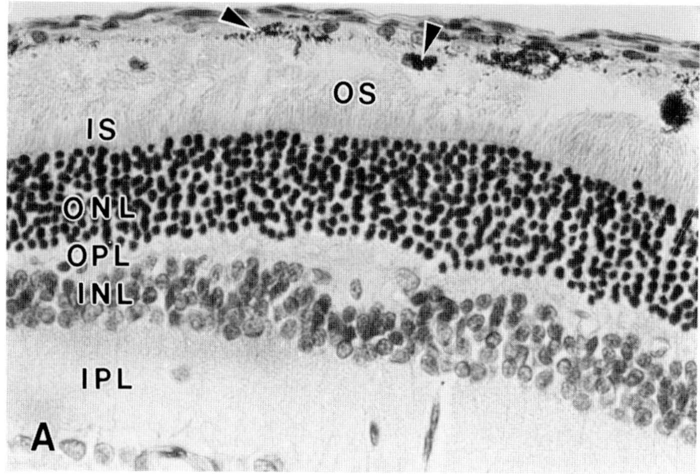

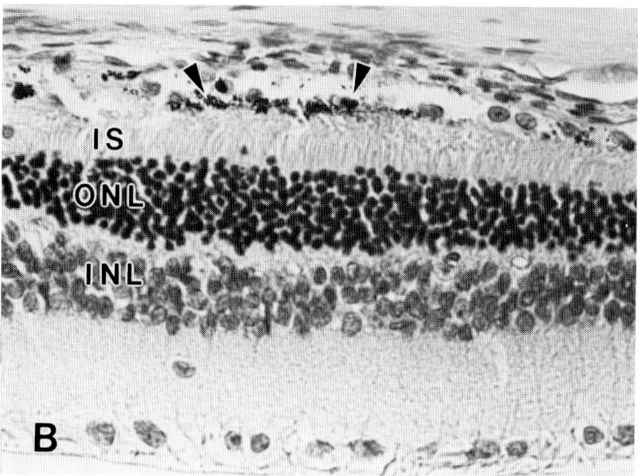

Figure 11.2 Comparison of the effects of transplanted RPE cells from neonatal and adult Long Evans rats in retinas of 2-month-old RCS dystrophic rats. *A*, the ONL beneath the transplanted neonatal RPE cells (*arrowheads*) is eight to ten cells in thickness. Also, the rescued photoreceptor cells (*RPCs*) have inner (*IS*) and outer (*OS*) segments. *IPL*, inner plexiform layer. *B*, the effect of transplants of adult normal RPE cells (*arrowheads*), however, is not as significant as seen in neonatal RPE cell–transplanted retinas. Note the ONL is maximally eight cells in thickness, but the beneficial effect of the transplant on PRC survival tapers off laterally. Although IS are present, it is difficult to distinguish OS. In this study, normal neonatal and adult RPE cells were transplanted at 26 days. Hematoxylin-eosin–stained sections. Magnification x375.

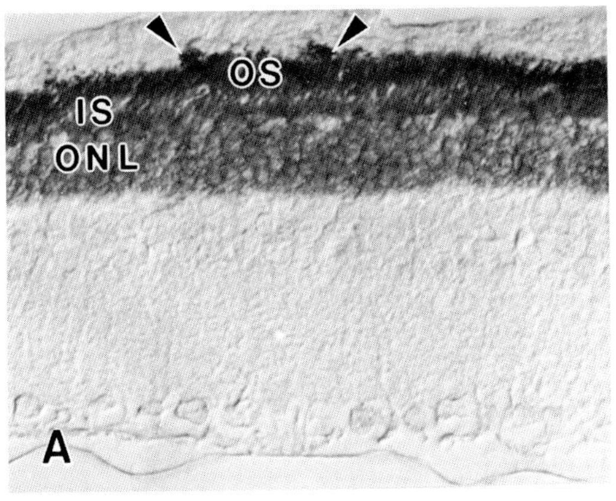

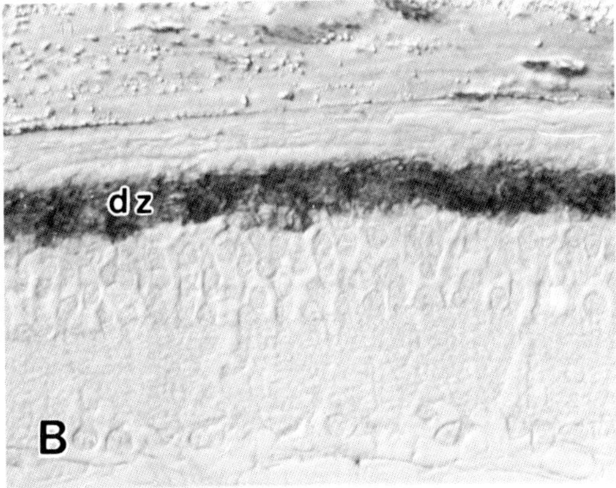

Figure 11.3 Opsin localization in RPE cell–transplanted and nontreated retinas of 4-month-old RCS dystrophic rats. *A*, in the RPE cell–transplanted dystrophic retinas, opsin is associated with photoreceptor cell bodies in the outer nuclear area (*ONL*) (five to six cells in thickness) and cell membranes of inner (*IS*) and outer (*OS*) segments. The *arrowheads* indicate the transplanted RPE cells. In this study, the RPE cells were transplanted at 10 days. *B*, in nontreated retinas of 4-month-old RCS dystrophic rats, opsin immunostain is restricted to the debris zone (*dz*). Magnification x375.

(IPL), and ganglion cells—continued to express Na^+, K^+-ATPase (Sheedlo et al., 1989a,b).

Also, RPE cell–transplanted retinas of young RCS dystrophic rats expressed messenger RNA (mRNA) for the photopigment opsin, detected in the four transcripts, 2, 2.8, 3.7, and 5.5 kb, as shown by Northern blotting. In this study it was shown that opsin mRNA was not detected in retinas of sham-injected and control 3-month-old RCS dystrophic rats. However, in RPE cell–transplanted dystrophic retinas, a high level of opsin mRNA was detected 3 months post transplantation.

As shown by immunocytochemistry and Northern blotting, rescued PRCs in RPE cell–transplanted dystrophic retinas retained their capacity to synthesize the photopigment opsin. Detection of a normal distribution of Na^+,

     Sheedlo et al.: RPE Cell Transplantation

K^+-ATPase beneath the RPE cell transplant would suggest that retinal integrity is also maintained.

Effects of RPE Transplants on Retinal Vasculature

RPE cell transplantation into retinas of 26-day-old RCS dystrophic rats affected maintenance of the deep retinal vessel bed, but not the superficial vessel bed, 3 months post transplantation. In transplanted retinas, the deep vessel bed, measured in units of millimeters per square millimeter, were 37% and 24% greater than retinas of either age-matched nontreated or sham control RCS dystrophic rats, respectively. Also, the number of neovascularization profiles in the deep retinal vessel bed were significantly reduced in the mid-peripheral region, which was the targeted transplant area, of transplanted retinas ($0.65/mm^2$), when compared with control normal retinas ($7.8-9.1/mm^2$) (figure 11.4). Furthermore, neovascularization profiles were reduced in transplanted retinas at 6 months, when contrasted with sham control retinas ($3.9/mm^2$ and $11.2/mm^2$, respectively). Retinas of normal Sprague-Dawley rats were devoid of new vessel growth at any age studied (4 and 6 months) (Seaton and Turner, 1991).

We propose two hypotheses to explain the results of this work. First, normal RPE cell transplants in retinas of young RCS dystrophic rats affect PRC survival, thus a normal retinal structure. Therefore, the vascularization of RPE cells and a decrease in the deep retinal vessel bed are prevented, at least up to 6 months. Second, normal RPE cells may secrete a factor(s) which directly affects the retinal vasculature. In this regard, an RPE cell factor(s) has been shown to inhibit retinal neovascularization (Glaser et al., 1985).

Sham and Macrophage Injections and Surgical Manipulations in Retinas of RCS Dystrophic Rats

When vehicle ($1-10$ μl of CMF-HBSS) was injected into the interphotoreceptor space of young RCS dystrophic rats, a short-term PRC survival effect was observed 1 month after injection. However, the beneficial effect on PRCs was significantly diminished by 2 months, and by 3 months no effect could be detected (Li and Turner, 1991). The same short-term rescue effect was also seen in saline-injected, dry needle insertion, and lesioned-only dystrophic retinas.

Retinas of young RCS dystrophic rats injected with rat macrophages showed no significant PRC survival 1 month post transplantation. However, the debris material in the area of the transplanted cells was significantly reduced by RPE cell phagocytic activity when compared with adjacent regions and in the corresponding region of nontreated retinas. Thus, removal of the debris zone, which may contain substances toxic to PRCs, between the RPE and PRCs, does not appear to significantly affect significant cell rescue (Turner et al., 1991).

     Retinal Responses to Injury and Transplantation

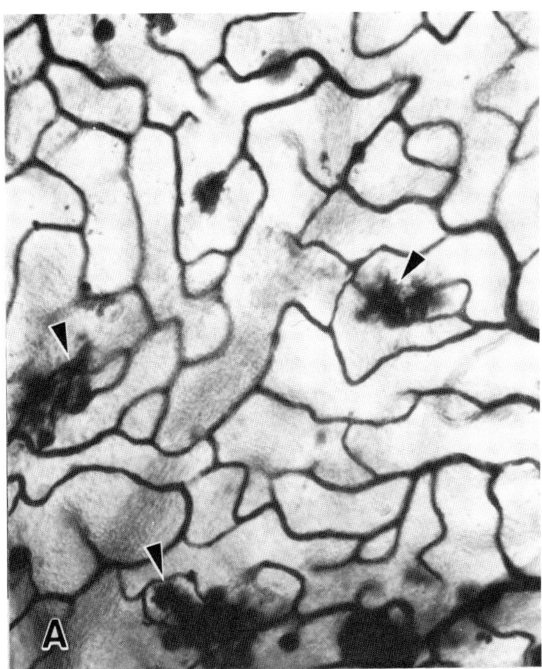

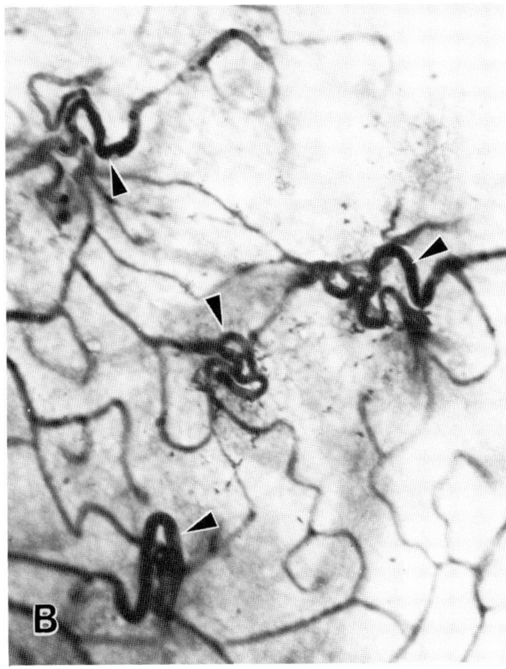

Figure 11.4 Horseradish peroxidase–injected retinas of 4-month-old RCS dystrophic rats: RPE cell–transplanted and nontreated. *A,* in those regions of RPE cell transplants (*arrowheads*), a normal retinal vasculature in the deep vessel bed is observed, as shown by horseradish peroxidase–stained blood vessels. *B,* in nontreated dystrophic retinas, neovascularization profiles (*arrowheads*) are apparent, which are rare in dystrophic retinas in regions of RPE cell transplants (see *A*). Magnification x200.

   Sheedlo et al.: RPE Cell Transplantation

EFFECTS OF RPE CELL–CONDITIONED MEDIUM AND GROWTH FACTOR INJECTIONS IN RETINAS OF RCS DYSTROPHIC RATS

Medium conditioned (10 μl) by RPE cells of normal neonatal rats when injected into the vitreous of young RCS dystrophic rats affected significant PRC rescue, when examined 1 month after treatment. This rescue was seen as a thickening of the ONL in the peripheral retina, which measured 15.9 $\pm$ 1.8 μm, while the ONL in the same region of a sham-injected retina measured only 5.71 $\pm$ 2.4 μm. These results would suggest that a trophic factor(s) secreted by cultured RPE cells affected the survival of PRCs.

Injection of 166 ng bFGF into the subretinal space and vitreous of young RCS dystrophic rats caused significant PRC rescue. When injected into the vitreous, the effect on PRCs was over a significant area of the retina. The beneficial effect of bFGF injected into dystrophic retinas was first reported by Faktorovich and co-workers (1990). Therefore, it is possible that a bFGF-like molecule is deficient in retinas of RCS dystrophic rats. A recent culture study reported the presence of bFGF in medium conditioned by human RPE cells (Schweigerer et al., 1987).

EFFECTS OF RPE CELL TRANSPLANTATION IN RETINAS OF FISCHER 344 RATS

Cell number in both the ONL and INL was significantly greater in RPE cell–transplanted retinas of aging Fischer 344 rats than in either sham-injected or nontreated retinas of these rats, all treated at 3 months of age, when examined 3 to 9 months after surgery. The ONL thickness of pigmented RPE cell–transplanted retinas of Fischer 344 rats when analyzed 3 months after transplantation was 138 $\pm$ 4.0 μm, while ONL thicknesses of sham control and nontreated retinas were 106 $\pm$ 2.0 μm and 103 $\pm$ 3.0 μm, respectively. Similar effects on cell survival in these layers were detected in retinas transplanted with either pigmented (Long Evans rats) or nonpigmented (Sprague-Dawley rats) normal RPE cells. A general decrease in ONL and INL cell number was observed in transplanted and control retinas during the 9-month posttransplantation period; however, RPE cell–transplanted retinas showed a 3-month delay in this decline in cell number.

Also, aging retinas of 6-month-old Fischer 344 rats transplanted at 3 months with normal RPE cells exhibited a thicker INL when compared with control nontransplanted retinas—45 $\pm$ 1.0 μm and 33 $\pm$ 1.0 μm, respectively. The beneficial effect of normal RPE cell transplants was also evident in the IPL in retinas of Fischer 344 rats.

These results reveal that PRC degeneration occurring as a result of the aging process appears to be delayed by replacement of old RPE cells with younger RPE cells, in this case from neonatal rats. Therefore, as RPE cells age, they may become less able to support the underlying PRCs, possibly through a trophic relationship.

     Retinal Responses to Injury and Transplantation

CONCLUSIONS

These studies have shown that transplantation of normal neonatal RPE cells are necessary for long-term survival of PRCs in retinas of RCS dystrophic rats. PRC rescue was maximal when transplantation was performed at 17 days, while no rescue was seen in retinas transplanted at 38 days. Less PRC rescue was detected in dystrophic retinas transplanted with RPE cells from adult normal rats, when compared with neonatal transplanted retinas. Although sham injections cause a short-term beneficial effect on PRCs, correction of the genetic defect is only produced by RPE cell transplants. The rescued PRCs in transplanted dystrophic retinas have a normal distribution and level of opsin and Na^+, K^+-ATPase and also express message for the photopigment opsin. Also, RPE cell transplants prevent the formation of new vessel growth in dystrophic retinas.

Although macrophages transplanted into the retina of young RCS dystrophic rats remove the debris material, no PRC rescue was detected. Also, injection of both conditioned medium of normal RPE cells and bFGF into retinas of young RCS dystrophic rats caused a delay in PRC degeneration.

Furthermore, the loss of PRCs in the aging rat retina can be reversed by transplantation of neonatal normal RPE cells, as shown in the Fischer 344 rat.

FUTURE RESEARCH

The principal objectives of RPE cell transplantation research are to develop models that will help understand RPE and PRC relationships in normal and diseased states and develop possible therapeutic strategies for possible use in human patients suffering from various retinal diseases such as retinitis pigmentosa and macular degeneration. Future studies leading to these goals will have to carefully consider minimizing ocular and retinal damage, eliminating surgically induced immunological responses and rejection, providing a long-term remedy for PRC loss, choosing the most effective RPE cell for transplantation, and supplementing RPE cell transplants with trophic factors to affect cell survival and possibly limited cell proliferation.

Age-related functional aspects of RPE cells will also have to be studied further, both in vitro and in vivo. Questions of whether older RPE cells function less effectively than their younger counterparts and whether the RPE aging phenomenon can be reversed in the culture environment prior to transplantation need to be addressed. In addition, the concept of an RPE cell trophic factor(s) and its effect on PRCs both in vitro and in vivo has to be further analyzed. The isolation, purification, and characterization of this factor(s) would be a primary goal of this research. Finally, another important consideration relates to the development of a universal RPE cell, that would function normally but lack the cell surface antigens that could result in RPE cell transplant rejection.

Acknowledgment

Support for this work was provided by NIH grant EY 04337 and the National RPE Foundation Fighting Blindness. We thank Ming Lei, Paula Mooney, and Lauren Clarkson for their excellent technical assistance.

REFERENCES

Bok, D., and Hall, M.O. (1971). The role of pigment epithelium in the etiology of inherited retinal dystrophy in the rat. *J. Cell Biol.* 49:664–682.

Bourne, M.C., Campbell, D.A., and Tansley, K. (1938). Hereditary degeneration of the rat. *Br. J. Ophthalmol.* 22:613–622.

Caldwell, R.B. (1989). Extracellular matrix alterations precede vascularization of the retinal pigment epithelium in dystrophic rats. *Curr. Eye Res.* 8:907–921.

Caldwell, R.B., Wade, L.A., and McLaughlin, B.J. (1984). A quantitative study of intramembrane changes during cell junctional breakdown in the dystrophic rat retinal pigment epithelium. *Exp. Eye Res.* 38:104–117.

Cano, J., Machado, A., and Reinoso-Suayez, J. (1986). Morphological changes in the retina of ageing rats. *Arch. Gerontol. Geriatr.* 5:41–50.

Chaitin, M.H., and Hall, M.O. (1983). Defective ingestion of rod outer segments by cultured dystrophic rat pigment epithelial cells. *Invest. Ophthalmol. Vis. Sci.* 24:812–820.

Chang, T.W. and Chang, N.T. (1982). Production of monoclonal antibodies by hybridoma method. In *Genetic Engineering Technique: Recent Developments*, ed. P.C. Huang, T.T. Kuo, and R. Wu, 299–333. New York: Academic Press.

Chirgwin, J.M., Przybula, A.E., MacDonald, R.J. and Rutter, W.J. (1979). Isolation of biologically active ribonucleic acid from sources enriched in ribonuclease. *Biochemistry* 18:5294–5299.

Dorey, C.K., Wu, G., Eberstein, D., Garsd, A., and Weiter, J.J. (1989). Cell loss in the aging retina: Relationship to lipofuscin accumulation and macular degeneration. *Trans. Amer. Acad. Ophthalmol. Otolaryngol.* 76:64–70.

Dowling, J.E., and Sidman, R.L., (1962). Inherited retinal dystrophy in the rat. *J. Cell Biol.* 14:73–109.

El-Hifnawi, E. (1987) Pathomorphology of the retina and its vasculature in hereditary retinal dystrophy in RCS rats. *Adv. Biosci.* 62:417–433.

Faktorovich, E.G., Steinberg, R.H., Yasumura, D., Matthes M.T., and LaVail, M.M. (1990). Photoreceptor degeneration in inherited retinal dystrophy delayed by basic fibroblast growth factor. *Nature* 347:83–86.

Gartner, S., and Kenkind, P. (1981). Aging and degeneration of the human macula. *Br. J. Ophthalmol.* 65:23–28.

Gerstein, D.D., and Dantzker, D.R. (1969). Retinal vascular changes in hereditary visual cell degeneration. *Arch. Ophthalmol.* 81:99–105.

Glaser, B.M., Campochiaro, P.A., Davis, J.L., and Sato, M (1985). Retinal pigment epithelial cells release an inhibitor of neovascularization. *Arch. Ophthalmol.* 103:1870–1878.

Katz, M.L., and W.G. Robison (1984). Age-related changes in the retinal pigment epithelium of pigment rats. *Exp. Eye Res.* 38:137–151.

   Retinal Responses to Injury and Transplantation

Lai, Y.L., Jacoby, O., and Jonas, A.M. (1978). Age-related and light-associated retinal changes in Fischer rat. *Invest. Ophthalmol. Vis. Sci.* 17:634−638.

LaVail, M.M. (1981). Analysis of neurological mutants with inherited retinal degeneration. *Invest. Ophthalmol. Vis. Sci.* 21:638−657.

Li, L., and Turner, J.E. (1988a). Transplantation of retinal pigment epithelial cells to mature and adult rat hosts: Short and long term survival characteristics. *Exp. Eye Res.* 47:771−785.

Li, L., and Turner, J.E. (1988b). Inherited retinal dystrophy in the RCS rat: Prevention of photoreceptor degeneration by pigment epithelial cell transplantation. *Exp. Eye Res.* 47:911−917.

Li, L., and Turner, J.E. (1991). Optimal conditions for long term photoreceptor cell rescue in RCS rats: The necessity for healthy RPE transplants. *Exp. Eye Res.* 52:669−679.

Li, L., Sheedlo, H.J., and Turner, J.E. (1990). Long-term rescue of photoreceptor cells in the retinas of RCS dystrophic rats by RPE cell transplantation. *Prog. Brain Res.* 82:179−185.

Lopez, P., Gouras, P., Kjeldbye, H., Sullivan, B., Reppucci, V., Brittis, M., Wapner, F., and Goluboff, E. (1989). Transplanted retinal pigment epithelium modifies the retinal degeneration in the RCS rat. *Invest. Ophthalmol. Vis. Sci.* 30:586−588.

Marshall, J., Grindle, J., Ansell, P.C., and Borwein, B. (1979). Convolution in human rods: An ageing process. *Br. J. Ophthalmol.* 63:181−187.

Mayerson, P.L., Hall, M.O., Clark, V., and Abrams, T. (1985). An improved method of isolation and culture of rat retinal pigment epithelial cells. *Invest. Ophthalmol. Vis. Sci.* 26:1599−1609.

Mullen, R.J., and LaVail, M.M. (1976). Inherited retinal dystrophy: Primary defect in pigment epithelium determined with experimental rat chimeras. *Science* 192:799−801.

Nathans, J., and Hogness, D.S. (1983). Isolation, sequence analysis and intro-exon arrangement of the gene encoding bovine rhodopsin. *Cell* 34:807−814.

Raviola, P., and Freddo, T.F. (1980). A simple staining method for blood vessels in flat preparations of ocular tissues. *Invest. Ophthalmol. Vis. Sci.* 19:1518−1523.

Schweigerer, L., Malerstein, B., Neufeld, B., and Gospodarowicz, D. (1987). Basic fibroblast growth factor is synthesized in cultured retinal pigment epithelial cells. *Biochem. Biophys. Res. Commun.* 143:934−940.

Seaton, A.D., and Turner, J.E. (1992). RPE transplants stabilize retinal vasculature and prevent neovasculization in the RCS rat. *Invest. Ophthalmol. Vis. Sci.* 33:83−91.

Sheedlo, H.J., and Siegel, G.J. (1987). Comparison of the distribution of Na^+, K^+-ATPase and myelin-associated glycoprotein (MAG) in the optic nerve, spinal cord and trigeminal ganglion of shiverer (shi/shi) and control ($+/+$) mice. *Brain Res.* 415:105−114.

Sheedlo, H.J., Li, L., and Turner, J.E. (1989a). Functional and structural characteristics of photoreceptor cells rescued in RPE-cell grafted retinas of RCS dystrophic rats. *Exp. Eye Res.* 48:841−854.

Sheedlo, H.J., Li, L., and Turner, J.E. (1989b). Na^+, K^+-ATPase and opsin in retinas of RCS dystrophic rats: Time course study. *Curr. Eye Res.* 8:741−750.

Sheedlo, H.J., Li, L., and Turner, J.E. (1990). Photoreceptor cell rescue at early and late RPE-cell transplantation periods during retinal disease in RCS dystrophic rats. *J. Neurol. Transplant.* 2:55−63.

Shinowara, N.L., London, E.D., and Rapoport, S.I. (1982). Changes in retinal morphology and glucose utilization in aging albino rats. *Exp. Eye Res.* 34:517−530.

Timmers, Ad.M.M., Dratz, E.A., deGrip, W.J., and Daemen, F.J.M. (1984). A new isolation procedure for retinal pigment epithelium. *Invest. Ophthalmol. Vis. Sci.* 25:1013–1018.

Turner, J.E., Li, L., Sheedlo, H.J., and Gaur, V. (1991). Saline injections, surgical manipulations do not substitute for the effect of RPE transplant mediated photoreceptor cell rescue in RCS dystrophic rats. *Invest. Ophthalmol. Vis. Sci.* 32:1219.

Weber, M.C., Mancini, M.A., and Frank, R.N. (1989). Retinovitreal neovascularization in the Royal College of Surgeons rat. *Curr. Eye Res.* 8:61–73.

     Retinal Responses to Injury and Transplantation

12 Retinal Transplants Improve Vision in Light-Blinded Rats: Behavioral Results from the Use of a New Retinal Transplantation Technique

Manuel P. del Cerro, James R. Ison, Eliot Lazar,
G. Peter Bowen, Donald A. Grover, and
Coca del Cerro

Since our introduction of intraocular retinal transplantation between unrelated individuals (del Cerro, et al., 1984), great progress has been made in the field. Light and electron microscopic evidence of the repopulation of photoreceptors through growth and differentiation of transplants, reports of synaptic connectivity, and rescue effects on the host retina, have been reported by us and by others to occur in light-damaged or genetically deficient visually impaired hosts (see del Cerro, 1990, for a review). In spite of all the morphological and histochemical data gathered, no documented evidence has come forward that any of these positive morphological changes have made any contribution whatsoever to the functional amelioration of the conditions they aim to improve. We consider that the credibility of the field, and the possibility of applying retinal transplantation to humans, hinges on the availability of compelling proof that intraretinal grafts function to improve the sensory abilities of the visually impaired recipient.

We have recently combined two experimental procedures in our initial attempt to begin to fill this important gap in our knowledge. We are starting on a road intended to take us to a description of the nature of the recovery that can be expected to result from retinal transplantation, using the principles that will be most effective in restoring functional vision. First, we resorted to a new transplantation method which allows multiple cell grafting into a single rodent eye (Lazar and del Cerro, 1991). Second, we tested the functional outcome of the grafts by means of a behavioral procedure, called reflex modification, that reflects both the sensitivity and the speed of sensorineural processing of the damaged or dystrophic eye (Ison, et al., 1991a; Wecker and Ison, 1986). This seemed to have the promise of showing objective evidence of functional recovery after the introduction of an intraretinal graft. As a result of the success of this collaboration, we report here, for the first time, quantitative data on functional recovery in severely visually impaired light-damaged eyes following intraretinal grafts.

METHODS

Donor Cells

The retinas of Fischer 344 rat embryos (E21) were subjected to mechanical-enzymatic dissociation to obtain single cell suspensions.

Cell Preparation

The eyes were collected in either Ca^{2+}, Mg^{2+}-free medium or in human plasma at 4°C, and were dissected open. The retinas were cut away, free of contamination from either the vitreous or the retinal pigment epithelium. Isolated retinas were trimmed into small fragments and then placed in ice-cold medium. Mechanical dissociation was used to obtain suspensions of retinal cells and cell clusters by aspirating the retinal fragments through a small-gauge needle and then releasing them through the same port. By varying the needle gauge and the number of aspiration-ejection cycles, it is possible to maintain fine control over the final degree of dissociation.

Hosts and Anesthesia

A total of 25 young male adult Fischer 344 rats were used in the experiment, of which 18 were the recipients of intraretinal transplants, which were performed at two points in different stages of the experimental design. Prior to the grafting of the host animals, they were anesthetized with a mixture of chloral hydrate and sodium pentobarbital at a dose of 3 ml/kg. Topical 1% proparacaine hydrochloride drops (Alcaine, Alcon Laboratories, Fort Worth, Tex.) were also used as an anesthetic. The eyes were dilated preoperatively with one drop each of 1% phenylephrine hydrochloride (Neo-Synephrine Hydrochloride) and 1% tropicamide (Mydriacyl, Alcon). All procedures adhered strictly to National Institutes of Health quidelines for animal care and use, and were approved by the University Committee for Animal Research.

Delivery System and Transplantation Procedure

A 30-gauge needle with a 15-degree bevel, tightly sheathed in plastic, with 1.1 to 1.4 mm of the needle tip left exposed, was connected to a Hamilton microliter syringe (Series 1700, Hamilton, Reno, Nev.), prior to the procedure. The plastic sheath placed on the needle serves as an adjustable regulator to limit the depth of penetration and provide protection against overpenetration. The plastic sheath is regulated so that only enough of the needle tip is exposed to reach the subretinal space without actually penetrating the retina. This prevents retinal holes or tears.

A stereomicroscope fitted with a 35-mm photographic camera is used for direct visualization of the injection, and it is important to note that the entire procedure is continuously monitored and under visual control. Collibri forceps

    Retinal Responses to Injury and Transplantation

(Storz, St. Louis, Mo.) are used to grasp the sclera at the limbus and rotate the globe anteriorly. Then, the needle of a 50-μl syringe, which has been pre-loaded with the suspension of neuroretinal cells, is manually inserted through the sclera, with its bevel facing the surgeon in order to afford the best view. The needle is gently rotated, without changing its angle, until the tip can be directly viewed through the retina. Then the tip is advanced further so as to slightly elevate the retina. At this point, with the bevel of the needle turned to face the wall of the globe, an injection of 2 to 4 μl of cells is made. The procedure is then repeated at a point 180 degrees opposite to the first injection site in the same eye. The needle is quickly withdrawn following each injection, and after the experiment is completed, a topical lubricant is placed on the cornea to prevent drying. Two microinjections were made into the equatorial region of each eye, one superiorly at the 12-o'clock position and the other at the 6-o'clock position. (We note that in other work as many as four penetrations have been performed in a single rat eye.) A macro-photograph obtained at the moment of injection is presented in figure 12.1.

Histological Procedures

Animals were sacrificed under deep anesthesia using intramuscular injections of ketamine at 90 mg/kg and xylazine hydrochloride (Rompun, Bayvet Division, Miles Laboratories, Shawnee, Kans.) at a dose of 8-mg/kg. The eyes were enucleated and fixed in 6% glutaraldehyde and split along a sagittal axis. The hemisected eyes were examined and photographed under a stereomicroscope and then embedded in plastic (Eponate 12, Ted Pella, Redding, Calif.). Sections 1 μl thick were cut and stained with Stevenel blue (del Cerro, et al., 1980a,b) for light microscopic study. Ultrathin sections were cut for electron microscopic studies. They were stained with lead acetate and studied under a Zeiss 10 electron microscope.

Behavioral Procedure

Sensory function was measured with the behavioral technique known as "reflex modification" (see Ison, 1984, 1990). After a minimum of 1-hour dark adaptation, the animal was placed in a small unilluminated cage, which was placed over the transducer that records the force of the startle response to a brief tone burst. Stimulus presentation and response measurement were entirely objective, controlled by a standard laboratory computer. Light flashes (20 ms in duration, 30 ft-c) were presented from 20 to 500 ms before the startle stimulus (10 kHz, 20 ms in duration, 120 dB), while in control trials the startle stimulus was presented by itself. Each stimulus condition was repeated ten times, in quasi-random order. In normal animals the reflex is inhibited by the light flash, with the degree of inhibition determined in part by light intensity and in part by its lead time (Hoffman and Ison, 1980). The animal's detection of the light flash is revealed by the reliable difference in reflex

    del Cerro et al.: Retinal Transplants in Light-Blinded Rats

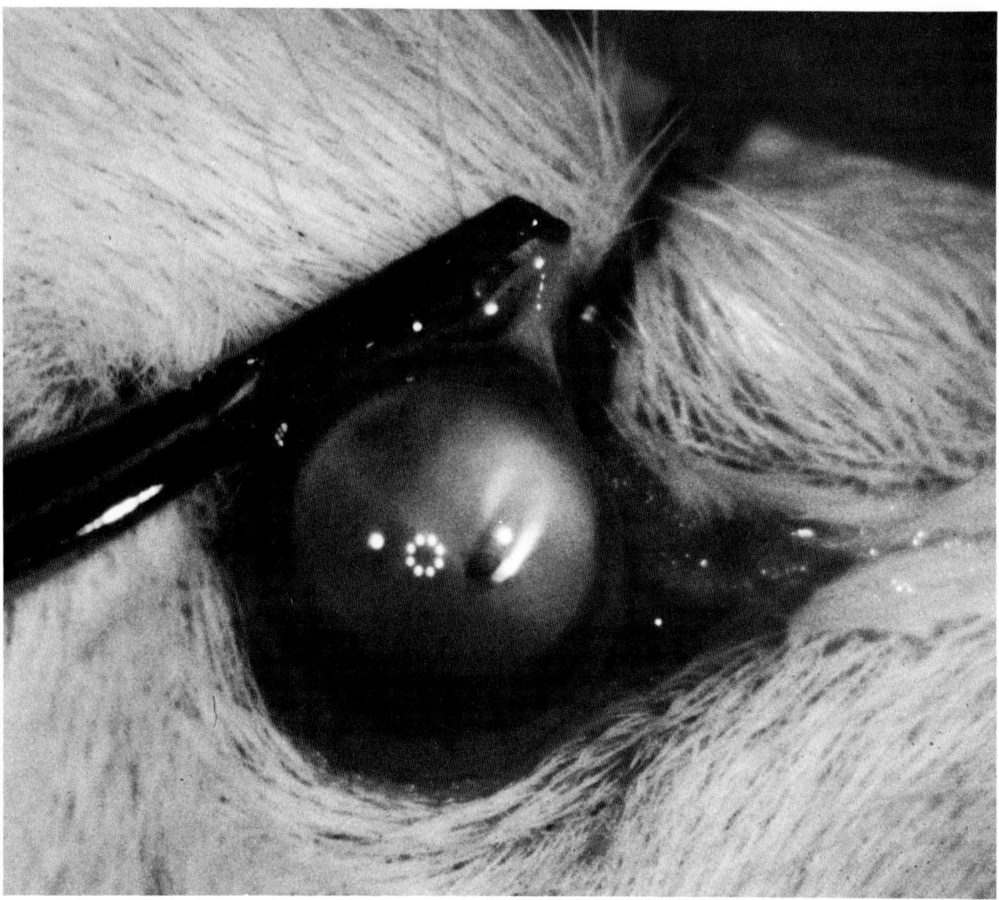

Figure 12.1 Macrophotograph obtained through the operating microscope at the moment of performing an injection in the subretinal space.

behavior on tone-alone baseline trials, as opposed to probe trials, in which the tone is preceded by the flash (figure 12.2).

Many experiments, performed in both laboratory animals and humans, have shown that reflex inhibition measures of sensory threshold approximate those determined by more conventional means (see Ison, 1990). Other experiments, again performed in both laboratory animals and in humans, indicate that cortical input is necessary for reflex inhibition at the short interstimulus intervals that are important in the present work (Hilgard and Wendt, 1933; Ison et al., 1991b). Finally, we have previously shown that the Royal College of Surgeons (RCS) rat, which serves as an animal model for retinitis pigmentosa, suffers a loss of light-produced reflex inhibition which is characterized first by a slowing of the point of maximal inhibition, and then by a progressive loss of absolute inhibition. These behavioral changes are more or less coincident with the progression of the disease state and the attendant loss of photoreceptors (Wecker and Ison, 1986). Thus, this method seemed appropriate to track the loss of visual function that followed light exposure in the

     Retinal Responses to Injury and Transplantation

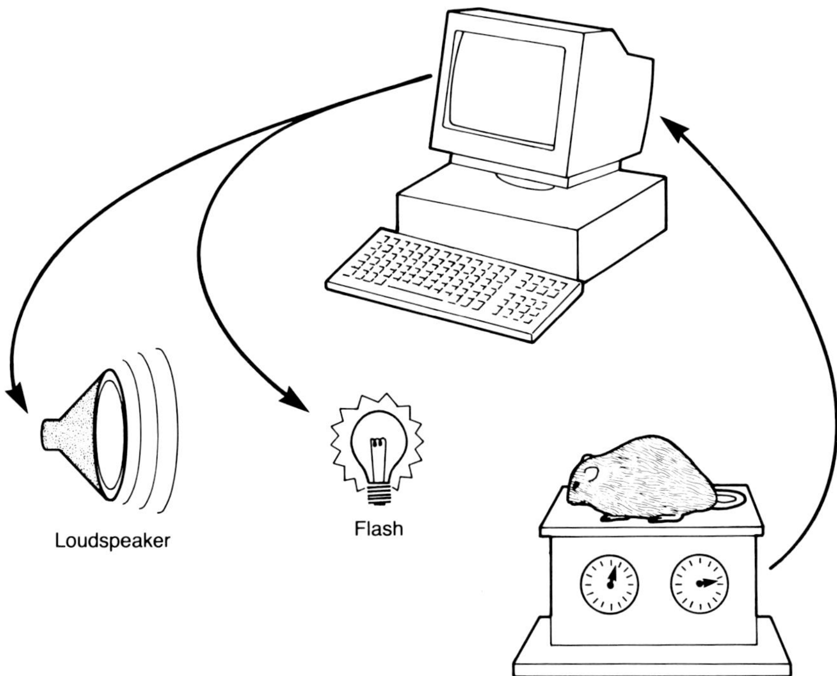

Figure 12.2 The experimental setup used to test the effects of the visually driven reflex modification procedure. The test animal sits on a platform mounted on an accelerometer. The accelerometer records the startle response and sends the data to the computer for storage and analysis. The computer also triggers the flash and the loudspeaker; variable interstimuli intervals are used according to a preprogrammed protocol.

rat. Furthermore, we could track the course of any functional recovery that might follow retinal transplantation.

Experimental Design

The experiment began with a behavioral pretest for all animals. Then, 18 rats were exposed to a bright light, 300 ft-c (approximately 3,000 lux) for 23 hours each day, while 7 animals were exposed on the same schedule to a very dim light, set at just 1 ft-c. For the 1 remaining hour each day, the animals were moved to the vivarium (which is kept at about 5 ft-c. in the light portion of the 12-hour light–12-hour dark [12/12 L/D] schedule) for routine maintenance. This exposure condition continued for 4 weeks, a treatment that we have previously shown to destroy over 99% of the photoreceptors in the rat eye, leaving none of the remaining photoreceptors with a normal morphological appearance (del Cerro, et al., 1989). At the end of the 4-week exposure period, all 25 animals were replaced into the 12/12 L/D schedule of the vivarium for a 4-week "rest period," which we thought might result in their having reached some stable level of retinal degeneration. Then, nine of the animals which had been exposed to the bright light received two injections of fetal retinal cells in one eye, while the nine other animals which had had this

     del Cerro et al.: Retinal Transplants in Light-Blinded Rats

exposure regimen were untouched. Behavioral testing continued weekly during the exposure series, then every 2 weeks in the postexposure rest period and in the posttransplant recovery period, which lasted for 10 weeks. Finally, the group that had been exposed to the bright light, but which had not received the transplant, received exactly the same grafting treatment as had its matched group of nine animals. These former control animals were run, on average, weekly for 4 more weeks after the transplantation procedure in order to determine the reproducibility of the findings noted in the first group of grafted animals.

RESULTS

The data, given as mean response amplitudes relative to the baseline control value, plus the standard error of the means, are given in table 12.1 for the critical intermediate of lead times of 40, 70, 110, and 160 ms. As is typical in these experiments, in the pretest, the light flash substantially inhibited the reflexive response to the loud tone burst. The strength of inhibition was determined by the lead time of the light. Beyond the 40-ms interval, inhibition rapidly increased to a maximum at the 70-ms interval, and then declined in strength. The second set of entries in the table gives the values for inhibition of the group which had been exposed to the bright light for 4 weeks, (n = 18) compared with the group (n = 7) that had been exposed to the dim light. Compared with the pretest results, the inhibition was minimally affected by the animals' having been kept in the dim light, but in sharp contrast to this, reflex inhibition was lost following exposure to the bright light. To this point in the experiment, the effect of exposure to bright light resulted in the same behavioral outcome as that which we have reported earlier to accompany the loss of photoreceptors in the dystrophic RCS rat (Wecker and Ison, 1986). The next set of values shows the changes in reflex inhibition that followed the 4-week period in which the animals were returned to the 12/12 L/D schedule of the vivarium. It is very interesting that in both groups, those exposed to the continuous dim light and those previously exposed to the continuous bright light, the light now showed a substantial and reliable effect on reflex expression. The group previously exposed to dim light showed an extraordinary increase in inhibition which suggests to us the very tentative hypothesis that some hypertrophy of the sensorimotor control mechanisms may have occurred, because these animals had been exposed to continuous illumination despite the fact that illumination was set at a very low level. In the group exposed to the very bright light, however, a completely opposite effect occurred. For these animals, there was no hint of an inhibitory effect of the light at the normal early inhibitory interval, but instead, the light flash now facilitated the reflex response, particularly at an interval of 110 ms. At the next longest interval, 160 ms, the light then provided a modest degree of reflex inhibition, which may be best characterized as a "postexcitatory depression." It certainly occurred at an unusual time period, and was seen primarily to follow the peak of excitation.

     Retinal Responses to Injury and Transplantation

Table 12.1 Quantitative Results of the Effect of Light Flashes on the Acoustic Startle Response at Five Stages of the Experiment*

| | Lead Time Intervals (ms) | | | |
Flash	40	70	110	220
Test A: Pre-Exposure test				
Control	56 ± 5	45 ± 4	64 ± 3	76 ± 3
(n = 25)				
Test B: Post-Exposure test				
Dim light	59 ± 5^a	49 ± 8^b	67 ± 6^c	79 ± 6^d
(n = 7)				
Bright light	109 ± 5^a	100 ± 5^b	107 ± 5^c	102 ± 5^d
(n = 18)				
Test C: Post-Rest test				
Dim light	33 ± 6^a	25 ± 5^b	58 ± 8^c	76 ± 5
(n = 7)				
Bright light	108 ± 5^a	107 ± 4^b	129 ± 6^c	87 ± 7
(n = 18)				
Test D: Post-Graft test 1				
Bright light	96 ± 5^a	92 ± 5	147 ± 13^b	75 ± 9
(n = 9)				
Grafted	81 ± 4^a	89 ± 5	107 ± 6^b	86 ± 6
(n = 9)				
Test E: Post-Graft test 2				
Pre-graft	92 ± 6	87 ± 5	142 ± 12^a	77 ± 7
Post-graft	79 ± 5	81 ± 4	106 ± 8^a	86 ± 7
(n = 9)				

* Each section shows mean reflex amplitudes (relative to the baseline control response, with no flash) at the noted flash lead times, with standard errors. Within each section differences between conditions that are significant ($P < .05$) are marked with a common superscript (i.e., a, b, c, or d). Test A shows pretest figures: note the rapid development of inhibition and slow recovery beyond 70 ms. Test B depicts the effect of 4 weeks' exposure to either 300 ft-c (bright light) or 1 ft-c illumination (dim light): inhibition is lost following the bright light exposure. Test C shows the effects of the 4-week recovery period, the return to the 12/12 L/D schedule. Inhibition increased in the animals exposed to the dim light but anomalous reflex facilitation appeared at 110-ms lead times in animals previously exposed to the bright light. Test D shows the test day of peak inhibition for all groups, following grafting for nine of the animals. Normal inhibition at 40 ms increased, and aberrant facilitation at 110 ms decreased in the grafted animals. Test E shows the effect of the grafting in the animals that had been exposed to the bright light but which had not previously received a graft. Again, modest inhibition appeared at the 40-ms and 70 ms intervals (significant at $p < 0.05$, one-tail), while facilitation at the 110-ms interval disappeared.

del Cerro et al.: Retinal Transplants in Light-Blinded Rats

We have never seen this facilitative effect in a normal animal, and its specific meaning is yet unknown. It may be significant, however, that this same light flash produces a wave of startle reflex excitation beginning at the same 110-ms interval (but not the following phase of reflex depression) in animals that are in a state of functional decortication (Ison et al., 1991b). It may then be a sign of some aberrant subcortical pathway that has developed in these animals once they had been removed from the continuous bright light. Although this particular hypothesis may not be correct, there should be no question that this behavior is grossly atypical, as it results in the light not only losing its normal moderating effect on the startle reaction but, in fact, the replacement of that effect by its exact opposite. It should be noted at this point that the inhibitory effect of a preliminary stimulus on reflex expression is a powerfully generalized phenomenon across animal species and is studied routinely not just in mammals—mice, rats, and humans, most commonly— but also in species as diverse as pigeons and frogs. Thus the replacement of reflex inhibition in the light-damaged animal by an equally strong facilitative effect is a sign that the visual system in the light-damaged rat, while somehow still responsive to light, has very badly rearranged itself.

Half of the animals that had been previously exposed to the bright light now received a transplant, and behavioral testing again was continued at 2-week intervals. In the nongrafted control animals the facilitatory effect of the light and the subsequent postexcitatory depression continued to increase over this period of continued testing. This effect was so strong that at its peak, observed at about 10 weeks after the end of the exposure period, these animals jumped with double their normal baseline force when the light preceded the startle stimulus by 110 ms. In contrast to this, the light flash in the animals exposed to the dim light had its usual inhibitory effect at this interval, so that for them the response was less than one-half of the baseline startle.

The most striking effect of the intraretinal transplantation was that of completely eliminating this abnormal facilitative effect of light on reflex expression. This was seen in all of the animals that received the monocular graft, and it occurred as early as 2 weeks post transplantation. By itself, this might only suggest that the graft resulted in further damage to the eye of the host, so that even the aberrant effect of photic input was now lost. Two facts, however, dispose of this argument in convincing fashion. Firstly, it should be remembered that only one eye received the graft. Thus, even if it had been the case that the graft was harmful to the registration of light in one eye, the animal would have had its other eye, at least, functioning at the same level as before. Secondly, it happens that the grafted animals went on to show a second significant change in their behavior. In every animal, there was at least a modest recovery of reflex inhibition produced by the light flash at the normal early and proper time for it to occur, namely at 40 and 70 ms. This effect was transitory, and occurred at different times in different animals, but for the group as a whole it occurred maximally with a mean of 4 weeks post grafting.

Because reflex inhibition peaked and then waned at different rates across these animals, we used the peak inhibitory performance at the 40- and 70-ms intervals to judge their recovery of function. Necessarily, we contrasted these measures against the comparable peak performance in the bright-light exposed control group in order to control for chance variation from test to test. These data are given in the next set of numbers in table 12.1. The group exposed to the continuous dim light showed profound inhibition at 40 and 70 ms, and inhibition even at 110 ms averaged about 70%. At its peak, the group that had been exposed to the bright light but had not received the transplants showed only 6% inhibition at 40 ms but 47% facilitation at the 110-ms interval. In marked contrast to this, it can be seen that the group that had received the transplants showed modest but reliable inhibition (19%) at 40 ms, and retained very little of the anomalous facilitatory effect of the light at 110 ms (just 7%).

To assess the reliability of these data, we tested the change in the effectiveness of the light in controlling reflex expression produced by the transplant, compared with the bright light–exposed group that had not had the transplant, in a mixed design ANOVA (analysis of variance). The most important finding was the significant three-way interaction between inter-stimulus interval (ISI), pre- vs. post-test, and transplant vs. control, $F(8/128) = 2.44$, $P < .02$, revealing that the influence of the light flash on reflex expression was different on the post-test, compared to the pre-test, in the two groups. Further ANOVAs showed no pretransplant difference between the two groups ($F < 1$), while their posttransplant ISI functions differed: $F(8,128) = 4.95$, $P < .01$. Subsequent posttransplant t-tests showed that peak inhibition at 40 ms was greater in the group that had received the transplant [$t(16) = 2.34$, $P < .005$], whereas reflex facilitation at 110 ms on that same test day was greater in the animals that had not received the transplant [$t(16) = 2.79$, $P < .005$].

Both groups of bright-light exposed animals showed flat electroretinogram (ERG) measures at the end of the final behavioral test, although reflex facilitation at the 110-ms interval was presumptive evidence for some measure of residual retinal function. In the histological analysis, the eyes with no transplant revealed a massive degeneration of the photoreceptor layer. In contrast to this, clusters of photoreceptors were seen at injection points in the grafted eyes, but the clusters were small and were regressing at the time of sacrifice.

Although the differences that were observed between animals that had received the transplant and those that had not were statistically significant at a conventionally satisfactory level, it must be confessed that the specific outline of the findings had not been anticipated, and thus none of the statistical analyses had been thought out in an a priori fashion. For this reason we decided it would be wise to repeat the grafting operation, now in the set of nine animals that had been exposed to the light but had not received a transplant. The one change in the testing protocol was that animals were tested once each week rather than every 2 weeks. Now, the same statistical

     del Cerro et al.: Retinal Transplants in Light-Blinded Rats

analyses could be done in the context of a set of a priori expectations concerning peak inhibitory performance following the operation, compared to peak performance on the tests prior to the transplant (which included an additional and independent pretransplant test). These data are given in the last set of numbers in table 12.1. Again, facilitation was eliminated following the transplant, and for the pre- versus post-transplant comparison, $t(16) = 2.80$, $P < 0.05$. A modest degree of reflex inhibition at 40 and 70 ms reappeared, and the pre- versus post-transplant comparison, combining 40 and 70 ms, $t(16) = 1.79$, $P < .005$, one-tail. Again the average time to the peak was 4 weeks. The change in reflex expression after the transplant again met the conventional levels of significance in the analysis of variance, and for the interaction between ISI and pre- versus post-transplant, $F(8.64) - 4.15$, $P < 0.01$. Even more important than these details of the inferential statistics is the fact that the data observed earlier were most clearly reproduced in the overall pattern of findings.

DISCUSSION

Retinal transplantation may one day provide a means of restoring function to visually impaired eyes. That possibility creates the need to develop methods that would allow the surgeon to seed a substantial portion of the host retina with donor cells, and other methods that would allow an objective and quantitative evaluation of posttransplantatiaton visual improvement. We have developed in laboratory animals the useful behavioral procedures that are sensitive to retinal damage and retinal repair (Ison, 1990) and the necessary surgical procedures which are relatively noninvasive yet effective (Lazar and del Cerro, 1991). Our aim in this study was to put these past developments to the test, to furnish unequivocal data on whether or not we had reached the goal of ameliorating a severe visual deficit by means of intraretinal transplants.

We have known for some time that perinatal retinal cells grafted into the light-damaged retina of adult rats provides the host with new photoreceptors that synapse on the adjacent plexiform layers (del Cerro et al., 1989). Moreover, light-produced activity of fetal cells transplanted to the anterior chamber of healthy rat eyes is detected in ERGs (Collier et al., 1989). The next logical research question was whether visually controlled behavior might reappear in blinded rats following intraretinal transplants. Our prior observations suggest there may be a positive answer to this important question: If the new photoreceptors are sensitive to light and their contacts are functional, then may light input once again influence behavior? Here, we provide evidence that light-damaged rats demonstrate reliable visual sensitivity following intraretinal transplants of fetal retinal cells in a way not evident in matched controls, thus revealing the potential contribution of transplantation to the amelioration of sensory dysfunction.

Strict temporal concordance of behavioral recovery and the structural repair produced by the grafts cannot be established in the present experimental design, but both measures are in substantial agreement in showing the effectiveness of intraretinal grafting. We may conclude that at least in some partial measure, this procedure does repair the structural damage and the functional deficit that follow light blinding in the rat. In sum, a measurable and objective functional benefit of intraretinal transplantation into the eye of a visually impaired animal has been achieved.

Acknowledgments

Support for this work was provided by National Eye Institute grants NEI-05262 (MdC), EY-01319, EY-02843, The Rochester Eye Bank (ESL), and anonymous donations.

REFERENCES

Collier, R.J., del Cerro, M., Yeh, H.H., del Cerro, C., Trojanczyk, L. A., and Westenberg, I. A. (1989). Electroretinographic assessment of intraocular retinal transplants. *Invest. Ophthalmol. Vis. Sci.* 30(suppl.):349.

del Cerro, M. (1990). Intraocular retinal transplantation. In *Progress in Retinal Research*, ed. N.N. Osborne and G. J. Chader, 229–272. Oxford, England: Pergamon Press.

del Cerro, M., Cogen, M. J., and del Cerro, C. (1980a). Stevenel's blue, an excellent stain for optical microscopical study of plastic embedded tissues. *Microscopica Acta* 83:117–121.

del Cerro, M., Standler, M. N., and del Cerro, C. (1980b). High resolution optical microscopy of animal tissues by the use of sub-micrometer thick sections and a new stain. *Microscopica Acta* 83:217–220.

del Cerro, M., Gash, D. M., Rao, G. N., Notter, M. F., Wiegand, S. J., and Gupta, M. (1984). Intraocular retinal transplants. *Invest. Ophthalmol. Vis. Sci.* 25(suppl.):62.

del Cerro, M., M. F. D. Notter, C. del Cerro, S. J. Wiegand, D. A. Grover, and Lazar, E. 1989). Intraretinal transplantation for rod-cell replacement in light-damaged retinas. *J. Neurol. Transplant.* 1:1–10.

Hilgard, E. R., and Wendt., G. R. (1933). The problem of reflex sensitivity to light studied in a case of hemianopsia. *Yale J. Biol. Med.* 5:373–385.

Hoffman, H. S., and Ison, J. R. (1980). Principles of reflex modification in the domain of startle: I. Some empirical findings and their implications for the interpretation of how the nervous system processes sensory input. *Psychol. Rev.* 87:175–189.

Ison, J.R. (1984). Reflex modification as an objective test for sensory processing following toxicant exposure. *J. Neurobehav. Toxicol. Teratol.* 6:437–445.

Ison, J. R. (1990). Behavioral methods applicable to laboratory animals and humans. In *Advances in Neurobehavioral Toxicology: Applications in Environmental and Occupational Health*, ed. B.L. Johnson, W.K. Anger, A. Durao, and C. Xintaras, 389–400. Chelsea, Mich.: Lewis Publishers.

Ison, J. R., Bowen, G.P., Collier, R.J., del Cerro, M., Lazar, E., Grover, D.A., and del Cerro, C. (1991a). Light damage increases the latency, then diminishes the amplitude of reflex inhibition by a light flash in the rat. *Invest. Ophthalmol. Vis. Sci.* 32(suppl.):1098.

Ison, J. R., Bowen, G.P., and O'Connor, K. (1991b). Reflex modification by visual stimuli in the rat following functional decortication. *Psychobiology* 19:122–126.

Lazar, E. and del Cerro, M. (1991). Intraretinal transplantation: An External Approach. In *Retinal Degenerations*, Boca Rator, Fla., CRC Press. ed. G. Anderson, J. Hollyfield, and M. LaVail, 313–320.

Wecker, J. R., and J. R. Ison. (1986). Visual function measured by reflex modification in rats with inherited retinal dystrophy. *Behav. Neurosci.* 100:679–684.

V   Plasticity of Connectivity in the Visual System

13 Regulation of Gene Expression by Afferent Activity in Adult Monkey Visual Cortex

Edward G. Jones

The influence of neural activity in the development of the nervous system is profound (Harris, 1981). The initiation and conduction of action potentials and the induction of membrane conductance and polarization changes appear to be key elements in the stabilization and maintenance of synaptic connections during critical phases of development. In the maturation of the mammalian central nervous system (CNS), balanced patterns of neural activity entering the CNS from the sense organs are considered to be the primary factors in the establishment of normal patterns of neural connections. Studies of the primate visual cortex have played an important role in the elucidation of the fundamental processes by which activity influences neural maturation. Anatomical and physiological plasticity of terminations can be induced by perturbed visual experience during a critical period in the first few months of life (Hubel and Wiesel, 1977; Hubel et al., 1977; LeVay et al., 1980) and effects may continue into the second year (Blakemore et al., 1978). Although originally considered as a developmentally regulated process, plasticity of this type appears to continue into adult life. Even in adult monkeys, a brief period of monocular deprivation brought about by eye removal, or by action potential blockade due to intraocular tetrodotoxin injections, quickly leads, in the deprived-eye columns of the visual cortex, to reductions in cellular and terminal levels of immunocytochemically detectable γ-aminobutyric acid (GABA); its synthesizing enzyme, glutamic acid decarboxylase (GAD); the $GABA_A$ receptors; and certain tachykinins (Hendry and Jones, 1986; Hendry et al., 1988, 1990). At the same time, immunocytochemically detectable levels of type II Ca^{2+}-calmodulin–dependent protein kinase (CaM II kinase), an enzyme associated with synaptic function, increase in the deprived-eye columns (Hendry and Kennedy, 1986). The effects are rapidly reversible, and thus the maintenance of normal levels of these and other molecules depends on action potentials in the optic nerve (Hendry and Jones, 1988).

Changes in levels of transmitter-, receptor-, and second messenger–related proteins under activity-dependent conditions can be expected to influence profoundly the functions of cortical neurons. Such influences should be evident in the central visual system after injuries to the peripheral visual apparatus, and the restoration of normal patterns after procedures such as optic nerve grafting. Detecting the resultant effects may provide a useful assay of the efficacy of such procedures. In recent investigations from our laboratory, efforts have been made to determine the underlying molecular basis of activity-dependent effects on transmitter-related cortical function, focusing on the genes coding for the enzyme involved in the production of the major cortical inhibitory transmitter, GABA, and for one of the most common second messenger–related proteins of the forebrain, CaM II kinase.

METHODS

Synthetic oligonuceotide primers that corresponded to conserved regions were used to isolate and amplify GAD and CaM II kinase complementary DNAs (cDNAs) derived from monkey messenger RNA (mRNA) by the polymerase chain reaction (PCR). Oligonucleotides for GAD PCR amplification contained 21 bases of sequence identical to cat (Kobayashi et al., 1987) and human GAD cDNAs (Benson et al., 1991). The 5′ sense oligonucleotide (5′-GGATCCCCTCACAAGAT-GATGGGCGTG-3′) contained a *Bam*HI site, corresponded to bases 1324-1344 of cat cDNA (Kobayashi et al. 1987), and encompassed the sequence encoding the pyridoxal phosphate–binding region of GAD. The 3′ antisense oligonucleotide (5′-GAGGCTTTGTGGAATATACCA-3′) corresponded to bases 1663-1683 of cat GAD cDNA.

Oligonucleotides for CaM II kinase amplification contained 21 bases flanking the region of greatest subunit variability between the α, β, and β' sequences of rat CaM II kinase (Bennett and Kennedy, 1987; Lin et al., 1987). The 5′ sense oligonucleotide (5′-GGATCCCTGAAGAAGTTCAATGCCAGG-3′) contained a *Sal*I site and corresponded to bases 1165-1185 of the α-subunit downstream from the region of greatest variability. All oligonucleotides contained restriction sites for cloning directly into pBluescribe (pBS, Stratagene) (Scharf et al., 1986).

RNA was extracted from monkey cerebral cortex by the method of Chirgwin et al. (1979); 10 μg was primed with oligo(dT) and reverse-transcribed with AMV reverse transcriptase (Boehringer Mannheim Biochemicals). Single-stranded cDNA was amplified by 35 cycles of PCR (Saiki et al. 1985, 1988). Amplified cDNA was restricted with *Bam*HI and *Eco*RI for GAD and with *Sal*I for CaM II kinase. It was purified by electroelution from a polyacrylamide gel, ligated to *Bam*HI/*Eco*RI- or *Bam*HI/*Sal*I-digested pBS, and transformed into 71.18 cells. Plasmids containing inserts were sequenced (Sanger et al., 1977; Tabor and Richardson, 1987).

Eight PCR-generated CaM II kinase α cDNA clones (CaM II kinase α) had 95% sequence identity with rat CaM II kinase in the comparable region (Lin et al., 1987). Two of the clones (CaM II kinase α^{33}) contained a 33-bp insert at the point where rat CaM II kinase α, β and β'-subunit sequences diverge (Bulleit et al., 1988), but were otherwise identical. Three 360-bp GAD cDNA clones contained the proposed pyridoxal phosphate–binding region at the 5′ end (Bossa et al., 1977). There was 97% sequence homology with a GAD cDNA (Kobayashi et al., 1987) in this region.

     Plasticity of Connectivity in the Visual System

GAD clones were linearized with *Bam*HI and transcribed with T7 RNA polymerase. This yielded a 365-nucleotide, antisense riboprobe which was transcription-labeled with $[\alpha\text{-}^{35}S]$UTP for in situ hybridization studies. Sense-strand control riboprobes were transcribed from the *Pvu*II-digested GAD plasmid using T3 RNA polymerase. CaM II kinase $\alpha\text{-}^{33}$ clones were linearized with *Bam*HI and transcribed with T3 RNA polymerase. This yielded a 373-nucleotide riboprobe that was labeled with $[\alpha\text{-}^{35}S]$UTP. Sense-strand control riboprobes were transcribed form the *Pvu*II-digested plasmid using T7 RNA polymerase.

For in situ hybridization, ten adult macaque monkeys ranging in age from 3 to 20 years were used. Six animals were deprived of vision in one eye for 48 hours to 5 days by injecting 15 μg of the Na$^+$ channel blocker tetrodotoxin (TTX) into the vitreous cavity under ketamine anesthesia. In one monkey retinal ganglion cells were destroyed by an intraocular injection of 0.3 ml of 100mM cobalt chloride 15 days before sacrifice (Malpeli and Schiller, 1979); in another monkey, one eye was removed 5 days prior to sacrifice. Twenty other animals from previous studies had been monocularly deprived for varying periods by the same methods. In these animals the visual cortex was stained immunocytochemically to show changes in GAD and CaM II kinase immunoreactivity (Hendry and Jones, 1986, 1988; Hendry and Kennedy, 1986) and in immunoreactive tachykinin (Hendry et al., 1988). Two normal animals served as controls. All animals for in situ hybridization studies were perfused with 4% paraformaldehyde in 0.5M phosphate buffer at pH 7.4. Brains were postfixed overnight in 4% paraformaldehyde and then immersed in 20% sucrose in 4% paraformaldehyde.

The visual cortex was frozen on dry ice, and 25 μm of serial sections were cut on a sliding microtome in the frontal plane or in a plane parallel to the surface and collected in cold 0.1M phosphate buffer. Series were labeled with the antisense GAD or the antisense CaM II kinase probes. Alternate series were stained with a 0.25% thionin or for cytochrome oxidase (CO) (Wong-Riley, 1979).

Sections were washed in 0.1M glycine in 0.1M phosphate buffer (pH 7.2) at room temperature, then treated with proteinase K (1 μg/ml in 50mM ethylenediaminetetraacetate (EDTA)/0.1M Tris, pH 8) for 30 minutes at 30°C, and 0.25% acetic anhydride in 2 × SSC (saline sodium citrate) at room temperature. They were incubated in hybridization buffer containing 50% deionized formamide, 10% dextran sulfate, 0.7% Ficoll, 0.7% polyvinylpyrrolidone, 350 mg/ml bovine serum albumin (BSA), 0.15 mg/ml yeast transfer RNA (tRNA), 0.33 mg/ml denatured herring sperm DNA, and 20mM dithiothreitol (DTT) for 1 hour at 60°C. Then they were transferred to fresh hybridization buffer containing additional 20mM DTT and 1×10^4 cpm/μl of $[\alpha\text{-}^{35}S]$ antisense riboprobe for 20 or more hours at 60°C.

Following hybridization, the sections were washed in 4 × SSC, digested with ribonuclease A in 10mM Tris-saline, pH 8, containing 1mM EDTA for 30 minutes at 45°C. They were finally washed through descending concentrations of SSC with 5mM DTT to a final stringency of 0.1 × SSC at 60°C for 1 hour. Sections were mounted on slides, dried, and exposed on Amersham βmax film for 1 to 4 days. After developing the film, lipids were extracted in chloroform and the slides were dipped in Kodak NTB2 emulsion, exposed for 7 to 15 days at 4°C, developed, fixed, and stained with cresyl violet. Optical density measurements were made from the films and calibrated to ^{14}C-labeled brain paste standards. Sense-strand radiolabeled RNA probes were hybridized to sections as controls. In these, the visual cortex showed no labeling above background.

RESULTS

Immunocytochemical Changes in Area 17 Following Monocular Deprivation

Monocular deprivation in adult monkeys affects immunocytochemically detectable levels of several transmitters, peptides, receptors and other proteins. All of the effects are most evident in layer IVC which contains large numbers of terminals of geniculocortical afferents, possesses a high density of $GABA_A$ receptors, and shows intense histochemical staining for CO. CO staining indicates a high level of metabolic activity and provides a marker for identifying deprived and nondeprived ocular dominance columns in sections adjacent to those stained by immunocytochemistry or showing localization of molecular probes.

In the immunocytochemical studies, after monocular deprivations, increased levels of immunoreactivity have been detected for the α-subunit of CaM II kinase, and decreased levels have been detected for GABA and its synthesizing enzyme GAD, as well as for tachykinins (Hendry and Jones, 1986, 1988; Hendry and Kennedy, 1986; Hendry et al., 1987, 1988). Decreases also occur in the $GABA_A$ receptor, as localized by immunocytochemistry, using a monoclonal antibody (Vitorica et al., 1988) and by ^{3}H-labeled flunitrazepam and ^{3}H-labeled muscimol binding (Hendry et al., 1990).

The effects detected after eye removal, after injection of TTX into an eye, and after monocular eyelid suture are identical and just as robust in each case. They appear within 4 days of eye removal or TTX injection, but only after 4 to 6 weeks of eyelid suture. The effects are most pronounced in layer IVC and are characterized by enhanced immunoreactive staining for CaM II kinase α in the deprived-eye dominance columns and by reductions in immunoreactive staining for GAD, GABA, and $GABA_A$ receptors and for tachykinins in the same columns.

GABA- and GAD-immunoreactive cells are affected to the extent that 50% of the GABA cells in layer IVC of a deprived column fail to stain (figures 13.1 and 13.2). It appears that all the GABA-tachykinin subpopulation fails to stain for tachykinin immunoreactivity. The effects on immunoreactive staining are not determined by cell death, for cell counts reveal that the total cell population is unchanged (see figure 3.2). Moreover, the effect is reversible: cessation of TTX injections or reopening of the eyelids returns the immunocytochemical

     Plasticity of Connectivity in the Visual System

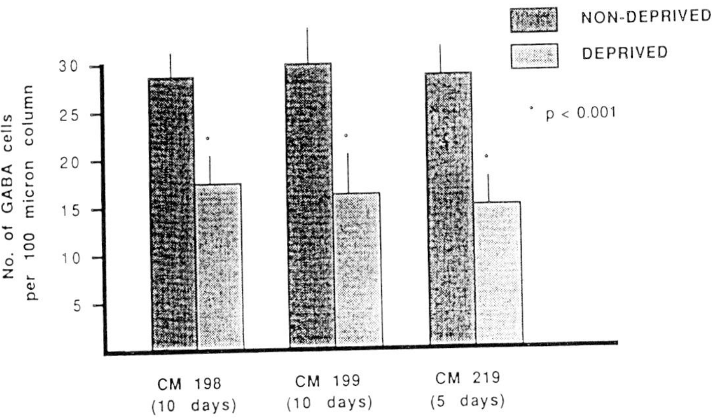

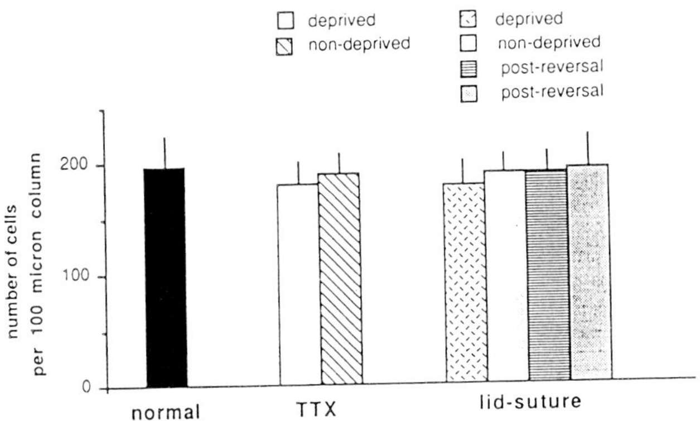

Figure 13.1 *Above*: reduction in GABA-immunoreactive cells in 100-μm-wide columns through layer IVC at the centers of deprived ocular dominance columns in two monkeys subjected to monocular tetrodotoxin (TTX) injection, showing statistically significant differences ($P < .001$) between the centers of deprived and nondeprived columns. *Below*: absence of significant cell death in layer IVC, demonstrated by counting the total number of thionin-stained neurons in 100-μm-wide columns through layer IVC in normal animals, in deprived and nondeprived ocular dominance columns of lid-sutured and TTX-injected animals, and in an animal subjected to lid reopening (two sets of counts). Counts were made from three different sections in each case. Differences are statistically insignificant. (Reproduced with permission from Hendry and Jones, 1988.)

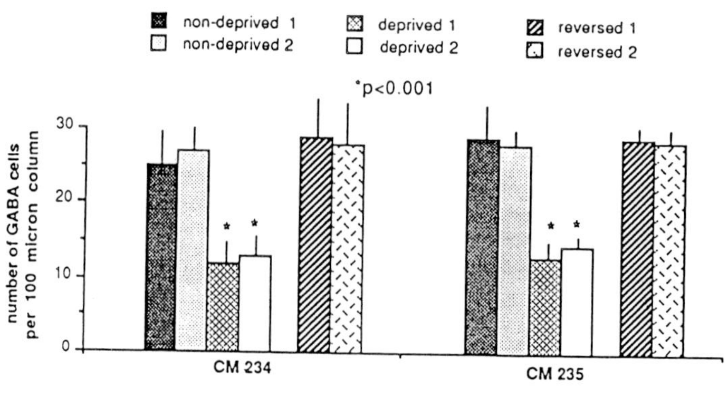

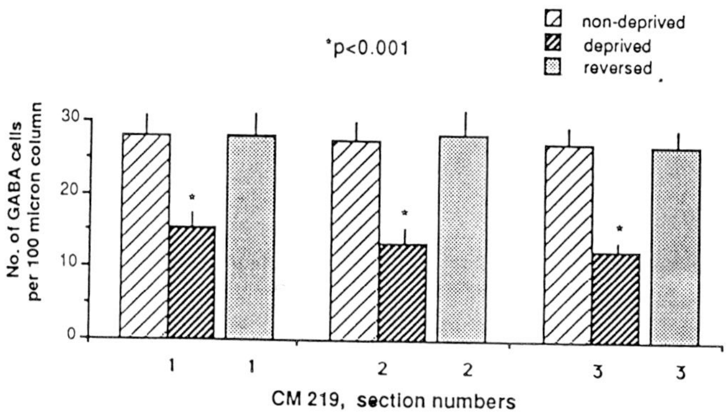

Figure 13.2 *Above*: number of GABA-immunoreactive cells in 100-μm-wide columns through the centers of deprived and nondeprived ocular dominance columns in layer IVCβ in biopsies from two TTX-injected animals, compared with comparable counts through layer IVCβ of the contralateral visual cortex after recovery. Two sets of counts are shown in each case. *Below*: number of GABA-immunoreactive cells in 100-μm-wide columns through the centers of deprived and nondeprived ocular dominance columns in layer IVCβ in a biopsy from a lid-sutured animal, compared with comparable counts through layer IVCβ of the contralateral visual cortex after reopening the eyelids. Data are from three different sections(1–3). (Reproduced with permission from Hendry and Jones, 1988.)

staining patterns to normal within 20 to 30 days (see figure 13.2). The deprivation effects are not age-dependent and have been induced as readily in monkeys at 2 years of age as in those 20 years or older.

In Situ Hybridization of CaM II Kinase and GAD mRNAs in Monkey Visual Cortex

CaM II kinase   In area 17 of normal monkey visual cortex, hybridization of the CaM II kinase riboprobes is very dense in layers II through VI. Differences in density enable individual cortical laminae to be discerned and their borders are clearly seen (figure 13.3). Layers II and IVB contain the greatest amount of label., layers III, IVCβ, and VI contain lesser amounts, although a narrow band

   Plasticity of Connectivity in the Visual System

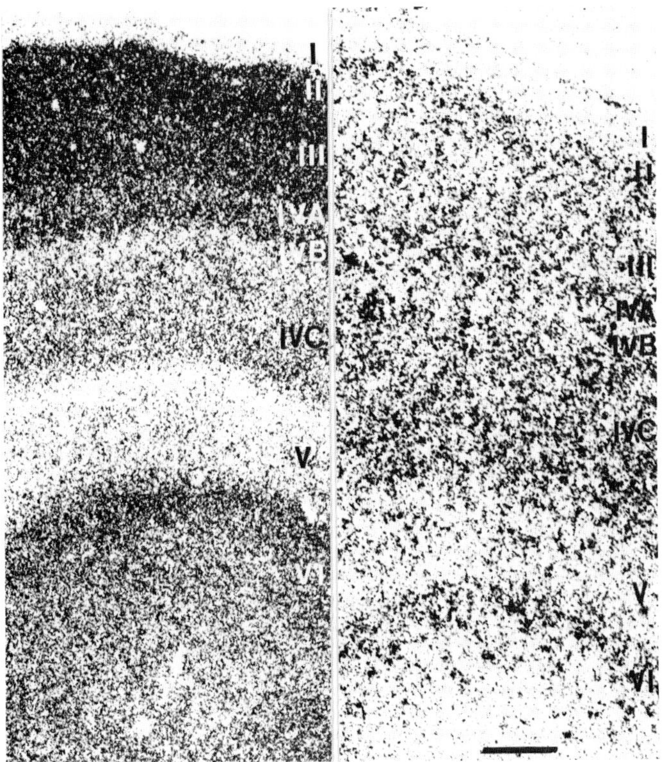

Figure 13.3 Autoradiographs showing in situ hybridization of CaM II kinase (*left*) and GAD (*right*) riboprobes in area 17 of a normal monkey. Note differences in lamination densities and the dense neuropil label in most layers on the left. Bar: 100 μm.

in the upper portion of layer VI is more densely labeled. Levels are low in layers IVCα and V, and the lowest levels are in layers IVA and I and in a narrow strip at the border between layers IVC and V. Within a layer, no periodicities can be detected in the labeling pattern that would conform to the well-known CO periodicities or "blobs." In each layer, the density of auto-radiographic grains is relatively homogeneous (see figure 13.3), and even at very short exposure times, the level of labeling is exceedingly high, with an unusually large amount of labeling over the neuropil, making it difficult to localize the grains to individual cell somata.

In area 18, CaM II kinase hybridization is dense in layers II and III. Layer IV is homogeneously labeled and approximately equal in density to layer IVCα of area 17. Levels of neuropil hybridization are also particularly high. No inhomogeneities corresponding to stripes in the CO staining pattern are visible.

After monocular deprivation by TTX injections, retinal destruction, or eye removal, the pattern of CaM II kinase mRNA localization changes dramatically, irrespective of the age of the animal. CaM II kinase cRNA hybridization becomes greatly enhanced in regular columns that extend through the thickness of layers II through VI in area 17. These alternate with columns of similar

    Jones: Regulation of Gene Expression

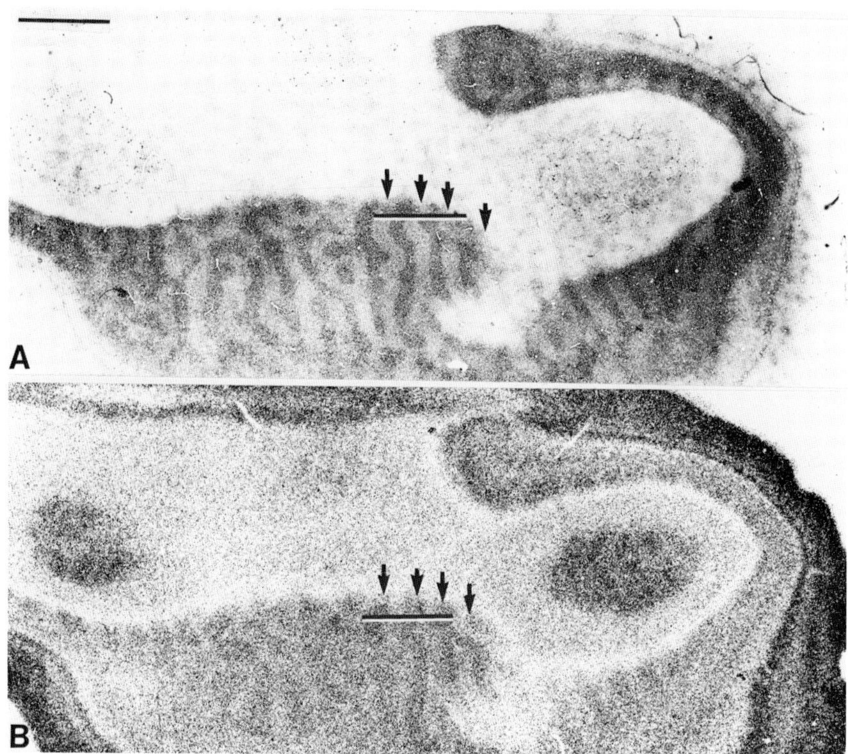

Figure 13.4 Paired cytochrome oxidase (*CO*)–stained (*A*) and autoradiographic (*B*) sections from areas 17 and 18 of a monocularly deprived monkey showing (*B*) enhanced levels of in situ hybridization that reveal increased levels of CaM II kinase mRNA in the deprived eye dominance columns. Line in **B** indicates region quantified in figure 13.5. Bar: 1 μm (Modified from Benson et al., 1991a.)

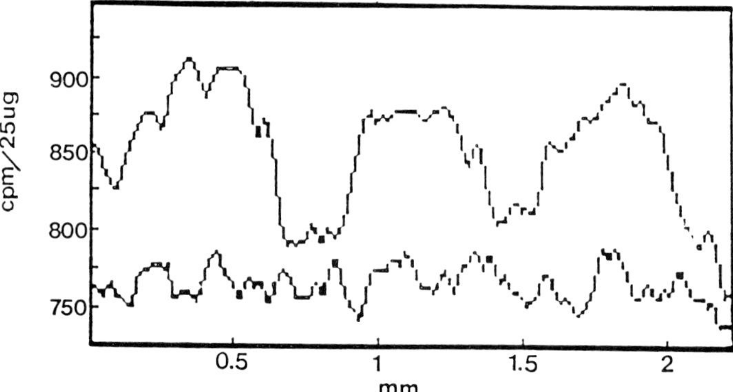

Figure 13.5 Comparison of CaM II kinase mRNA levels in the region indicated by the line in figure 13.4. The *upper trace* shows enhanced levels (*peaks*) over the three deprived columns included in the traverse. Valleys, representing normal columns, show levels close to normal. Normal levels are shown by the lower trace taken from section of a similar region of area 17 of a normal monkey, hybridized at the same time, and exposed on the same sheet of x-ray film. (Reproduced with permission from Benson et al., 1991a.)

     Plasticity of Connectivity in the Visual System

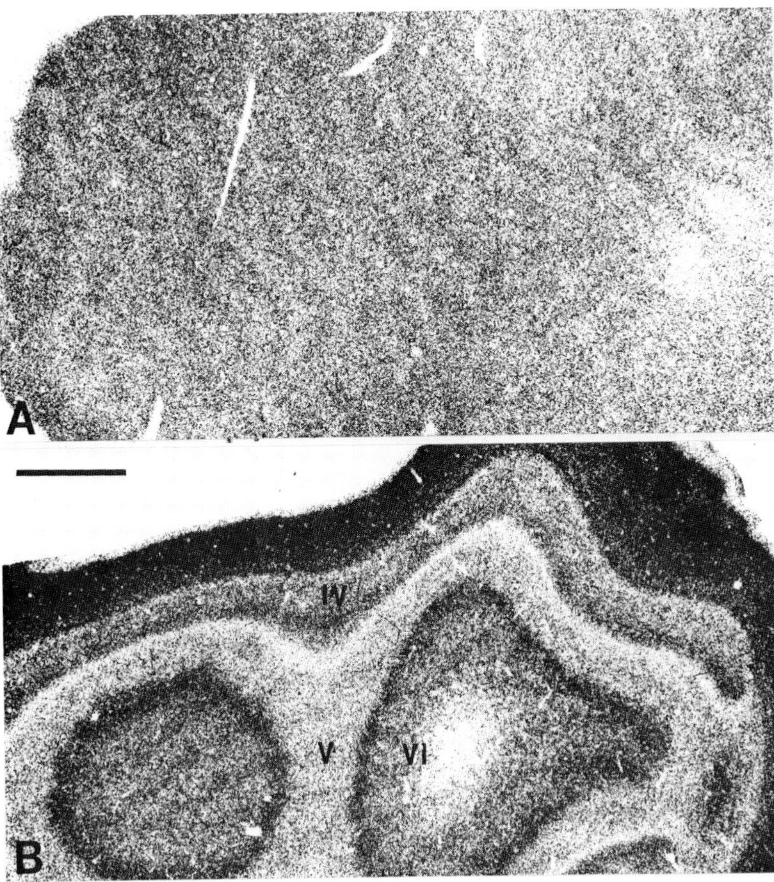

Figure 13.6 *A*, enhanced CaM II kinase hybridization signal in stripes that correspond to rows of deprived eye blobs and adjacent inter-rows in layer III of a TTX-injected monkey. *B*, enhanced CaM II kinase hybridization signal in stripes that correspond to rows of deprived blobs in layers V and VI of the same monkey. Bars: 1 mm.

size that show lower levels of labeling (figures 13.4, 13.5, and 13.6). In sections cut parallel to the pial surface, the alternating dense and less-dense columns appear as long stripes that are very distinct in layer IVC where they correlate closely with the ocular dominance stripes seen in adjacent CO-stained sections. When CO sections are superimposed on adjacent auto-radiographs using the cut profiles of blood vessels as guides, the stripes of enhanced in situ hybridization correspond to the lightly stained CO stripes, and thus to deprived ocular dominance columns. The stripes showing weaker hybridization correspond to the darker CO stripes, and thus to nondeprived columns (Wong-Riley 1979; Horton and Hubel, 1981). Enhanced CaM II kinase mRNA levels in the deprived-eye columns are apparent 3 to 4 days after monocular deprivation and are maintained after 15 days of monocular deprivation. Optical density analysis shows that label over deprived-eye columns is four to five times denser than that over normal eye columns (see figure 13.5). Beyond 15 days, however, although the CO-stained sections

     Jones: Regulation of Gene Expression

show maximal deprivation effects, there is less distinction between deprived and nondeprived columns in the CaM II kinase autoradiographs.

In layers II and III in the monocularly deprived animals, continuous stripes of higher autoradiographic grain density, approximately 500 μm wide alternate with less-dense stripes approximately 300 μm wide (see figure 13.6). Superimposition of adjacent CO-stained sections shows that the denser stripes of hybridization lie over rows of CO-stained blobs that lie at the centers of ocular dominance columns in layers outside layer IVC (Horton and Hubel, 1981; Horton, 1984). In the rows of deprived-eye blobs, the CO patches become shrunken in longer-deprived animals (Horton, 1984), and this reveals that the wider, denser stripes of hybridization label lie in rows of blobs that represent the deprived eye and adjacent CO weak regions. The narrower, less-dense stripes of label lie over the intervening rows of nonshrunken co-blobs that represent the nondeprived eye (Benson et al., 1991a).

In layers IVB, V, and VI, slightly wider stripes of enhanced label also alternate with narrower stripes of less-dense label and are also aligned with rows of CO-stained blobs (Horton, 1984). The denser stripes of label correspond to rows of blobs that lie above (layer IVB) or below (layers V and VI) the dense stripes of label that define the deprived-eye dominance columns in layer IVC. No inhomogeneities in the hybridization pattern are detected in area 18 of monocularly deprived animals.

GAD Autoradiographic grains associated with hybridized GAD riboprobes are distinctly localized over cell somata, contrasting with the more homogeneous CaM II kinase hybridization pattern. Large or small clusters of silver grains are clearly associated with underlying Nissl-stained cell nuclei, and correspond to large (c. 21 μm) and small (c. 10 μm) cells, respectively. Laminae of differential grain density correspond to laminae and sublaminae of normal area 17 (see figure 13.3). Infrequent small clusters with few grains are observed throughout layer I. Large and small clusters occur through layers II and III. Layer IVA shows a thin, densely labeled band of cells. Layer IVB has a line of large clusters forming a strip in the middle of the layer. Layer IVC has many small clusters indicative of lightly labeled small cells and sublaminae of different labeling density are revealed, two in layers IVCα and three in IVCβ. Layer V has less overall grain density but many large clusters of grains. Layer VI is subdivided into three laminae with superficial and deep less-dense bands flanking an intermediate less-dense band.

In area 18, grain density in layers I, II, and III is approximately equal to that in area 17. Layer IV is slightly denser than overlying layers, but with no sublaminae. Layers V and VI resemble area 17. Sections of areas 17 and 18 cut parallel to the pial surface show no periodicities in the GAD mRNA localization pattern.

The same animals that revealed increases in CaM II kinase mRNA levels in deprived-eye dominance columns showed no detectable change levels of GAD mRNA hybridization in areas 17 or 18 and no irregularitites associated with deprived- or nondeprived-eye dominance columns or CO blobs (figure

  Plasticity of Connectivity in the Visual System

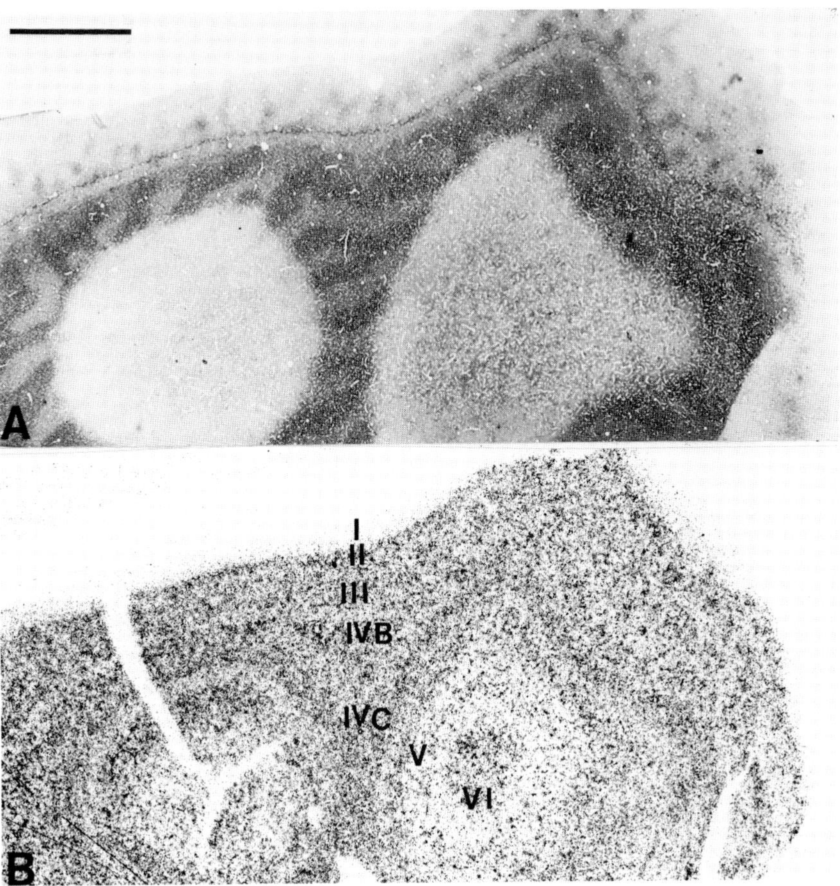

Figure 13.7 Paired CO-stained (*A*) and autoradiographic (*B*) sections from a monocularly deprived monkey showing lack of change in glutamic acid decarboxylase (GAD) mRNA levels, as indicated by in situ hybridization. Bar: 1 mm. (Modified from Benson et al., 1991a.)

13.7). No statistical difference between hybridization in deprived and non-deprived ocular dominance columns was detected in layer IV by quantitative image analysis (level of significance = 0.01).

DISCUSSION

Immunocytochemical studies of adult monkey visual cortex have shown that brief periods of monocular deprivation are associated with large changes in levels of many neuroactive molecules. Among these, the second messenger–related protein CaM II kinase is of particular interest since cells containing it show increases in immunoreactivity. The present study shows that these changes in protein levels are likely to be due to reduced gene expression under conditions in which afferent input to the cells is reduced. This implies that levels of CaM II kinase are normally maintained by an activity-dependent effect acting at transcriptional levels. By contrast, the large decreases in GAD immunoreactivity that occur in deprived-eye columns of adult monkey visual

     Jones: Regulation of Gene Expression

cortex following monocular deprivation (Hendry and Jones, 1986, 1988), and which result in large reductions in GABA levels, are not accompanied by detectable changes in GAD mRNA. This implies that regulations of GAD protein levels by activity is likely to be mediated at a posttranscriptional level.

CaM II kinase makes up at least 1% of all forebrain protein in the rat (Erondu and Kennedy, 1985). An apparently similar abundance in monkeys is reflected in the high CaM II kinase mRNA levels revealed by in situ hybridization. The high levels in the neuropil are most likely in the large, densely packed apical and basal dendritic systems of cortical pyramidal cells, which are stained by CaM II kinase immunoreactivity (Benson et al., 1992). Dendrites of the pyramidal cells contain significant amounts of free and attached ribosomes (Peters et al., 1976) and CaM II kinase mRNA may be translated at these sites as well as in the somata. CaM II kinase protein is one of the major components of postsynaptic densities (Kennedy et al., 1983; Kelly et al., 1984), so its mRNA may be specifically associated with the large numbers of dendritic spines on the pyramidal cells, each receiving asymmetrical synapses. Dendritic ribosomes have previously been associated with dendritic spine synapses on pyramidal cells of the rat hippocampus. There, both may show plastic changes during reinnervation following deafferentation (Steward, 1983).

Regulation of CaM II Kinase by Neural Activity

Immunoreactivity for CaM II kinase α increases in deprived-eye dominance columns of layer IVC as early as 4 days following eye removal or monocular TTX injections and 9 weeks after monocular eyelid suture (Hendry and Kennedy, 1986; D.L. Benson et al., unpublished observations). The present results imply that the increase in immunocytochemically detectable protein levels results from an increase in CaM II kinase α gene transcription in cells of the deprived-eye columns, although increased mRNA stability cannot be ruled out. The increase in immunoreactivity seen under deprived conditions could have reflected increased phosphorylation of the enzyme (Erondu and Kennedy 1985), but the increase in mRNA levels appears to confirm that a true increase in protein levels is actually induced. Increased CaM II kinase mRNA in the deprived columns can be distinguished as late as 15 days following monocular deprivation, but is less apparent at this greater deprivation time. The more prolonged increase in CaM II kinase protein as revealed by immunocytochemistry might be maintained by increased protein stability or other mechanism rather than by a continued increase in transcription.

Neuronal activity plays an important role in regulating transmitter-related gene transcription in the peripheral nervous system. Increases in presynaptic activity in explanted sympathetic ganglia resulting in depolarization of the cells elicit increases in mRNA for tyrosine hydroxylase (TH) and subsequent increases in TH protein levels. This is accompanied by decreases in preprotachykinin mRNA and hence in substance P levels (Kessler and Black, 1982; Black et al., 1985; Roach et al., 1987). Reductions in presynaptic activity, on the other hand, are accompanied by increases in preprotachykinin mRNA but with no change in TH mRNA (Roach et al., 1987). TH and proenkephalin and their mRNAs appear to be differentially regulated along similar lines in the adrenal medulla (Kilpatrick et al., 1984; LaGamma et al., 1984; Kanamatsu et al., 1986; LaGamma and Black, 1989). In the CNS, epileptiform activity, which causes widespread depolarization of hippocampal neurons, causes increases in proenkephalin and preproneuropeptide Y mRNAs and changes in immuno-cytochemically detectable levels of the relevant peptides (White et al., 1987; White and Gall 1987; Gall and Isackson, 1989). All of these results suggest that changes in the balance of normal neural activity are critical determinants in the regulation of transmitter-related gene expression in neurons.

In the visual cortex of the monocularly deprived monkeys, the increase in CaM II kinase gene expression revealed by in situ hybridization extends from layer IVC deprived-eye dominance columns into layers II through VI (Hendry and Kennedy, 1986). The earlier immunocytochemical observations showed changes only in layer IVC (Hendry and Kennedy, 1986). The evidence for effects extending beyond layer IVC probably reflects differences in the sensi-tivity of the techniques. In regions corresponding to rows of CO-stained, deprived-eye blobs, and in parts of the inter-row regions adjacent to them, CaM II kinase mRNA is enhanced relative to the alternating rows of non-deprived eye blobs. CaM II kinase mRNA levels thus increase in regions of decreased CO activity. The decreases in CO staining are thought to re-flect reduced metabolic activity carried along the vertically oriented synaptic circuits that connect layer IVC to over- and underlying layers.

CaM II kinase can phosphorylate many substrates so changes in CaM II kinase levels are likely to have long-lasting effects. Known substrates in-clude structural proteins, and transmitter-related and other neuronal enzymes (Bennet et al., 1983; Yamaguchi and Fujisawa, 1983; Schulman, 1984; Bulleit et al., 1988). By phosphorylating synapsin I, and enhancing synaptic vesicle mobility, it enhances transmitter release at the squid giant synapse (Llinás et al., 1985; McGuinness et al., 1989). It is a major postsynaptic density protein (Kennedy et al., 1983; Kelly et al., 1984), and is associated mainly with asymmetrical (i.e., excitatory) synapses (see Benson et al., 1991b). In the hippocampus, it is thought to be essential for the induction of long-term potentiation at certain excitatory synapses (Malenka et al., 1989; Malinow et al., 1989). Monocular deprivation effects on CaM II kinase may therefore affect synapse function in both the short and long term and may have struc-tural consequences. Increases in CaM II kinase transcription resulting from visual deprivation in adult monkeys are likely to be indicative of a cascade of intracellular events set in motion by reduced activity in cells of the deprived-eye dominance columns. These events probably play a role in the regulation of levels of the other proteins and peptides found by immunocytochemistry, but verification of this is required. Several immediate-early genes are induced in response to increased neuronal activity in other systems as well as by mitogens and growth factors (Greenberg et al., 1985; Morgan and Curran, 1986; Kujubu et al., 1987; Milbrandt, 1987). These may yield clues to the nature of the relevant intracellular mediators.

Distribution of GAD-Expressing Cells

GAD and GABA immunoreactivity is confined to nonpyramidal neurons of large and small size in all layers of the primate cerebral cortex (Hendrickson, et al. 1981; Hendry and Jones, 1986; Fitzpatrick et al., 1987; Hendry et al., 1987). The distribution of large and small grain clusters seen with in situ hybridization using GAD riboprobes reflects the immunocytochemical pattern. Distinct sublaminae were revealed in layers IVCα, IVCβ, and VI. The two subdivisions of layer IVCα are the same as those shown immunocytochemically by Fitzpatrick et al. (1987). No subdivisions comparable to those detected by in situ hybridization in layers IVCβ or VI have previously been described by immunocytochemistry. The nature of the in situ labeling for GAD mRNA localization is clearly somal and more typical of mRNA localization for most other cellular proteins. This serves to emphasize the uniqueness of the pattern of presumed dendritic localization of CaM II kinase α mRNA.

Monocular Deprivation Effects on GAD Expression

Levels of GAD mRNA are maintained in deprived-eye columns following monocular deprivation, contrasting with the CaM II kinase effect and with the huge reduction in immunoreactive GAD seen under identical conditions. The apparent maintenance of GAD gene expression in the face of monocular deprivation is also seen in adult cat visual cortex (Benson et al., 1989).

Failure to detect changes in GAD mRNA levels in the present experiments may be due to three factors. First, GAD enzyme levels could be regulated by neuronal activity at a posttranslational level. Deamidation, methylation, or limited proteolysis, for example, could render the enzyme undetectable by immunocytochemistry (see Benyon, 1980). Second, GAD levels could be regulated by activity-dependent events occurring between DNA transcription and posttranslational processing. Covalent modification of mRNA, transcript splicing, and blocking the initiation of mRNA translation are all potential regulatory mechanisms. Third, changes in mRNA maturation are not likely to cause the changes in GAD protein levels, since changes in polyadenylation or 5′ capping would affect mRNA stability and would therefore be detected by an increase or decrease in hybridization levels. GAD gene expression could be regulated by alternative splicing but there is no present evidence that cells use alternative splicing to regulate protein levels. Instead, mature functional GAD mRNA may be prevented from being translated, thus leading to the reduction in GAD detectable by immunocytochemistry protein levels.

Two GAD genes, one encoding a 65-kD protein and the other encoding a 67-kD protein, are known (Kaufman et al., 1989; A.J. Tobin, personal communication, 1989). Immunocytochemical studies indicate that both proteins are localized in GABA cells, but with different intracellular distributions (Houser et al., 1989). The GAD probes used in the present study would localize the transcript of the GAD gene that corresponds to the 67-kD protein. Although it is conceivable that the GAD gene coding for the 67-kD protein maintains normal transcriptional levels and that coding for the 65-kD protein shows reduced transcription in response to monocular deprivation, this is unlikely. Polyclonal antisera used in earlier studies to demonstrate a decrease in GAD protein immunoreactivity following monocular deprivation preferentially localize the larger GAD protein. Therefore, it is unlikely that changes in the 65-kD protein alone could be responsible for the decrease in GAD immunoreactivity. However, additional GAD mRNAs have been identified in cats and mice. These may represent alternative splicing products or additional GAD genes that could be differentially regulated (Bond et al., 1988; Benson et al., 1989; Katarova et al., 1990).

SUMMARY AND CONCLUSIONS

Immunocytochemistry and receptor binding reveal that levels of a large number of neuroactive molecules are regulated in an activity-dependent manner in the adult primate visual cortex. The large, reversible changes evident under conditions in which afferent activity is reduced in deprived-eye dominance columns by monocular deprivation are likely to be manifestations of a general effect whereby neural activity regulates transmitter-, receptor-, and second messenger—related functions throughout the nervous system. The regulatory mechanisms are likely to be complex and varied. The present results, for example, suggest that activity-dependent changes may be effected at both transcriptional and posttranscriptional levels. Changes in protein levels associated with changes in neural activity, and detectable by immunocytochemistry, cannot therefore be attributed in the first instance to changes in gene transcription. Interplay among many potential mechanisms is probably involved and holds the key to understanding how neural activity regulates neuronal gene expression under activity-dependent conditions. The implications for normal visual cortical function await further study, but the results show that the adult cortex is far from unresponsive to perturbations of retinal functions that are probably excessive manifestations of a normally fine-tuned system whereby afferent activity regulates cortical neuronal function throughout the life of the individual.

Acknowledgments

This work was supported by grant No. EY-07193 from the National Institutes of Health, U.S. Public Health Service. I am grateful for the many contributions of my colleagues Drs. D.L. Benson, S.H.C. Hendry, and P.J. Isackson.

REFERENCES

Bennett, M.K., and Kennedy, M.B. (1987). Deduced primary structure of the α subunit of brain type II Ca^{++} calmodulin-dependent protein kinase determined by molecular cloning. *Proc. Natl. Acad. Sci.* 84:1794.

Bennett, M.K, Erondu, N.E., and Kennedy, M.B. (1983). Purification and characterization of a calmodulin-dependent protein kinase that is highly concentrated in brain. *J. Biol. Chem.* 258:12735.

Benson, D.L., Isackson, P.J., Hendry, S.H.C., and Jones, E.G. (1989). Expression of glutamic acid decarboxylase mRNA in normal and monocularly deprived cat visual cortex. *Mol. Brain Res.* 5:279.

Benson, D.L., Isackson, P.J., Gall, C., and Jones, E.G. (1991a). Differential effects of monocular deprivation on glutamic acid decarboxylase and type II calcium-calmodulin dependent protein kinase gene expression in adult monkey visual cortex. *J. Neurosci.* 11:31.

Benson, D.L., Isackson, P.J., Hendry, S.H.C., and Jones, E.G. (1991b). Differential gene expression for glutamic acid decarboxylase and type II calcium-calmodulin—dependent protein kinase in basal ganglia, thalamus, and hypothalamus of the monkey. *J. Neurosci.* 11:1540.

Benson, D.L., Isackson, P.J., Gall, C.M., and Jones, E G. (1992). Contrasting patterns in the localization of glutamic acid decarboxylase and Ca^{2+}/calmodulin protein kinase gene expression in the rat central nervous system. *Neuroscience* 46:825–849.

Benyon, R.J. (1980). Protein modification and the control of intracellular protein degradation. In *The Enzymology of Post-Translational Modification of Proteins,* ed. R.F. Freedman and H.C. Hawkins, 363–389. New York: Academic Press.

Black, I.B., Chikaraishi, D.M., and Lewis, E.J. (1985). Trans-synaptic increase in RNA coding for tyrosine hydroxylase in a rat sympathetic ganglion. *Brain Res.* 339:151.

Blakemore, C., Garey, L.J., and Vital-Durant, F. (1978). The physiological effects of monocular deprivation and their reversal in the monkey's visual cortex. *J. Physiol. (Lond.)* 283:223.

Bond, R.W., Jansen, K.R., and Gottleib, D.J. (1988). Pattern of expression of glutamic acid decarboxylase mRNA in the developing rat brain. *Proc. Natl. Acad. Sci. U.S.A.* 85:3231.

Bossa, R., Martini, F., Barra, D., Borri Voltattorni, C., Minelli, A., and Turano, C. (1977). The chymotryptic phosphopyridoxyl peptide of dopa decarboxylase from pig kidney. *Biochem. Biophys. Res. Commun.* 78:177.

Bulleit, R.F., Bennett, M.K., Malloy, S.S., Hurley, J.B., and Kennedy, M.B. (1988). Conserved and variable regions in the subunits of brain type II Ca^{2+}/calmodulin-dependent protein kinase. *Neuron* 1:63.

Chirgwin, J.M., Przblya, A.E., MacDonald, R.J., and Rutter, W.J. (1979). Isolation of biologically active ribonucleic acid from sources enriched in ribonuclease. *Biochemistry* 18:5294.

Erondu, N.E., and Kennedy, M.B. (1985). Regional distribution of type II Ca^{2+}/calmodulin dependent protein kinase in rat brain. *J. Neurosci.* 5:3270.

Fitzpatrick, D., Lund, J.S., Schmechel, D.E., and Towles, A.C. (1987). Distribution of GABAergic neurons and axon terminals in the macaque striate cortex. *J. Comp. Neurol.* 264:73.

Gall, C.M., and Isackson, P.J. (1989). Limbic seizures increase neuronal production of messenger RNA for nerve-growth factor. *Science* 245:758.

Greenberg, M.E., Greene, L.A., and Ziff, E.B. (1985). Nerve growth factor and epidermal growth factor induce rapid transient changes in proto-oncogene transcription in PC12 cells. *J. Biol. Chem.* 260:14101.

Harris, W.A.C. (1981). Neural activity and development. *Ann. Rev. Physiol.* 43:689.

Hendrickson, A.E., Hunt, S.P., and Wu, J.-Y. (1981). Immunocytochemical localization of glutamic acid decarboxylase in monkey striate cortex. *Nature* 292:605.

Hendry, S.H.C., and Jones, E.G. (1986). Reduction in number of immunostained GABAergic neurons in deprived-eye dominance columns of monkey area 17. *Nature* 320:750.

Hendry, S.H.C., and Jones, E.G. (1988). Activity dependent regulation of GABA expression in the visual cortex of adult monkeys. *Neuron* 1:701.

Hendry, S.H.C., and Kennedy, M.B. (1986). Immunoreactivity for a calmodulin-dependent protein kinase is selectively increased in macaque striate cortex after monocular deprivation. *Proc. Natl. Acad. Sci. U.S.A.* 83:1536.

Hendry, S.H.C., Schwark, H.D., Jones, E.G., and Yan, J. (1987). Numbers and proportions of GABA immunoreactive neurons in different areas of monkey cerebral cortex. *J. Neurosci.* 7:1503.

Hendry, S.H.C., Jones, E.G., and Burstein, N. (1988). Activity-dependent regulation of tachykinin-like immunoreactivity in neurons of monkey visual cortex. *J. Neurosci.* 8:1225.

Hendry, S.H.C., Fuchs, J., De Blas, A.L., Jones, E.G. (1990). Organization and plasticity of immunocytochemically localized GABA$_A$ receptors in adult monkey visual cortex. *J. Neurosci.* 10:2438.

Horton, J.C. (1984). Cytochrome oxidase patches: A new cytoarchitectonic feature of monkey visual cortex. *Philos. Trans. R. Soc. Lond. [Biol.]* 304:199–253.

Horton, J.C., and Hubel, D.H. (1981). Regular patchy distribution of cytochrome oxidase staining in primary visual cortex of macaque monkey. *Nature* 292:762.

Houser, C.R., Miyashiro, J.E., Kaufman, D.L., and Tobin, A.J. (1989). Immunocytochemical studies using a new antiserum against bacterially produced feline glutamate decarboxylase. *Soc. Neurosci. Abstr.* 15:488.

Hubel, D.H., and Wiesel, T.N. (1977). Functional architecture of macaque monkey visual cortex. *Proc. R. Soc. Lond. [Biol.]* 198:1.

Hubel, D.H., Wiesel, T.N., and LeVay, S. (1977). Plasticity of ocular dominance columns in monkey striate cortex. *Philos. Trans. R. Soc. Lond. [Biol.]* 278:377.

Kanamatsu, T., Unsworth, C.D., Diliberto, E.J., Jr., Viveros, O.H., and Hong, J.S. (1986). Reflex splanchnic nerve stimulation increases levels of proenkephalin A mRNA and proenkephalin A related peptides in the rat adrenal medulla. *Proc. Natl. Acad. Sci. U.S.A.* 83:9245.

Katarova, Z., Szabo, G., Mugnaini, E., Greenspan, R.J. (1990). Molecular identification of a 62 Kd form of glutamic acid decarboxylase from the mouse. *Eur. J. Neurosci.* 2:190.

Kaufman, D.L., Houser, C.R., and Tobin, A.J. (1989). Two forms of glutamic acid decarboxylase (GAD), with different *N*-terminal sequences, have distinct intraneuronal distributions. *Soc. Neurosci. Abstr.* 15:487.

Kelly, P.T., McGuinness, T.L., and Greengard, P. (1984). Evidence that the major postsynaptic density protein is a component of a Ca^{2+}/calmodulin dependent protein kinase. *Proc. Natl. Acad. Sci. U.S.A.* 81:945.

Kennedy, M.B., Bennett, M.K., and Erondu, N.E. (1983). Biochemical and immunochemical evidence that the "major postsynaptic density protein" is a subunit of a calmodulin-dependent protein kinase. Proc. Natl. Acad. Sci. U.S.A. 80:7357.

Kessler, J.A., and Black, I.B. (1982). Regulation of substance P in adult rat sympathetic ganglia. *Brain Res.* 234:182.

Kilpatrick, D.L., Howells, I.B., Fleminger, G., and Udenfriend, S. (1984). Denervation of rat adrenal glands markedly increases preproenkaphalin mRNA. *Proc. Natl. Acad. Sci. U.S.A.* 81:7221.

Kobayashi, Y., Kaufman, D.L., and Tobin, A.J. (1987). Glutamic acid decarboxylase cDNA: Nucleotide sequence encoding an enzymatically active fusion protein. *J. Neurosci.* 7:2769.

Kujubu, D.A., Lim, R.W., Varnum, B.C., and Herschman, H.R. (1987). Induction of transiently expressed genes in PC12 pheochromocytoma cells. *Oncogene* 1:257.

LaGamma, E.F., and Black, I.B. (1989). Transcriptional control of adrenal catecholamine and opiate transmitter genes. *Mol. Brain Res.* 5:17.

LaGamma, E.F., Adler, J.E., and Black, I.B. (1984). Impulse activity differentially regulates [Leu] enkephalin and catecholamine characters in the adrenal medulla. *Science* 224:1102.

LeVay, S., Wiesel, T.N., and Hubel, D.H. (1980). The development of ocular dominance columns in normal and visually deprived monkeys. *J. Comp. Neurol.* 191:1.

Lin, C.R., Kapiloff, M.S., Durgerain, S., Tatemoto, K., Russo, A.F., Hanson, P., Schulman, H., and Rosenfeld, M.G. (1987). Molecular cloning of a brain-specific calcium-calmodulin–dependent protein kinase. *Proc. Natl. Acad. Sci. U.S.A.* 84:5962.

Llinás, R., McGuinness, T.L., Leonard, C.S., Sugimori, M., and Greengard, P. (1985). Intra-terminal injection of synapsin I or calcium/calmodulin–dependent protein kinase II alters neurotransmitter release at the squid giant synapse. *Proc. Natl. Acad. Sci. U.S.A.* 82:3035.

Malenka, R.C., Kauer, J.A., Perkel, D.J., Mauk, M.D., Kelly, P.T., Nicoll, R.A., and Waxham, M.N. (1989). An essential role for postsynaptic calmodulin and protein kinase activity in long-term potentiation. *Nature* 340:554.

Malinow, R., Schulman, H., and Tsien, R.W. (1989). Inhibition of postsynaptic PKC or CaMKII blocks induction but not expression of LTP. *Science* 245:862.

Malpeli, J.G., and Schiller, P.H. (1979). A method of reversible inactivation of small regions of brain tissue. *J. Neurosci. Methods.* 1:143.

McGuinness, T.L., Brady, S.T., Gruner, J.A., Sugimori, M., Llinas, R., and Greengard, P. (1989). Phosphorylation-dependent inhibition by synapsin I of organelle movement in squid axoplasm. *J. Neurosci.* 9:4139.

Milbrandt, J. (1987). A nerve growth factor–induced gene encodes a possible transcriptional regulatory factor. *Science* 238:797.

Morgan, J.I., and Curran, T. (1986). Role of ion flux in the control of c-fos expression. *Nature* 322:552.

Peters, A., Palay, S.L., and Webster, H.deF. (1976). *The Fine Structure of the Nervous System: The Neurons and Supporting Cells.* Philadelphia: WB Saunders.

Roach, A., Adler, J.E., and Black, I.B. (1987). Depolarizing influences regulate preprotachykinin mRNA in sympathetic neurons. *Proc. Natl. Acad. Sci. U.S.A.* 84:5078.

Saiki, R.K., Scharf, S., Faloona, F., Mullis, K.B., Horn, G.T., Erlich, H.A., and Arnheim, N. (1985). Enzymatic amplification of beta-globin genomic sequences and restriction site analysis for diagnosis of sickle-cell anemia. *Science* 230:1350.

Saiki, R.K., Gelfand, D.H., Stoffel, S., Scharf, S.J., Higuchi, R., Horn, G.T., Mullis, K.B., and Erlich, H.A. (1988). Primer directed enzymatic amplificaton of DNA with a thermostable DNA polymerase. *Science* 239:487.

Sanger, F., Nicklen, S., and Coulson, A.R. (1977). DNA sequencing with chain terminating inhibitors. *Proc. Natl. Acad. Sci. U.S.A.* 74:5463.

Scharf, S.J., Horn, G.T., and Erlich, H.A. (1986). Direct cloning and sequence analysis of enzymatically amplified genomic sequences. *Science* 233:1076.

Schulman, H. (1984). Phosphorylation of microtubule-associated proteins by a Ca^{2+}/calmodulin-dependent protein kinase. *J. Cell Biol.* 99:11.

Steward, O. (1983). Alterations in polyribosomes associated with dendritic spines during reinnervation of the dentate gyrus of the adult rat. *J. Neurosci.* 3:177.

     Plasticity of Connectivity in the Visual System

Tabor, S., and Richardson, C.C. (1987). DNA sequence analysis with a modified bacteriophage T7 DNA polymerase. *Proc. Natl. Acad. Sci. U.S.A.* 84:4767.

Vitorica, J., Park, D., Chin, G., and deBlas, A.L. (1988). Monoclonal antibodies and conventional antisera to the $GABA_A$ receptor/benzodiazepine receptor/Cl^- channel complex. *J. Neurosci.* 8:615.

White, J.D., and Gall, C.M. (1987). Differential regulation of neuropeptide and proto-oncogene mRNA content in the hippocampus following recurrent seizures. *Mol. Brain Res.* 3:21.

White, J.D., Gall, C.M., and McKelvy, J.F. (1987). Enkephalin biosynthesis and enkephalin gene expression are increased in hippocampal mossy fibers following a unilateral lesion of the hilus. *J. Neurosci.* 7:753.

Wong-Riley, M.T.T. (1979). Changes in the visual system of monocularly sutured or enucleated kittens demonstrable with cytochrome oxidase histochemistry. *Brain Res.* 171:11.

Yamauchi, T., and Fujisawa, H. (1983). Purification and characterization of the brain calmodulin-dependent protein kinase (kinase II), which is involved in the activation of tryptophan 5-monooxygenase. *Eur. J. Biochem.* 132:15.

14 Visual Processing by Novel, Surgically Created Neural Circuits

Douglas O. Frost

A major goal of contemporary neurobiological research is to devise means of repairing damaged neural circuits. One obstacle to achieving this goal has been the seeming refractoriness of severed, mature central nervous system (CNS) axons to regeneration; recent experiments (reviewed in Aguayo et al., 1990; Savio et al., 1990) are beginning to suggest means for the resolution of this problem. A second difficulty has been the creation of new neural circuits that might be used to replace damaged ones. Recently, we have performed surgery on developing mammals that has permitted us to permanently connect the retina with the auditory and somatosensory systems. With respect to many of their essential morphological and functional features, the novel circuits thus formed resemble those of the normal visual system. The recent progress in the induction of regeneration suggests that similar results might be achieved in the mature CNS. Thus, our techniques may eventually provide a paradigm for the replacement of damaged sensory circuits.

SURGICAL CREATION OF NOVEL SENSORY CIRCUITS

In newborn hamsters, we ablated two of the principal targets of retinal ganglion cell (RGC) axons, the superior colliculus (SC) and the dorsolateral geniculate nucleus (LGd). We also partially deafferented the main somatosensory (ventrobasal, VB) or auditory (medial geniculate, MG) thalamic nuclei by ablation of their specific, ascending sensory afferents. Under these conditions, RGC axons form permanent connections in VB or MG, nuclei to which they do not project in normal, adult animals (see figure 14.1; Frost, 1981, 1982; Schneider, 1973). These results suggest that the choice of targets by growing RGC axons depends on multiple factors and can be altered by changes in the axonal environment. Among the factors influencing the axons' choice of targets are: (1) their tendency to conserve their total amount of axonal arbor or synaptic connections (Frost, 1981, 1982; Schneider, 1973); (2) competition among developing axons for terminal space or for a trophic factor present in their regions of termination (Frost, 1981, 1982; Gouzé et al., 1983; Schneider, 1973; and (3) the proximity of growing axons to a potential terminal site (Frost, 1986; Zimmer, 1974).

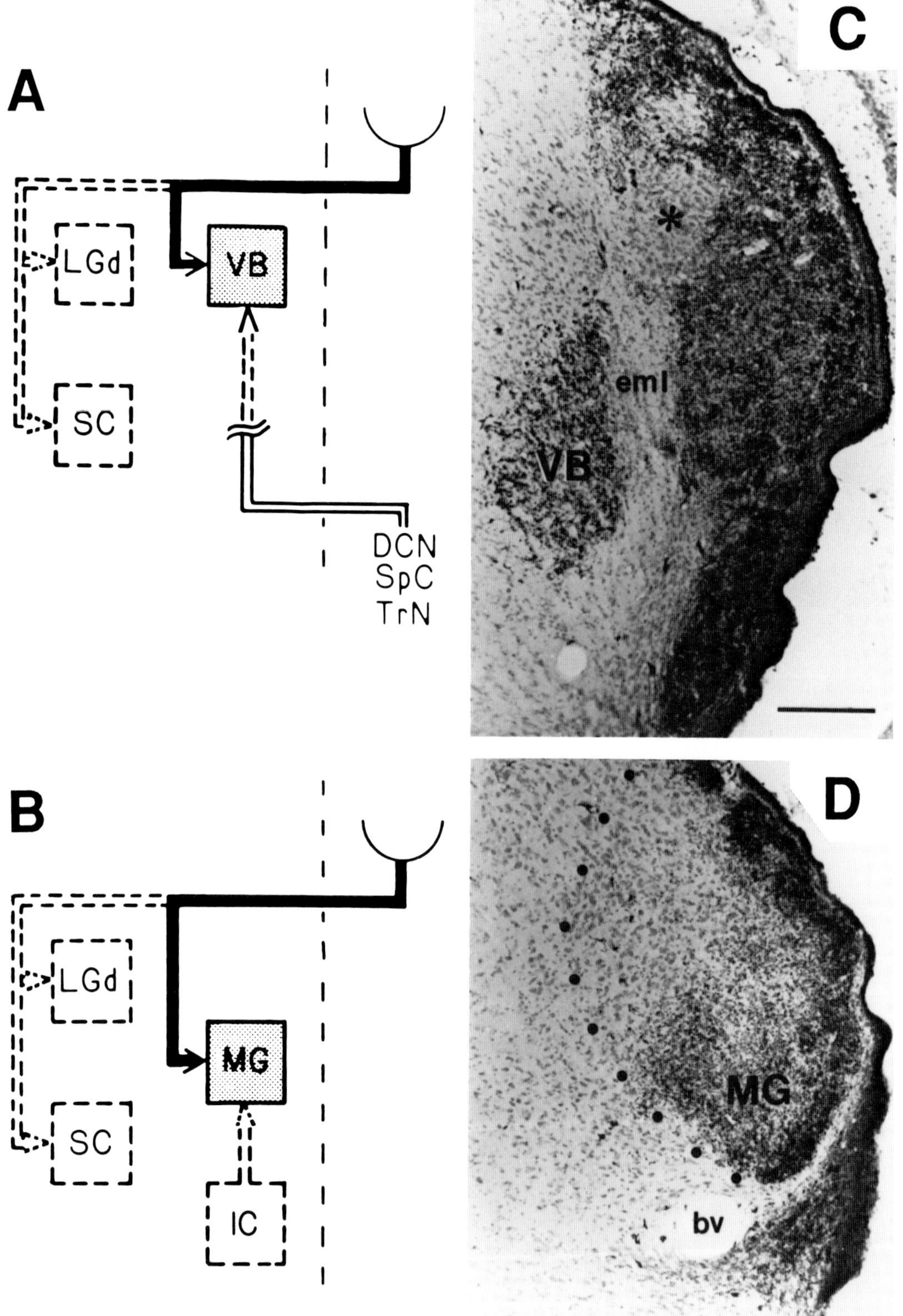

A
LGd
SC
VB
DCN
SpC
TrN
B
LGd
SC
MG
IC
C
*
eml
VB
D
MG
bv

ULTRASTRUCTURE OF NOVEL SYNAPTIC CONNECTIONS

The terminals of many CNS axons, including those of ascending specific sensory axons in the thalamus, participate in "synaptic glomeruli"—regions containing numerous neuronal elements engaged in multiple synaptic contacts and isolated from areas of simpler neuropil by sheets of astrocyte cytoplasm. The organization of the synaptic glomeruli presumably has an important influence on the transmission and processing of information within the regions where they are present. In LGd of normal animals, the morphology of these terminals and the synaptic organization of their glomeruli differ from those in VB and MG with respect to multiple features (reviewed in Campbell and Frost, 1988). The novel retinal projections to VB and MG provide an opportunity to investigate how terminal morphology and glomerular synaptic organization are determined. The terminals and synaptic glomeruli of retino-VB and retino-MG axons can be compared with those of normal afferents to LGd, VB, and MG. Features of normal retino-LGd afferents that are not shared with the normal somatosensory and auditory afferents to VB and MG, respectively, and that are conserved by retino-VB and retino-MG axons, are likely to be determined by the afferent axons. Features of retino-VB and retino-MG axons that more closely resemble those of normal specific sensory afferents to VB and MG, respectively, are likely to be determined by their targets.

Using the electron microscope, we examined normal retino-LGd projections, normal ascending sensory projections to VB and MG, and anomalous retino-VB and retino-MG projections (Campbell and Frost, 1987; Campbell and Frost, 1988). RGC axon terminals were identified by anterograde labeling with horseradish peroxidase (HRP). Retino-LGd axon terminals and their glomeruli differ from those of the normal, specific sensory afferents to VB and MG with respect to: (1) the position of glomeruli on target neurons; (2) the types and synaptic relationships of the neural elements constituting the glomeruli; (3) the number of specific sensory terminals per glomerulus; (4) the size of the specific sensory terminals; (5) the number of dendritic or somatic appendages contacted by each bouton; and (6) the mitochondrial morphology of the specific sensory afferent boutons (figure 14.2). In operated hamsters, with respect to all these features except mitochondrial morphology, the termi-

---

Figure 14.1 *A, B,* experimental design. *Semicircles* represent retina. Fiber tracts and nuclei indicated by *dashed lines* were destroyed by neonatal surgery. Resultant anomalous pathways (*solid lines*) form permanent connections in ventrobasal (*VB*) and medial geniculatethalamic (*MG*) (*stipped*) nuclei. *Dashed vertical lines* indicate midline. DCN, dorsal column nuclei; *SpC*, spinal cord; *TrN*, trigeminal nuclei; *IC*, inferior colliculus. C, D, Horseradish peroxidase–labeled, anomalous retinal projections to VB (*C*) and MG (*D*) as seen in bright-field micrographs of coronal sections through the thalamus ipsilateral to the neonatal lesions and contralateral to the injected eye; young adult hamster (aged 11 weeks). Frozen sections 40 μm thick reacted with TMB and counterstained with neutral red. The remnant of the dorsolateral geniculate nucleus (*LGd*) (which is large, due to an incomplete lesion) contains a volid (*asterisk*) which represents the projection zone of axons originating in the ipsilateral, uninjected retina. *bv*, blood vessel; *eml*, external medullary lamina. Scale bar: 180 μm.

Frost: Processing by Surgically Created Neural Circuits

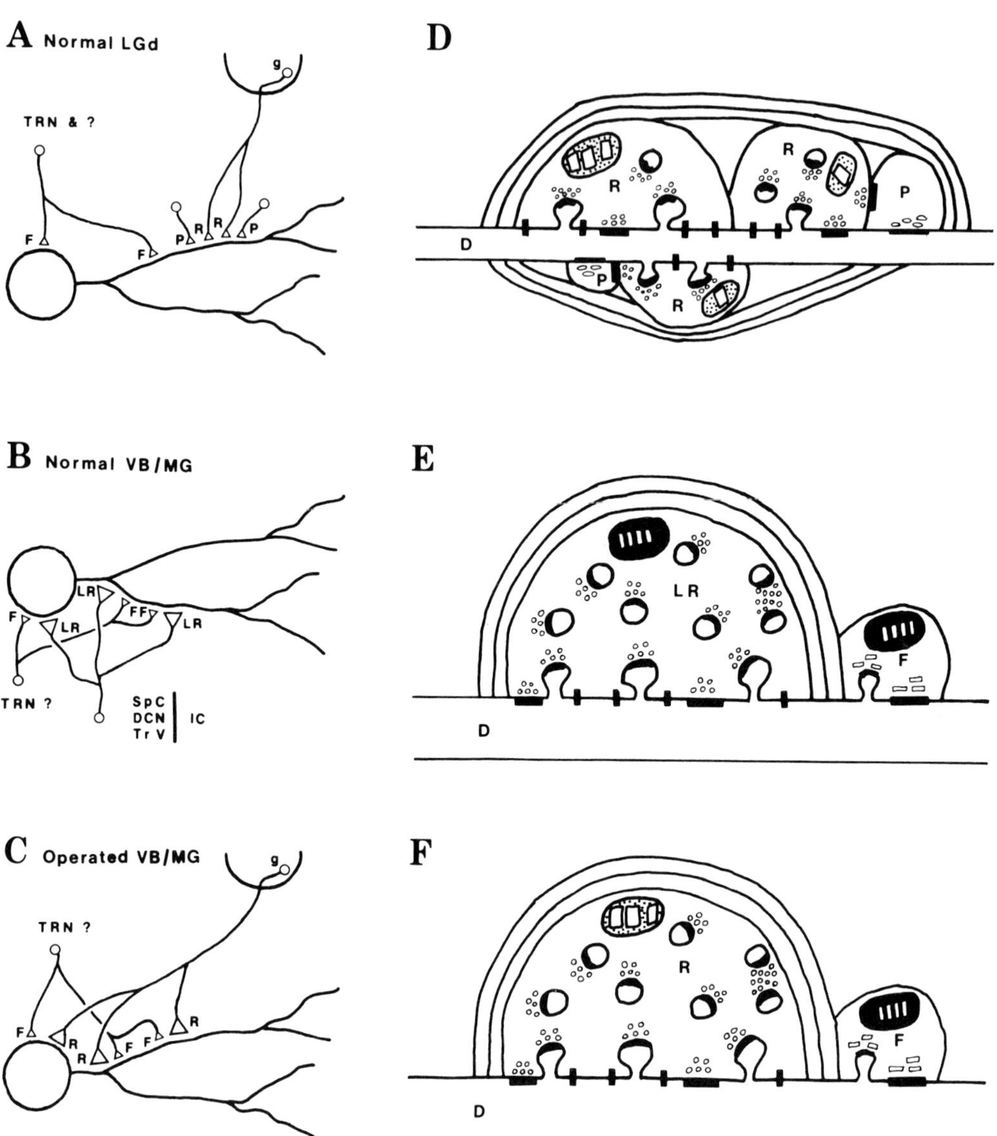

Figure 14.2 Morphology of synaptic complexes. *A–C* show glomerulus constitutents, their sources, and the location of the glomeruli on the target neurons. *D–F* show the detailed morphological features of the glomerulus constituents and their synaptic relationships in "reconstructed" glomeruli. *A*, the R-boutons of retinal ganglion cell (RGC) axons (cells of origin labeled *g* in *A* and *C*) participate in glomeruli on intermediate to proximal dendritic regions of relay neurons in *LGd*. P-boutons of presynaptic dendrites and (sometimes) F-boutons (some of which arise from reticulothalamic axons) are also present *B*, in *normal VB* or *MG* the LR-boutons of somatosensory axons (ascending from *SpC, DCN*, and trigeminal [*TRN*] nuclei) or auditory axons (ascending from the inferior colliculus [*IC*]) participate in glomeruli on more proximal dendritic regions or on relay neuron somata in VB or MG, respectively. P-boutons are rare, but F-boutons (of unknown origin; from reticulothalamic axons?) are nearly always present. *C*, in the glomeruli of retinorecipient regions of VB or MG in operated hamsters, R-boutons of RGC axons replace LR-boutons as the specific sensory axon terminals. The glomeruli are on more proximal dendritic regions or on relay neuron somata in VB or MG, respectively. Other bouton types are as in normal VB or MG. *D*, synaptic organization of glomeruli in normal LGd.

    Plasticity of Connectivity in the Visual System

nals and synaptic glomeruli of retino-MG and retino-VB axons more nearly resembled those of normal auditory and somatosensory afferent axons, respectively, than they did those of normal retino-LGd axons (see figure 14.2). Thus, all the features we examined, except mitochondrial morphology, are determined by factors in target neurons or their environment. The ultrastructural localization and biochemical nature of the determining factors are not known. A more general hypothesis suggested by our data is that the morphological differentiation of *interneuronal contacts*, which mediate communication among neurons, responds to interactions among the connected elements, or to interactions between those elements and their environment (e.g., glia, extracellular matrix), whereas the differentiation of structures that reflect *intrinsic functions* of individual neuronal elements (e.g., mitochondria) does not respond to such interactions. This interpretation is supported by numerous observations in the normal, adult CNS on the morphology of the terminals and synaptic contacts made by axons that project to multiple target nuclei (see Campbell and Frost, 1988, for review).

NUMBER AND TYPE OF RETINAL GANGLION CELLS

The mammalian retina contains multiple types of RGCs that differ with respect to their soma and dendritic morphologies, visual response properties, and cerebral projections (Stone, 1983). In rodents, neonatal lesions of the SC (but not of the visual cortex) cause retrograde degeneration of developing RGCs (Perry and Cowey, 1979; Udin and Schneider, 1981; Wickler et al.,

---

Each glomerulus usually contains multiple R-boutons that make asymmetrical synapses on dendritic shafts or appendages. The R-boutons also make filamentous contacts with the dendritic shafts. The R-boutons also synapse upon P-boutons that are themselves presynaptic to conventional dendrites. F-boutons, when present, are equally likely to be within or just outside the glial capsule and make symmetrical synapses on dendritic shafts and neuronal somata. The R-boutons are small-to large-seized, contact a limited number (0–6) of synaptic appendages, and have pale mitochondria with dilated cristae. E, synaptic organization of glomeruli in normal VB or MG. Each glomerulus usually contains a single LR-bouton that makes asymmetrical synapses on dendritic shafts or appendages, or somatic appendages. The LR-boutons also make filamentous contacts with dendritic shafts or neuronal somata. P-boutons are extremely rare. Glomeruli are nearly always associated with F-boutons, which are most often just outside the glial capsule and make symmetrical synapses on dendritic shafts and neuronal somata. The LR-boutons are medium-sized to extremely large, contact numerous (often 10–16) dendritic or somatic appendages, and have dark mitochondria with narrow cristae. F, synaptic organization of glomeruli in the retinorecipient zone of VB or MG in operated hamsters. Each glomerulus usually contains a single R-bouton that makes asymmetrical synapses on dendritic shafts or appendages or somatic appendages. The R-boutons also make filamentous contacts with dendritic shafts or neuronal somata. P-boutons are extremely rare. Glomeruli are nearly always associated with F-boutons, which are most often just outside the glial capsule and make symmetrical synapses on dendritic shafts and neuronal somata. The R-boutons are medium-sized to extremely large, contact numerous (often 10–16) dendritic or somatic appendages, and have pale mitochondria with dilated cristae. (Reproduced with permission from Campbell and Frost 1988.)

     Frost: Processing by Surgically Created Neural Circuits

1986; Raabe et al., 1986). Different RGC types may vary in their susceptibility to retrograde degeneration following cerebral lesions. Therefore, the interpretation of functional studies of the novel retinal projections, and the assessment of the utility of such projections in alleviating the deleterious consequences of damage to the visual system, depends, in part, on determining: (1) the number and type of RGCs that survive in the retinas of hamsters with novel retinal projections; and (2) which RGCs give rise to the novel retinothalamic projections.

In normal adult hamsters (Métin and Frost, 1989, and unpublished data), there are about 55,000 RGCs in each retina. The density of RGCs varies systematically across the retinal surface; there appear to be two local maxima of RGC density displaced inferotemporally and superonasally from the optic disc and connected to each other by a region of somewhat lower density. This may correspond to a sort of "visual streak" along the part of the retina that views the horizon, as is commonly found in lagamorphs and ungulates (Slonaker, 1897; Hughes, 1977). RGC density falls progressively in increasingly more peripheral retinal regions. The distribution of RGC soma diameter is unimodal with an elongated tail toward larger sizes; the distribution shifts toward larger cell sizes in retinal regions of progressively lower RGC density. Backfilling of RGCs with HRP injected into the optic tract suggests three broad classes of RGCs as defined by soma-dendritic morphology, although we are currently refining our data on RGC morphology by injecting RGCs intracellularly with Lucifer Yellow (Yamasaki et al., 1991), since retrograde labeling with HRP incompletely fills RGC dendrites.

Preliminary data obtained by retrograde labeling of RGCs following HRP injections into the optic tract of adult hamsters with neonatal ablations of SC and LGd to produce novel retinal projections (Irons et al., 1990, and unpublished data) suggest that although the overall number of RGCs in the retinas of these hamsters is reduced to about 23% of normal values, the shape of the distribution of RGC density across the retinal surface and the increase in RGC size with decreasing RGC density are maintained. The reduction in RGC density suggests that the visual acuity of these animals is likely to be reduced compared to that of normal hamsters. Despite the reduction in RGC density, all of the three broad morphological types of RGCs identified in the retinas of normal hamsters appear to be present in the retinas of the hamsters that were operated on (Irons et al., 1990, and unpublished data). (Similarly, when the optic nerve is cut in *adult rats* and RGCs are permitted to *regenerate* their cerebral projections through peripheral nerve grafts, although only 15% of the damaged RGCs regenerate their axons, the form of the size distribution of these RGCs is normal [Aguayo, 1985]).

In normal rodents, virtually all RGCs project to the midbrain (Linden and Perry, 1983; Linden and Esbérard, 1987). However, it is not known which types of RGCs project to the thalamus in normal hamsters or which types give rise to the novel retino-MG or retino-VB projections in operated hamsters. These questions are currently under investigation in our laboratory and are significant to the interpretation of our data on the function of the novel

     Plasticity of Connectivity in the Visual System

pathways (see below). However, the maintenance, in these hamsters, of the same three types of RGCs found in normal hamsters, as well as additional data on the types of RGC axons that make the novel retino-VB and retino-MG projections (see below), suggest that the same populations of RGCs may give rise to the normal and novel retinothalamic projections. This contrasts with the finding that novel retino-MG projections in ferrets arise from a different class of RGCs than the ones that normally relay visually information through LGd to area 17 (Sur et al., 1988). The reasons for the differences between the results obtained in hamsters and ferrets are unknown.

REPRESENTATION OF SENSORY FIELDS

In normal, adult hamsters, the entire contralateral retina (and therefore the entire contralateral visual field) is represented retinotopically on the surfaces of SC, LGd, and the ventral lateral geniculate nucleus (LGv). Each point on the retinal surface projects to cylinders of tissue that extend into each of these structures from its surface (Frost and Schneider, 1979); these cylinders correspond to "lines of projection" of points in the visual field, as defined neurophysiologically (Kaas et al., 1972). Using anatomical techniques, we mapped the retino-VB and retino-MG projections (Frost, 1981). In each nucleus, a given pole of the retina was consistently represented at a particular end of the overall retinal projection, and different retinal poles were systematically mapped around the circumference of the projection (figure 14.3). Thus, as for the visual nuclei of normal animals, in operated hamsters, the surface of the retina is mapped in a retinotopic fashion onto the surfaces of VB and MG and each retinal point is represented along a cylinder of tissue extending into VB or MG. This suggests that RGC axons may be "self-organizing": their receptotopic organization may come about by interactions among the developing axons themselves, with only the orientation of the projection within the target nucleus being determined by interactions between the axons and their targets. For further discussion of this problem, see Frost and Schneider (1979) and Frost (1981).

In normal, adult hamsters, there is also an orderly representation of the contralateral retina and visual field in the primary visual cortex (VI, area 17; Tiao and Blakemore, 1976). Visual stimulation within well-defined receptive fields (RFs) reliably evokes multi-unit responses in the first and second somatosensory cortices (SI and SII, respectively) of adult hamsters operated on as neonates (as described above) but not of normal hamsters (Frost and Métin, 1985). Since the synapses between retino-VB axons and VB neurons are interposed between the retina and the neurons from which we recorded, this finding demonstrates that these synapses are functional. The representations of the visual field in SI and SII (figure 14.4) are partially retinotopic in that there is an orderly representation of the lower to upper (or lower temporal to upper nasal) visual field axis, but not of the orthogonal axis; this organization can be explained on the basis of the way in which the visual field and body maps in VB intersect (Frost and Métin, 1985): in normal mammals, orderly

     Frost: Processing by Surgically Created Neural Circuits

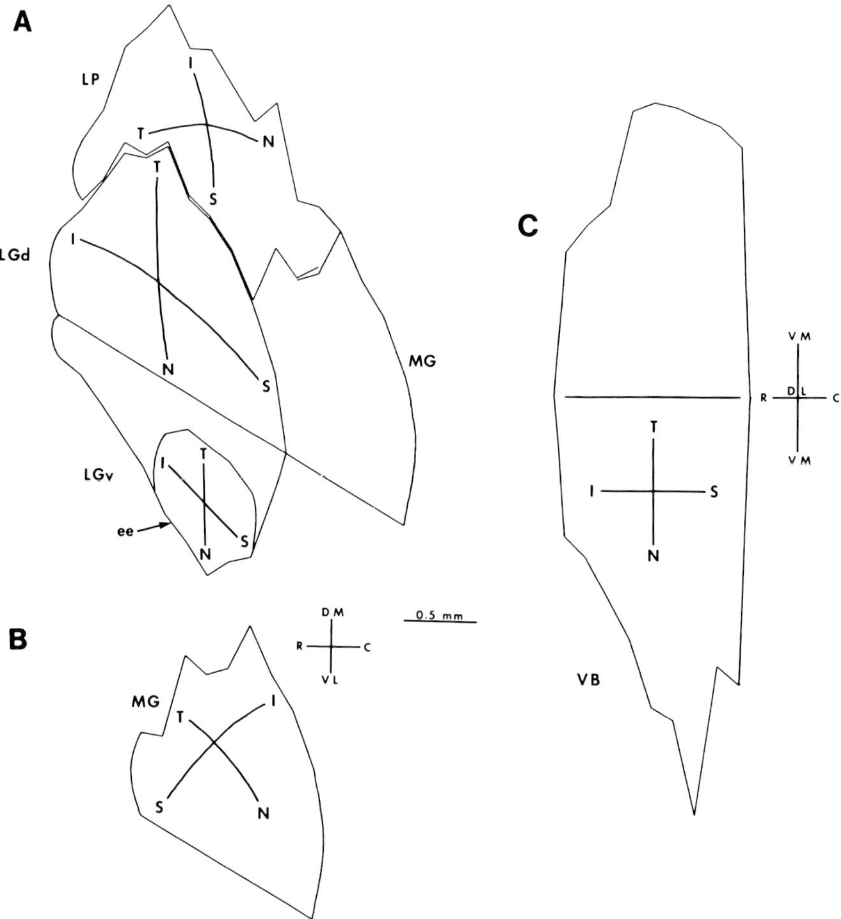

Figure 14.3 Computer reconstructions of the diencephalon of the hamster (see Frost, 1981), for methods) showing the polarity of retinal projections to the *LGd* and ventral lateral geniculate nucleus (*LGv*) of normal hamsters and the lateral posterior nucleus (*LP*), *MG*, and *VB* of neonatally operated hamsters. *A*, lateral surfaces of LGd, LGv, and LP. Part of the lateral surface of *MG* is also shown but its rostral extremity is separated from the thalamic surface by the caudal tip of LGd. The axes drawn on the surfaces of LGd and the *ee* lamina of LGv (Frost et al., 1979) indicate the polarities of the normal retinal representation on those areas (Frost and Schneider, 1979). *S*, superior; *I*, inferior; *N*, nasal; *T*, temporal. *B*, lateral surface of MG. The rostral extremity of MG, covered by LGd in A, is exposed in this view. All other conventions are as in *A*. *C*, surface of VB unrolled into a plane. The *horizontal line* represents the dorsolateral extremity of the nucleus. The areas above and below the line correspond, respectively, to the dorsomedial and lateral surfaces of VB. The axes drawn on the surfaces of LP, MG, and VB summarize data on the polarities of the anomalous representations of the retina formed on those areas as a result of neonatal surgery. Scale applies to all parts of this figures. Axes of reconstruction are identical for *A* and *B*, different for *C*: *C*, caudal; *DL*, dorsolateral; *DM*, dorsomedial; *R*, rostral; *VL*, ventrolateral; *VM*, ventromedial. (Reproduced with permission from Frost, 1981.)

     Plasticity of Connectivity in the Visual System

maps of the retina and the body in VI and SI-SII, respectively, arise because in LGd and VB, the "lines of projection" representing a restricted region of the receptor surface are congruent with the set of relay neurons that project beneath a single locus on the cortical surface (reviewed in Caviness and Frost, 1980; Frost and Caviness, 1980). In operated hamsters, VB relay neurons projecting beneath a single cortical locus are distributed in arcs that lie in a plane approximately orthogonal to the lines of projection defined by retino-VB afferents (Frost, 1981) and therefore intercept multiple, but not necessarily contiguous, lines of projection. Thus, unlike in LGd and VB of normal animals, in which relay neurons that project to the same cortical loci get input from the same point on the receptor surface, in VB of operated animals, neurons projecting to the same cortical locus get input from multiple retinal loci.

A somewhat different result has recently been reported in the auditory cortex of neonatally operated ferrets with retinal projections to MG (Sur et al., 1990). In these animals, as in hamsters with retino-VB projections, consideration of the patterns of retinal projections and of thalamocortical projections would predict that the novel cortical representation of the visual field contains an orderly representation of only one visual field axis; however, an orderly cortical representation of both visual field axes was observed. A tentative interpretation of these data is that changes in the patterns of intracortical excitation and inhibition occurred which synthesized a representation of the second axis of the visual field. We do not yet know if a similar phenomenon occurs in hamsters with retino-MG projections.

SENSORY RESPONSE PROPERTIES OF SINGLE NEURONS

In the visual, somatosensory, and auditory systems, single neurons respond preferentially to particular values of one or more parameters of sensory stimulation. This selectivity of neuronal responsiveness is the basis for sensory information processing in the CNS. Our single unit recordings show that neurons in SI-SII of neonatally operated hamsters respond to visual stimulation of distinct RFs and that their response properties resemble, in several characteristic features, those of neurons in VI of normal hamsters (Métin and Frost, 1989).

When single units were activated by the presentation of stationary, flashed stimuli, their RFs showed the same three types of spatial organization in VI of normal hamsters and SI-SII of the hamsters that were operated on: (1) "unizone" RFs had one on, off, or on or off zone (figure 14.5, RFs 1b, 2a, 2b, 3b); (2) "concentric" RFs had ON or OFF centers and antagonistic surrounds (see figure 14.5, RF 3a); (3) "multizone" RFs had adjacent, nonconcentric zones of on and off, or on and on or off response (see figure 14.5, RF 1a). The spatial organization of unit RFs in SI-SII of operated hamsters differed from that of unit RFs in VI of normal hamsters in two respects. First, unit RFs in VI consist of a single responsive region; 57% of the visual RFs in SI-SII of operated animals consisted of two responsive regions. Second, units in SI-SII had visual RFs that were larger than those of units in VI. These two differences probably

     Frost: Processing by Surgically Created Neural Circuits

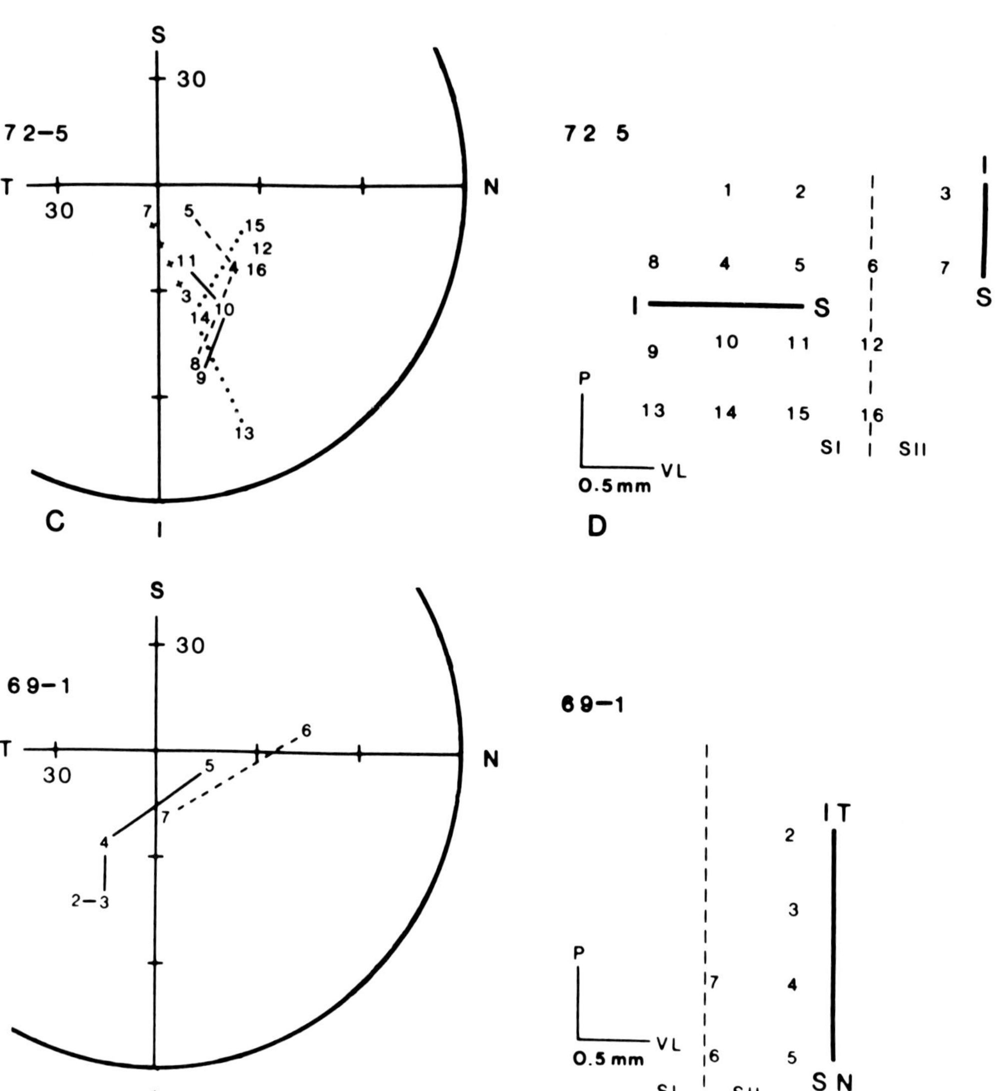
A
S
30
7 2—5
T
30
N
7
5
15
12
11
4 16
3
14 10
8
9
13
C
I
B
7 2 5
1 2 3
8 4 5 6 7
I S S
9 10 11 12
P
13 14 15 16
SI SII
0.5 mm VL
S
30
6 9—1
T
30
N
6
5
7
4
2—3
I
D
6 9—1
I T
2
3
P
4
7
VL
0.5 mm 6
5
SI SII
S N

have the same cause as the loss of nasal-temporal field order in the visual representations in SI-SII, namely that the VB neurons that project to the same cortical locus receive their visual input from multiple retinal loci.

We distinguished three functional categories of neurons in VI of normal hamsters (see figure 14.5, lower frames 1a–3a); the same three types of visually responsive neurons were present in SI-SII of operated hamsters (see figure 14.5, lower frames 1b–3b) in proportions not statistically different from those in VI: (1) *Orientation-selective* (see figure 14.5, 1a, 1b) units had a preferred orientation when stimulated with a stationary, flashed bar. There was no statistically significant difference in orientation bias (defined in the legend to figure 14.5) between orientation-selective units in VI and in SI-SII. The best response to a moving bar was obtained when a bar of the preferred orientation moved along one direction (for unidirectional units, e.g., 1a) or both directions (for bidirectional units, e.g., 1b) orthogonal to the preferred orientation. These units gave stronger responses to optimally oriented bars than to spots with the same area, intensity, and velocity of motion (not shown), but preferred directions were similar for bars and spots. (2) *Nonoriented, direction-selective* (see figure 14.5, 2a, 2b) units had no orientation preference for stationary bars (2b) or gratings (not shown), nor did they give stronger responses to a moving bar than to a moving spot of the same area, intensity, and velocity (2a). However, these units preferred movement in one (2a, 2b) or both (not shown) directions along a particular axis. (3) *Nonoriented, nondirection-selective* (see figure 14.5, 3a, 3b) units had no preferred orientation when stimulated with stationary gratings (3a) or bars (3b), and no preferred direction of movement when stimulated with moving gratings (3a), bars (3b), or spots (not shown). In normal and operated hamsters, the distributions of preferred orientations and directions of movement were both random. The depth distributions of the different types of visually responsive neurons are similar in both

---

Figure 14.4 Multi-unit visual receptive fields (RFs) recorded in SI and SII from two neonatally operated adult hamsters. RFs were mapped using bars and spots of light presented to the contralateral eye. Intersection of the horizontal and vertical axes indicates the projection of the optic disk. *S, N, I,* and *T* represent poles of the visual field, rather than retinal poles as in figure 14.3. The numbers *30* and *60* indicate degrees of eccentricity in the polar coordinate system. For clarity, the part of the visual field containing the RFs is magnified, while the rest is not shown. *A, B,* hamster 72-5. *C, D,* hamster 69-1. *A,* The positions of RF centers for three medial-to-lateral rows of electrode penetrations in SI (*8-4-5, 9-10-11,* and *13-14-15*) and one posterior-to-anterior row (*3-7*). RFs of penetrations in the same row are connected. The RFs recorded in penetrations *12* and *16* are not connected to the others as those penetrations were right on the SI-SII border, and are not certain to be part of the SI map. *B,* positions of all electrode penetrations in the parietal cortex; all but *2* and *6* yielded clear visual RFs. *Heavy lines* indicate the polarities of the Inferior(*I*)-superior (*S*) visual axis representations in SI and SII. *Broken line* indicates the SI-SII border. Scale bars: 0.5 mm. *P* and *VL* indicate the posterior and ventrolateral directions, respectively. *C,* positions of RF centers for two posterior-to-anterior rows of electrode penetrations in SII (*2-3-4-5* and *7-6*). Conventions are as in *A. D,* Positions of all electrode penetrations yielding visual RFs in the parietal cortex. *Heavy line* indicates the polarity of the inferotemporal (*IT*)-superonasal (*SN*) visual axis representation in SII. Scale bars and axes are as for *B.* (Reproduced with permission from Frost and Métin, 1985.)

     Frost: Processing by Surgically Created Neural Circuits

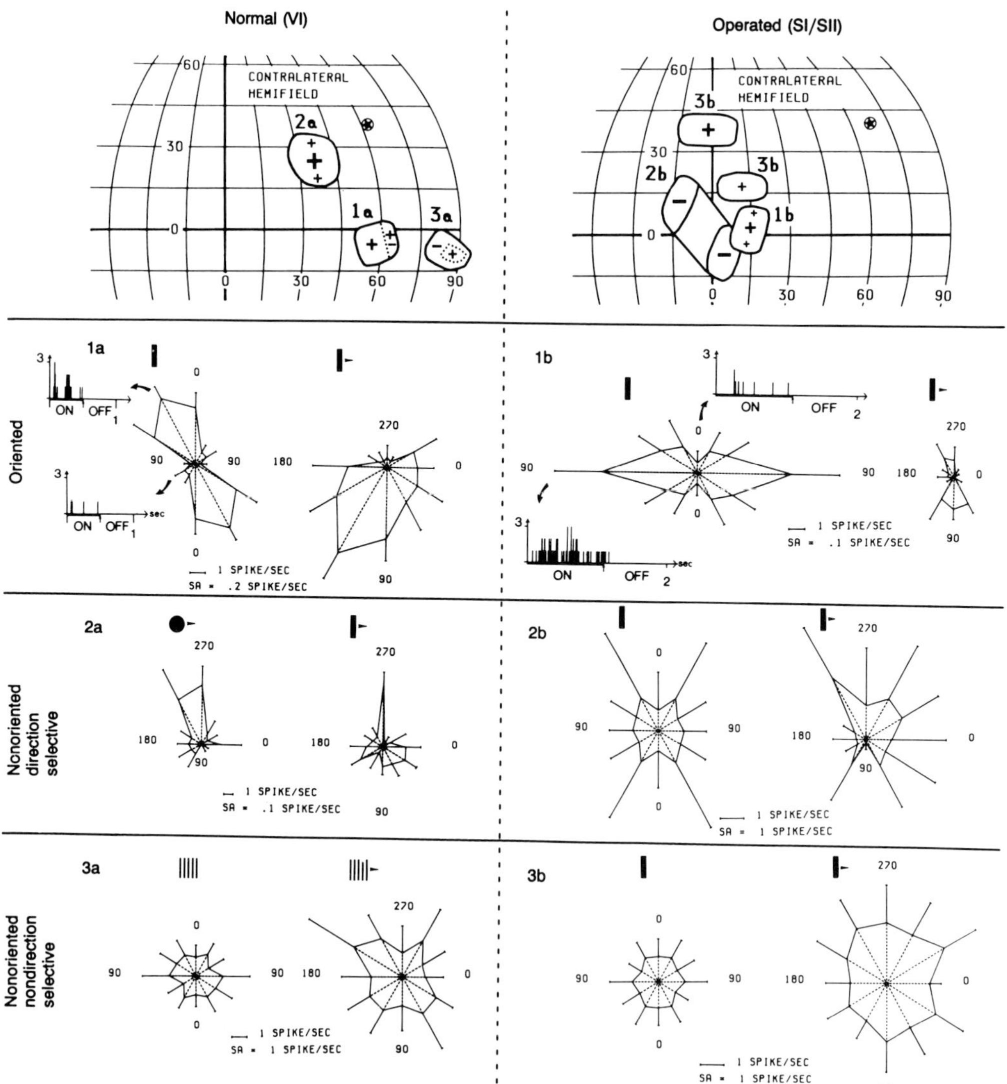

Plasticity of Connectivity in the Visual System

Figure 14.5 Visual RFs and response properties of three neurons in VI of normal hamsters and three neurons in SI-SII of operated hamsters, stimulated through the contralateral eye. RFs and polar histograms with the same number were obtained from the same neuron. *Top frames: spatial organization of visual RFs*. Spherical representations of part of the visual field; vertical meridian (0) is the projection of the body plane of symmetry; horizontal meridian (0) is the projection of the horizontal plane containing the eyes. Numbers *30, 60,* and *90* are eccentricities of meridians and elevation lines in degrees. *Circled star* is the projection of the optic disk. RF borders were determined using small, stationary, flashed stimuli. The *plus, minus,* and *plus or minus* symbols indicate zones in which responses were evoked by luminous stimuli turned on, off or on, and off, respectively. Response intensity in unizone RFs occasionally varied with position in the RF, as indicated in *2a* and *1b* by large and small symbols. *Six lower frames: three functional categories of visual RFs (see text)*. Same neurons as above in VI (*1a–3a*) and SI-II (*1b–3b*). Symbols above each polar histogram indicate stimulus used to evoke responses illustrated. *Black bars* and *gratings* correspond, respectively, to *stationary,* flashed bars and to stationary, alternating phase gratings of six orientations separated by 30 degrees (0 degrees = vertical, 90 degrees = horizontal) and presented randomly in a sequence repeated five times or more. Orientation of each *dotted radius* on the polar plot indicates stimulus orientation; the length of the dotted radius gives the mean response rate (spikes sec^{-1}) at that orientation. *Solid line* segments show the standard deviation of each response. Bars, spots, and sinusoidal gratings *move* in 12 directions separated by 30 degrees (0 degrees = nasal to temporal, 90 degrees = superior to inferior) and repeatedly present in a random sequence. Bars and gratings move in directions perpendicular to their long axes. Orientations of radii on polar plots indicate direction of stimulus movement; lengths of radii give mean response rate; *solid line segments* = standard deviation. *SA* = mean spontaneous activity rate. (*1a* and *1b*) Orientation-selective units. Units were considered to be orientation-selective if their orientation bias, B, was equal to or greater than 0.7. (B = 1 − R$_{min}$/R$_{max}$; R$_{min}$ and R$_{max}$ are the mean firing rates evoked by stationary bars at orientations producing the weakest and strongest responses, respectively. For units responding equally at all orientations, B = 0, while for those giving no response at the least effective orientation, B = 1.) Poststimulus time histograms (PSTHs) are for responses to stationary flashed bars with the preferred orientations (150 and 90 degrees, respectively) and with orthogonal orientations (60 and 0 degrees, respectively). PSTHs show that the *ON* response to an optimally oriented, flashed bar was phasic in unit *1a* and more tonic in unit *1b*. In both cases, the *ON* response strongly decreased when the units were stimulated with bars orthogonal to the preferred orientation. (*2a* and *2b*) Nonoriented, direction-selective units. Both were unidirectional. Unit *2a* preferred 270 degree movement while unit *2b* preferred upward nasal movement. (*3a* and *3b*) Nonoriented, nondirection-selective units. They showed no preferred orientation when stimulated with stationary gratings (*3a*) or bars (*3b*), and no preferred direction of movement when stimulated with moving gratings (*3a*) or bars (*3b*). (Reproduced with permission from Métin and Frost, 1989.)

     Frost: Processing by Surgically Created Neural Circuits

groups: orientation-selective neurons predominated in the supragranular cortical layers of both VI and SI-SII, whereas units that were only direction-selective or that were neither orientation nor direction-selective predominated in the granular and infragranular layers.

Subsequent to their neonatal transection, the ascending somatosensory afferent pathways grow rostral to the level of the cut and reinvade VB (Frost, unpublished data). Thus, 22 visually responsive neurons in SI-SII were tested for somatosensory responsiveness. Eight (36%) responded to somatosensory stimulation; their response properties were qualitatively similar (Métin and Frost, unpublished data) to those of neurons in SI-SII of normal animals.

We have not yet recorded the visually evoked responses of neurons in the auditory systems of our neonatally operated hamsters. However, we would anticipate results similar to those we obtained in SI-SII. In adult ferrets with surgically induced retino-MG projections, neurons of the primary auditory cortex respond to visual stimulation; however, they are not as sharply tuned for the parameters of visual stimuli as are those in VI of normal ferrets because the retino-MG projection arises from a different class of RGCs than the ones that normally relay visual information to VI via the LGd (Sur et al., 1988).

Our data suggest two hypotheses that are not mutually exclusive:

1. *The "developmental" hypothesis.* In sensory thalamic nuclei and cortical areas, the differentiation of some biochemical and morphological features underlying normal function may reflect the modality of the sensory input. While sensory input of the appropriate modality clearly influences the development of sensory systems (Fregnac and Imbert, 1984; Sherman and Spear, 1982), there are few data on how the differentiation of sensory systems depends on the *modality* of their input. Available evidence, namely our electron microscopic studies of the retinal projections to VB and MG, has not demonstrated such a dependence: retino-VB and retino-MG axons participate in synaptic complexes that morphologically resemble those of normal, somatosensory, and auditory thalamic afferents, respectively, rather than visual ones (Campbell and Frost, 1988). (These data also suggest that the morphological features of thalamic synaptic complexes may not determine the parameters of cortical neuronal responses assayed in our visual RF studies.) However, computer models demonstrate the plausibility of neuronal networks whose connection strengths are modifiable in such a way that the response properties of their constituent neurons develop particular features as a result of their sensory input (Lehky and Sejnowski, 1988; Linsker, 1988); the visual and somatosensory cortices may contain such networks. Furthermore, it has been demonstrated for both lagomorphs (Levick, 1967) and birds (Maturana and Frenk, 1963), and suggested by indirect evidence for carnivores (Spinelli, 1966), that there are small populations of RGCs that have strong preferences for stimulus orientation; if similar RGCs are present during development in rodents, carnivores and primates, it is possible that during development in normal or neonatally operated animals, the cortical activity evoked by these RGCs could instruct the cortex (via an activity-dependent mechanism [e.g.,

     Plasticity of Connectivity in the Visual System

Bear et al., 1987]) to form circuits appropriate for the analysis of contour orientation.

2. *The "systems theoretic" hypothesis.* Three lines of evidence support the hypothesis that thalamic nuclei and cortical areas at corresponding levels in the visual and somatosensory systems perform similar transformations on their inputs: (a) The visual and somatosensory systems of normal animals appear to use similar information processing strategies, based on similar morphological substrates. (b) Orientation-selective neurons occur with equal frequency, are equally sharply tuned, and have similar depth distributions in VI of normal hamsters and SI-SII of operated hamsters. (c) The similarity of the visual and somatosensory response properties of *bimodal* neurons in SI-SII of operated hamsters to those of single neurons in VI and SI-SII, respectively, of normal hamsters suggests that similar circuits in the visual and somatosensory thalamic nuclei and cortices can generate both visual and somatosensory responses. The data supporting this hypothesis are discussed more thoroughly in our original report (Métin and Frost, 1989).

It is not known if the visual and somatosensory systems use similar strategies to accomplish similar tasks. While neurons in somatosensory cortex of normal animals are selective for the direction and velocity of tactile stimulus movement (Essick and Whitsel, 1985), orientation selectivity is rare (Hyvarinen and Poranen, 1978) and these features may not be abstracted by the same mechanisms as in the visual system. Even if these stimulus parameters are not analyzed similarly in the two systems, the visual and somatosensory cortices may perform a common operation, e.g., selectively filtering their inputs so as to emphasize changes in the spatial or temporal domains. The hypothesis that visual and somatosensory forebrain structures perform similar transformations on their inputs implies that differences in information processing strategy between the two systems occur principally at prethalamic levels.

DEVELOPMENT OF NOVEL CONNECTIONS

The preceding text focuses on novel, permanent, surgically induced retinal projections to "nonvisual" structures. This is not the only instance of the retina projecting to such targets. During *normal development*, the retina projects *transiently* to multiple nonvisual structures: in hamsters, the connections between the retina and its target nuclei have just begun to form on the day of birth (day 0 = 15.5 days post conception; Bhide et al., 1988; Bhide and Frost, 1991; Frost et al., 1979; Schneider and Jhaveri, 1983). In neonatal hamsters, the retina projects to such nonvisual targets as the VB, the main midbrain auditory nucleus (inferior colliculus, IC), the substantia nigra, the pons, the mesencephalic tegmentum, and the periventricular and anterior nuclei of the hypothalamus (Frost, 1984). The projection to VB disappears completely by postnatal day 4; the projection to IC (which also occurs in rats [Kato, 1983]) is largely eliminated by the end of the first postnatal week, although a remnant persists permanently in a restricted region of IC adjacent to SC.

     Frost: Processing by Surgically Created Neural Circuits

We have examined the ultrastructure of anterograde-labeled, transient, retino-VB and retino-IC axons in neonatal hamsters (Freeman and Frost, 1987). Both sets of axons make immature synapses on their target neurons; the synapses are indistinguishable from others in these nuclei, presumably including those made by permanent afferents. Thus, the elimination of transient retino-VB and retino-IC axons is not due to their inability to make synapses. In fact, the formation of synapses by transient retino-VB and retino-IC axons allows the possibility that these axons are eliminated by a mechanism that depends on the pattern or overall level of their synaptic activity (Stent, 1973; Changeux and Danchin, 1976; Bear et al., 1987).

Studies of the branching patterns of individual RGC axons filled with HRP or the fluorescent dye DiI in neonatal hamsters (Langdon et al., 1987; Langdon and Frost, 1991; Bhide et al., 1988; Bhide and Frost, 1991) and mice (Sachs et al., 1986) confirm previous suggestions (Frost, 1984; Schneider and Jhaveri, 1983; Schneider et al., 1985) that RGC axons go through three morphologically distinguishable growth states (figure 14.6, A, B): (1) *elongation*, during which RGC axons extend along the optic tract from the eye to the mesencephalon, but do not send collaterals into their target nuclei; (2) *collateralization*, during which unbranched or poorly branched processes extend from the main axonal trunks into the targets of RGC axons; and (3) *arborization*, during which the RGC axons elaborate their terminal arbors within their target nuclei (and form synapses at an accelerated rate [Campbell et al., 1984]). Additional data on the development of other long axon systems suggest that these three stages of growth are common to many different types of axons (reviewed in Bhide and Frost, 1991).

Different transient projections are formed by RGC axons in different growth states (Langdon et al., 1987; Langdon and Frost, 1991): The transient retino-IC projection is probably due to "exuberant" *elongation* of RGC axons,

---

Figure 14.6 Schematic representations of developing RGC axons in normal and neonatally operated hamsters. *A*, representation of three growth states in the development of RGC axons as observed at the level of the thalamus in the coronal plane. The elongation and collateralization states are common to both superficial optic tract (*SOT*) and internal optic tract (*IOT*) axons, but only SOT axons arborize fully in the thalamus. Even though the IOT collaterals enter the arborization state and make primitive terminal-terminal arbors, these arbors and the collaterals that bear them regress virtually completely. The transient retino-VB projection arises exclusively from IOT axons during the collateralization state. *B*, representation of three growth states in the development of RGC axons as observed at the level of the midbrain in the parasagittal plane. The transient retino-IC projection arises during the elongation state, but is subsequently eliminated as RGC axons from collaterals, then arbors, in the superior colliculus (*SC*) *C*, development of the novel retino-VB projection in neonatally operated hamsters as observed in the coronal plane. (*a*) Retinal projections on P$_0$, prior to surgery. (*b–d*) Three possible ways of forming a permanent retino-VB projection in hamsters neonatally operated on. (*b*) IOT axon collaterals may be anomalously stabilized, without sprouting of SOT collaterals into VB. (*c*) SOT axons may sprout into VB whereas IOT axon collaterals are eliminated or (*d*) both sprouting of SOT collaterals and anomalous stabilization of IOT collaterals can occur. Our data show that the novel retino-VB projection actually arises by sprouting of SOT axons without stabilization of the normally transient IOT axon collaterals (*c*).

    Plasticity of Connectivity in the Visual System

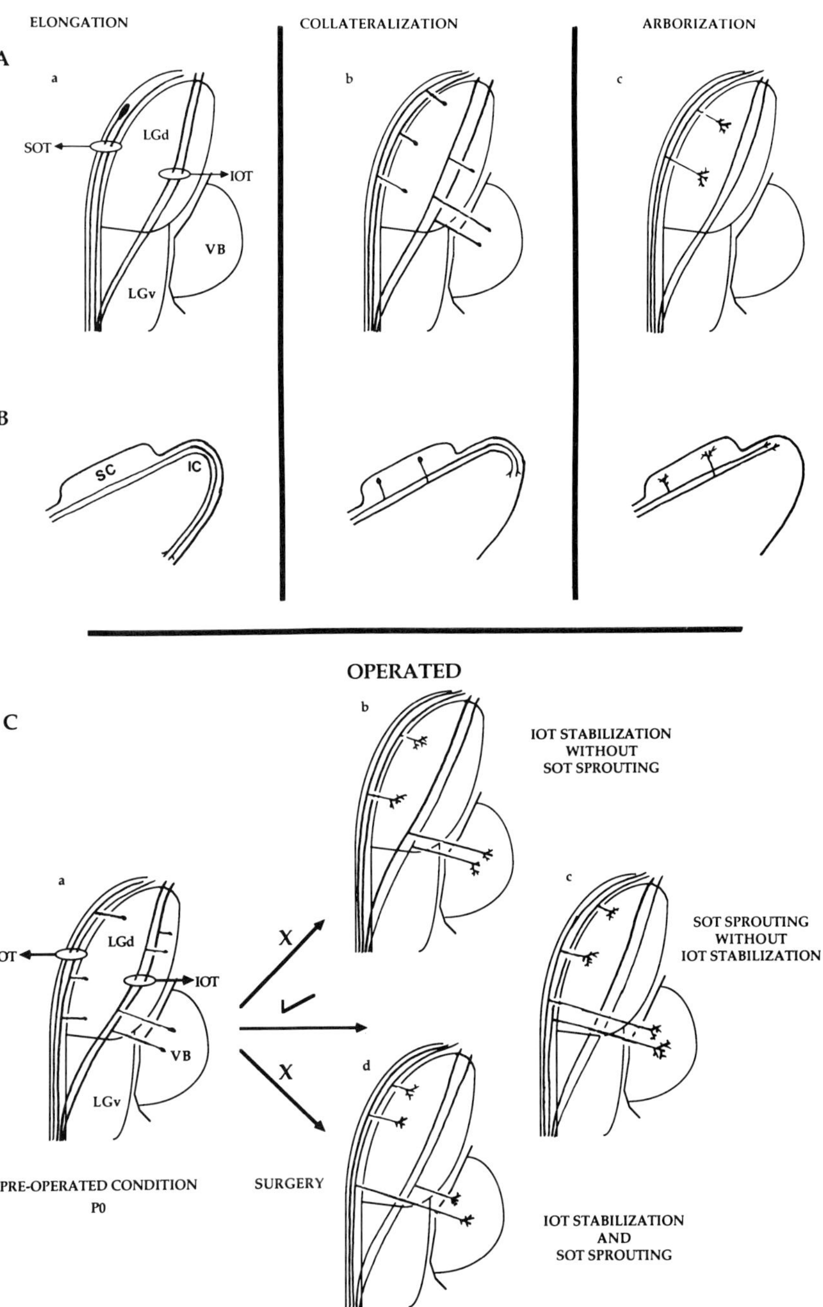

NORMAL
ELONGATION
COLLATERALIZATION
ARBORIZATION
A
a
SOT
LGd
IOT
VB
LGv
b
c
B
SC
IC
OPERATED
C
b
IOT STABILIZATION
WITHOUT
SOT SPROUTING
a
SOT
LGd
IOT
VB
LGv
c
SOT SPROUTING
WITHOUT
IOT STABILIZATION
d
PRE-OPERATED CONDITION
P0
SURGERY
IOT STABILIZATION
AND
SOT SPROUTING

whose trunks grow through SC and continue into IC (see figure 14.6, B). This is not the case for the retino-VB projection. In normal, *adult* rodents, RGC axons passing to the midbrain on the surface of the diencephalon in the superficial optic tract (SOT) send collaterals to the thalamus (where they terminate in the dLGN), whereas RGC axons that traverse the thalamus deeper in the internal optic tract (IOT), do not have thalamic collaterals (see figure 14.6, A, "arborization"; Bhide and Frost, 1991; Schneider and Jhaveri, 1983). During development, both SOT and IOT axons form thalamic collaterals. The immature SOT collaterals are restricted to LGd, whereas the IOT collaterals project to both LGd and VB (see figure 14.6, A, "collateralization"); the IOT axons subsequently lose their thalamic collaterals (Bhide and Frost, 1991; Langdon et al., 1987; Langdon and Frost, 1991). Thus, the transient retino-VB projection is due to the exuberant collateralization of RGC axons. It is not known whether the normal, transient retinal projections are eliminated by the death of the RGCs from which they originate or by the elimination of the transitory axonal processes from which they arise, with survival of the parent RGCs.

In light of the preceding data, we asked whether normal, transient retinal projections might contribute to the formation of the novel retinal projections to VB or MG. Transient projections may, in some instances, serve as substrates for the formation of novel neural connections (reviewed in Innocenti, 1981; Frost, 1991). Our data indicate that in the case of the novel retinal projections to VB and MG, this is a more complex issue than was originally appreciated. Whereas in normal hamsters, retino-VB projections are absent after day 3, in the hamsters operated on, they are present at all ages and occupy increasing proportions of VB between birth and 122 days (Frost, 1986). These data, obtained using techniques that did not permit the resolution of individual axons, suggested that the permanent retino-VB projection arises by the abnormal stabilization of normally transient retino-VB axons. Subsequent studies employing techniques that permit the visualization of individual axons and their branches demonstrate that the retino-VB projection initially consists exclusively of the IOT axon collaterals that are the source of the normal, transient projection (see above), but by 5 days of age, SOT axon collaterals also invade VB, and by 20 days of age and later, all the IOT collaterals are eliminated from VB and only SOT collaterals remain (figure 14.6, Cc; Bhide and Frost, in preparation). Thus, in the hamsters operated on even under conditions which cause retinal axons to make novel, permanent projections to the somatosensory thalamus, the IOT axons which initially project there still lose their thalamic collaterals and are replaced by the collaterals of SOT axons that are the sole source of retinothalamic input in normal mature animals. An even more remarkable sequence of events occurs in MG: In operated hamsters, retino-MG projections arise de novo by rapid, reactive sprouting of RGC axons—retino-MG axons are not present in normal animals at any age, but appear by 48 hours postoperatively (Frost, 1986). Studies of single axons in operated hamsters demonstrate that the retino-MG projection initially consists of novel IOT axon collaterals that form in re-

     Plasticity of Connectivity in the Visual System

sponse to the surgery. These are then joined by SOT axon collaterals and the IOT collaterals are then eliminated so that only the SOT collaterals persist (Bhide and Frost, manuscript in preparation).

These observations are doubly significant. First, they suggest that there may be intrinsic differences among RGCs in their capacity to form thalamic projections. Second, they suggest that the RGCs that give rise to the novel retinothalamic projections (to VB or MG) are restricted to a subset of the RGCs that are the origin of the normal retinothalamic projection (to LGd). Both these possibilities are currently under investigation in our laboratory.

CONCLUSIONS

We have demonstrated that when the retina makes novel projections to the auditory or somatosensory systems, the resultant retinothalamocortical pathway resembles that of the normal visual system with respect to a number of important anatomical and neurophysiological properties, thus permitting meaningful processing of visual sensory input. We are now investigating the capacity of these novel circuits to mediate visually guided behavior. Our results suggest the feasability of using novel, surgically created neural circuits to take over the function of damaged brain regions. However, it should be emphasized that the functional changes produced by novel neural circuits formed as a consequence of early lesions or surgery are not invariably adaptive (Schneider, 1979). Anomalous circuits formed as a consequence of early lesions probably underlie the neural dysfunction occurring in some disease states. For example, congenitally deaf patients exhibit abnormally large visually evoked responses in the auditory cortex (Neville et al., 1983); these changes may be mediated by anomalous stabilization of the normally transient retino-IC projection as a consequence of early cochlear degeneration. For these reasons, and because the effects of morphological or functional anomalies can be cascaded through multiple, interconnected brain regions, the use of novel circuits for the treatment of brain injuries will have to be evaluated extremely cautiously.

The novel retinal projections to the auditory and somatosensory systems described here were created in the developing nervous system. We believe, however, that these circuits will prove to be paradigms for novel circuits that are created surgically in mature brains. In adult animals, severed, regenerating CNS axons can be directed into novel targets using "bridges" made from grafted segments of peripheral nerves (reviewed in Aguayo, 1985). The morphology of the synaptic complexes formed by the regenerated axons appears to be determined by mechanisms similar to those we have described in the developing CNS (Aguayo et al., 1990). To date, it has proved extremely difficult to demonstrate electrical activity evoked by regenerated CNS axons in their target neurons (Aguayo et al., 1990). This is most likely due to the fact that the extent and density of the terminal arbors formed by the axons when they leave the environment of the peripheral nerve bridge and reenter the CNS are limited. Chemical factors that inhibit axonal growth have recently been identified in the mature CNS (Caroni and Schwab, 1988). Thus, the regenerated projections may possibly be made more robust (and thus more capable of driving their target neurons) by countering the action of those factors. If this proves to be so, then it should be possible to use peripheral nerve bridges to create novel circuits in the mature CNS that are analogous to the retino-MG and retino-VB projections created in the developing CNS and to examine their functional capabilities. The "systems theoretic" hypothesis that visual and somatosensory forebrain structures perform similar transformations on their inputs predicts that regenerated retino-MG or retino-VB pathways would also mediate visual processing.

Acknowledgment

This work was supported by grants EY03465 and NS22807 from NIH, 5-417 and 1-1060 from the March of Dimes Birth Defects Foundation, UA1199 from the CNRS (France), 0212/87 from NATO, from La Fondation de France, from the Burroughs-Wellcome Foundation, and from the Medical Foundation.

REFERENCES

Aguayo, A.J. (1985). Axonal regeneration from injured neurons in the adult mammalian central nervous system. In *Synaptic Plasticity and Remodeling*, ed. C.W. Cotman, 457–483. New York: Guilford Press.

Aguayo, A.J., Carter, D.A., Zwimpfer, T.J., Vidal-Sanz, M., and Bray, G.M. (1990). Axonal regeneration and synapse formation in the injured CNS of adult mammals. In *Brain Repair, Wenner-Gren International Symposium Series*, Vol. 56, ed. A. Björklund, A.J. Aguayo, and D. Ottoson, 251–271. London: Macmillan Press.

Bear, M.F., Cooper, L.N., and Ebner, F.F. (1987). A physiological basis for a theory of synapse modification. *Science* 237:42–48.

Bhide, P.G., and Frost, D.O. (1991). Stages of growth of hamster retinofugal axons: Implications for developing axonal pathways with multiple targets. *J. Neurosci.* 11:485–504.

Bhide, P.G., Lieberman, A.R., and Frost, D.O. (1988). Postnatal development of neurons and optic tract axon arbors in the hamster dorsal lateral geniculate nucleus: In vitro HRP study. *Soc. Neurosci. Abstr.* 14:1111.

Campbell, G., and Frost, D.O. (1987). Target-controlled differentiation of axon terminals and synaptic organization. *Proc. Natl. Acad. Sci. U.S.A.* 84:6929–6933.

Campbell, G., and Frost, D.O. (1988). Synaptic organization of anomalous retinal projections to somatosensory and auditory thalamus: Target-controled morphogenesis of axon terminals and synaptic glomeruli. *J. Comp. Neurol.* 272:383–408.

Campbell, G., So, K.-F., and Lieberman, A.R. (1984). Normal post-natal development of retino-geniculate axons and terminals and identification of inappropriately-located transient synapses. *Neuroscience* 13:743–759.

Caroni, P., and Schwab, M.E. (1988). Antibody against myelin-associated inhibitor of neurite growth neutralizes nonpermissive substrate properties of CNS white matter. *Neuron* 1:85–96.

Caviness, V.S., Jr., and Frost, D.O. (1980). Tangential organization of thalamic projections to the neocortex in the mouse. *J. Comp. Neurol.* 194:335–367.

     Plasticity of Connectivity in the Visual System

Changeux, J.P., and Danchin, A. (1976). Selective stabilisation of developing synapses as a mechanism for the specification of neuronal networks. *Nature* 264:705–712.

Essick, G.K., and Whitsel, B.L. (1985). Factors influencing cutaneous direction sensitivity: A correlative psychophysical and neurophysiological investigation. *Brain Res. Rev.* 10:213–230.

Freeman, J.M., and Frost, D.O. (1987). Synapse formation by optic tract axons that project transiently to somatosensory and auditory nuclei in the neonatal hamster. *Soc. Neurosci. Abstr.* 13:1023.

Fregnac, Y., and Imbert, M. (1984). Development of neuronal selectivity in primary visual cortex of cat. *Physiol. Rev.* 64:325–434.

Frost, D.O. (1981). Orderly anomalous retinal projections to the medial geniculate, ventrobasal and lateral posterior nuclei of the hamster. *J. Comp. Neurol.* 203:227–256.

Frost, D.O. (1982). Anomalous visual connections to somatosensory and auditory systems following brain lesions in early life. *Dev. Brain Res.* 3:627–635.

Frost, D.O. (1984). Axonal growth and target selection during development: Retinal projections to the ventrobasal complex and other "nonvisual" structures in neonatal Syrian hamsters. *J. Comp. Neurol.* 230:576–592.

Frost, D.O. (1986). Development of surgically induced retinal projections to the medial geniculate, ventrobasal and lateral posterior nuclei in Syrian hamsters: A quantitative study. *J. Comp. Neurol.* 252:95–105.

Frost, D.O. (1991). Cross-modal projections in the study of central nervous system development. In *Advances in Neural and Behavioral Development*, ed. V.A. Casagrande and P. Shinkman. Norwood, N.J.: Ablex (in press).

Frost, D.O., and Caviness, V.S., Jr. (1980). Radial organization of thalamic projections to the neocortex in the mouse. *J. Comp. Neurol.* 194:369–393.

Frost, D.O., and Métin, C. (1985). Induction of functional retinal projections to the somatosensory system. *Nature* 317:162–164.

Frost, D.O., and Schneider, G.E., (1979). Plasticity of retinofugal projections after partial lesions of the retina in newborn Syrian hamsters. *J. Comp. Neurol.* 185:517–568.

Frost, D.O., So, K.-F., and Schneider, G.E. (1979). Postnatal development of retinal projections in Syrian hamsters: A study using autoradiographic and anterograde degeneration techniques. *Neuroscience* 4:1649–1677.

Gouzé, J.-L., Lasry, J.-M., and Changeux, J.-P. (1983). Selective stabilization of muscle innervation during development: A mathematical model. *Biol. Cybern.* 46:207–215.

Hughes, A. (1977). The topography of vision in mammals of contrasting life style: Comparative optics and retinal organization. In *Handbook of Sensory Physiology*, Vol. VII/5: *The Visual System in Vertebrates*, ed. F. Crescitelli, 613–756. Berlin: Springer-Verlag.

Hyvarinen, J., and Poranen, A. (1978). Movement-sensitive and direction and orientation-selective cutaneous receptive fields in the hand area of the post-central gyrus in monkeys. *J. Physiol. (Lond.)* 283:523–537.

Innocenti, G.M. (1981). Transitory structures as substrates for developmental plasticity of the brain. *Dev. Neurosci.* 13:305–333.

Irons, A., Métin, C., and Frost, D.O. (1990). Retinal ganglion cells in hamsters with retinal projections to the ventrobasal and medial geniculate nuclei. *Soc. Neurosci. Abstr.* 16:336.

Kaas, J.H., Guillery, R.W., and Allman, J.M. (1972). Some principles of organization in the dorsal lateral geniculate nucleus. *Brain Behav. Evol.* 6:253–299.

Kato, T. (1983). Transient retinal fibers to the inferior colliculus in the newborn albino rat. *Neurosci. Lett* 37:7–9.

Langdon, R.B., Freeman, J.M., and Frost, D.O. (1987). Trajectories and branching patterns of optic tract axons that project transiently to somatosensory thalamus in the neonatal hamster. *Soc. Neurosci. Abstr.* 13:1023.

Langdon, R.B., and Frost, D.O. (1991). Development of optic tract axons that project transiently to somatosensory thalamus in the neonatal hamster. *J. Comp. Neurol.* 310:200–214.

Lehky, S.R., and Sejnowski, T.J. (1988). Network model of shape-from-shading: Neural function arises from both receptive and projective fields. *Nature* 333:452–454.

Levick, W.R. (1967). Receptive fields and trigger features of ganglion cells in the visual streak of the rabbit's retina. *J. Physiol. (Lond.)* 188:285–307.

Linden, R., and Esbérard, E.L. (1987). Displaced amacrine cells in the ganglion cell layer of the hamster retina. *Vision Res.* 27:1071–1076.

Linden, R., and Perry, V.H. (1983). Massive retinotectal projection in rats. *Brain Res.* 272:145–149.

Linsker, R. (1988). Self-organization in a perceptual network. *Computer* 21:105–117.

Maturana, H.R., and Frenk, S. (1963). Directional movement and horizontal edge detectors in the pigeon retina. *Science* 142:977–979.

Métin, C., and Frost, D.O. (1989). Visual responses of neurons in somatosensory cortex of hamsters with experimentally induced retinal projections to somatosensory thalamus. *Proc. Natl. Acad. Sci. U.S.A.* 86:357–361.

Neville, H.J., Schmidt, A., and Kutas, M. (1983). Altered visual-evoked potentials in congenitally deaf adults. *Brain Res.* 266:127–132.

Perry, V.H., and Cowey, A. (1979). The effects of unilateral cortical and tectal lesions on retinal ganglion cells in rats. *Exp. Brain Res.* 35:85–95.

Raabe, J.I., Windrem, M.S., and Finlay, B.L. (1986). Control of cell number in the developing visual system. III. Effects of visual cortex ablation. *Dev. Brain Res.* 28:23–31.

Sachs, G.M., Jacobson, M., and Caviness, V.S., Jr. (1986). Postnatal changes in the pattern of arborization of murine retinocollicular axons. *J. Comp. Neurol.* 246:395–408.

Savio, T., Schnell, L., and Schwab, M.E. (1990). Myelin-associated inhibitory substrate components: Role in CNS regeneration. In *Brain Repair*, ed. A. Björklund, A.J. Aguayo, and D. Ottoson, 145–153. London: Macmillan Press.

Schneider, G.E. (1973). Early lesions of the superior colliculus: Factors affecting the formation of abnormal retinal projections. *Brain Behav. Evol.* 8:73–109.

Schneider, G.E. (1979). Is it really better to have your brain lesion early? A revision of the "Kennard principle." *Neuropsychologia* 17:557–583.

Schneider, G.E., and Jhaveri, S. (1983). Projections of the internal optic tract: Retinal projections which survive superficial thalamic lesions in hamsters. *Soc. Neurosci. Abstr.* 9:809.

Schneider, G.E., Jhaveri, S.R., Edwards, M.A., and So, K.-.F. (1985). Regeneration, rerouting and redistribution of axons after early lesions: Changes with age, and functional impact. In *Recent Achievements in Restorative Neurology. Upper Motor Neuron Function and Dysfunction (Advances in Neurology)*, ed. M. Dimitrijenc and J. Eccles, 291–310. New York: Raven Press.

Sherman, S.M., and Spear, P.D. (1982). Organization of visual pathways in normal and visually deprived cats. *Physiol. Rev.* 62:738–855.

Slonaker, J.R. (1897). A comparative study of the area of acute vision in vertebrates. *R. Soc. Cat.* 13:445–502.

Spinelli, D.N. (1966). Visual receptive fields in the cat's retina: Complications. *Science* 152:1768–1769.

Stent, G.S. (1973). A physiological mechanism for Hebb's postulate of learning. *Proc. Natl. Acad. Sci. U.S.A.* 70:997–1001.

Stone, J. (1983). *Parallel Processing in the Visual System,* New York: Plenum Press.

Sur, M., Garraghty, P.E., and Roe, A.W. (1988). Experimentally induced visual projections into auditory thalamus and cortex. *Science* 242:1437–1441.

Sur, M., Pallas, S.L., and Roe, A.W. (1990). Cross-modal plasticity in cortical development: Differentiation and specification of sensory neocortex. *Trends Neurosci.* 13:227–233.

Tiao, Y.C., and Blakemore, C. (1976). Functional organization in the visual cortex of the golden hamster. *J. Comp. Neurol.* 168:459–482.

Udin, S.B., and Schneider, G.E. (1981). Compressed retinotectal projection in hamsters: Fewer ganglion cells project to tectum after neonatal tectal lesions. *Exp. Brain Res.* 43:261–269.

Wickler, K.C., Kirn, J., Windrem, M.S., and Finlay, B.L. (1986). Control of cell number in the developing visual system. II. Effects of partial tectal ablation. *Dev. Brain Res.* 28:11–21.

Yamasaki, E.N., Schätz, C.R., and Frost, D.O. (1991). Morphology of hamster retinal ganglion cells. *Soc. Neurosci. Abstr.* 17:1374.

Zimmer, J. (1974). Proximity as a factor in the regulation of aberrant axonal growth in postnatally deafferented fascia dentata. *Brain Res.* 72:137–142.

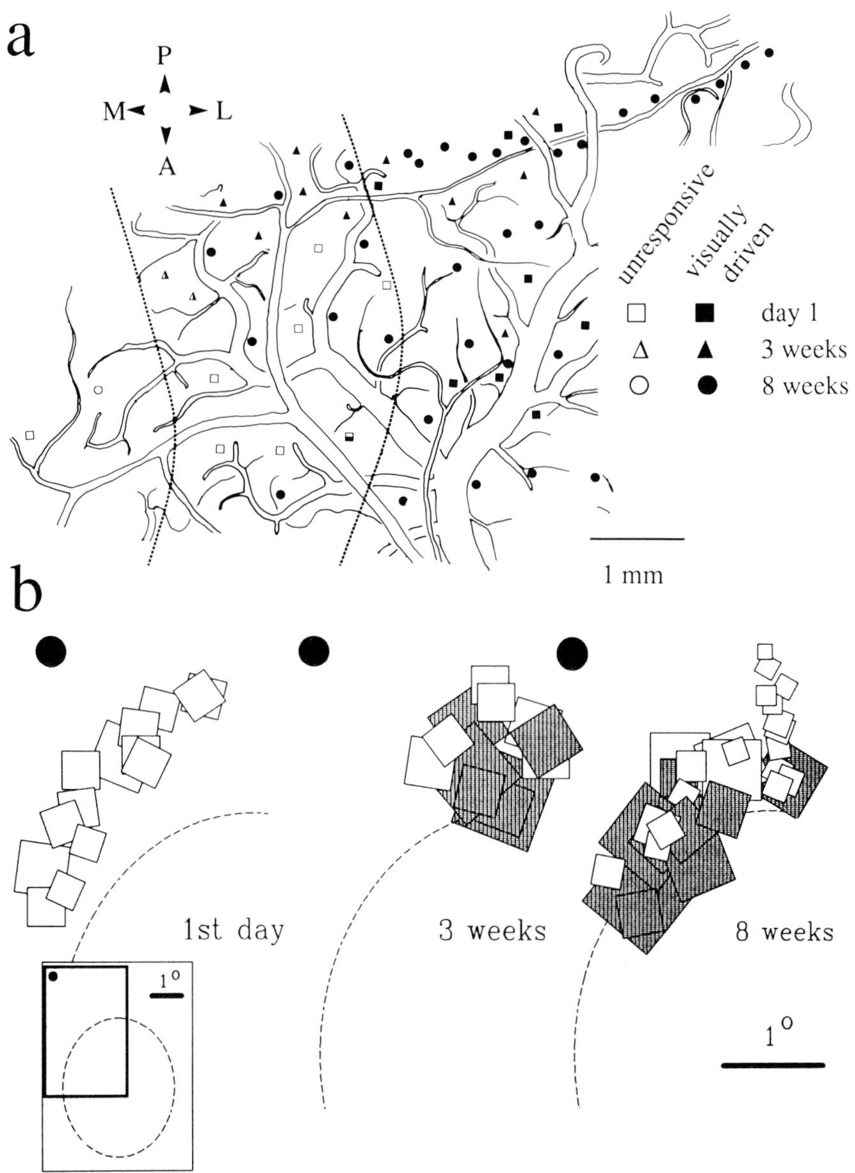

a
P
M L
A
unresponsive
visually
driven
day 1
3 weeks
8 weeks
1 mm
b
1st day
3 weeks
8 weeks
1°
1°

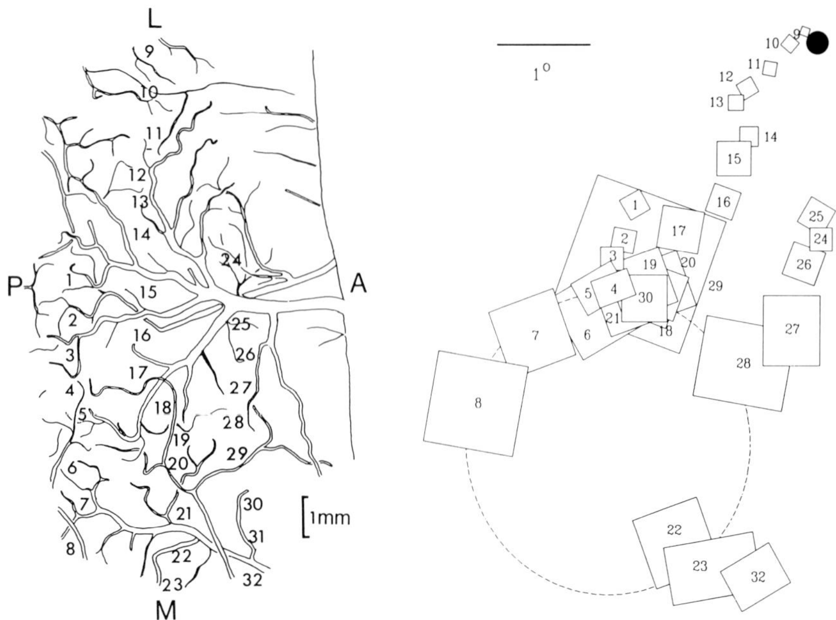

Figure 15.3 Progression in receptive field position with regular shifts in cortical recording sites in striate cortex, 8 weeks following binocular retinal lesion. *Left*, surface map of the cortical vasculature, with the sites of the electrode penetrations indicated by numbers. *Right*, the boundary of the lesion is indicated by the *dashed line*. The receptive fields tend to slow in their progression as they approach the visuotopic representation of the lesion boundary (cf. *9 to 21*), and then hop over to the other side of lesion (cf. *22 to 23*). In other sequences the fields tend to bend around the side of the lesion (cf. *1 to 8*). At this stage nearly all cortex received visual input, with no silent gaps. A, anterior; P, posterior; L, lateral; M, medial. (Reproduced with permission from Gilbert et al., 1990.)

The second example, shown in figure 15.3, shows a similar distortion of cortical topography, with the shift in receptive field position slowing as the fields approached the lesion; in some progessions, the sequence twisted around the side of the lesion. Here, a small shift in recording position (site 21 to site 22) was associated with a jump in receptive field position from one side of the lesion to the other, indicating that the cortical scotoma had completely filled in. In these experiments, the receptive fields in the reactivated cortex were somewhat larger than their counterparts at the same retinotopic position in normal cortex, but were still orientation-selective. In other experiments (not shown), we observed a number of bizarre behaviors in the receptive field maps of cells, some with bipartite fields spanning the lesion, some with shifts in different directions for the two eyes, and some within the ipsilateral visual field, indicating information transmitted across the corpus callosum.

In a subsequent series of experiments we mapped the same cortical territory before, immediately after, and a few months after making the lesion. This enabled us to determine the effects of making retinal lesions on cells at the same cortical site. The long-term changes were the same as those observed in the earlier experiments, though we were surprised to find shifts in receptive

     Plasticity of Connectivity in the Visual System

field position, even for cells with receptive fields originally outside the lesioned area. One possible explanation of this is that cortical topography is normally dependent on neighboring interactions, and when the cells with receptive fields originally within the lesioned retina change their receptive fields to outside the lesioned area, they cause a shift in topography in the surrounding cortex.

In this study and in the work done in somatosensory and motor cortex, one must ask whether the site of initial reorganization is in the cortex or at antecedent levels in the sensorimotor pathways. Earlier studies have shown topographical shifts in the spinal cord as a result of deafferentation (Devor and Wall, 1978). In our results, when the cortical scotoma fills in, is there a comparable fill-in at the level of the lateral geniculate nucleus? Retinal lesions had previously been shown to result in topographical shifts in the LGN, though the changes were small, on the order of 100 to 200 μm (Eysel et al., 1981). By comparing the topographical changes in the LGN and cortex in the same animal, at the same time, and with the same type of lesion, we were able to determine that the large part of the long-term conical changes seen in our experiments was due to a reorganization intrinsic to the cortex. In one cat and one monkey, at a time when the cortical scotoma had disappeared, there was a large unresponsive area in the LGN (approximately 1 mm in diameter, corresponding topographically to the size of the retinal scotoma). None of the other features of the cortical reorganization, such as an enlarged representation of perilesion retina, or enlarged or bipartite fields, were observed in the LGN. These results indicate that the topographical shifts resulted from synaptic changes intrinsic to the cortex, rather than at earlier stages.

In these experiments, a striking phenomenon was observed when we compared receptive fields before the lesion to those immediately after (Gilbert and Wiesel, 1991b). The cells with fields near the boundary of the lesion greatly expanded in diameter, many having fields three to four times the diameter of the cells recorded at the same site before the lesion was made. In addition to the changes in receptive field size, there was an apparent shift in receptive field position, moving centrifugally from the center of the lesion, though to a much smaller extent than we observed at longer times following the lesion. These findings suggested that the influence of the horizontal connections was potentiated to suprathreshold levels over a very short time scale, and that receptive field dimensions may be regulated dynamically by normal visual input. We are presently exploring the basis of these rapid increases in receptive field size and their possible role in normal visual processing.

A likely source of the transmission of visual information from one visual field locus to another, taking place in both the immediate and long term in the cortex, are the long-range horizontal connections (Gilbert and Wiesel, 1979, 1983; Rockland and Lund, 1982, 1983; Martin and Whitteridge, 1984). The effects of the horizontal inputs, bringing in visual information from an extended visual field area, are superimposed on those of the vertical connections, which provide more local retinal input (figure 15.4). Ordinarily, the horizontal input is modulatory, changing the response properties of cells to stimuli

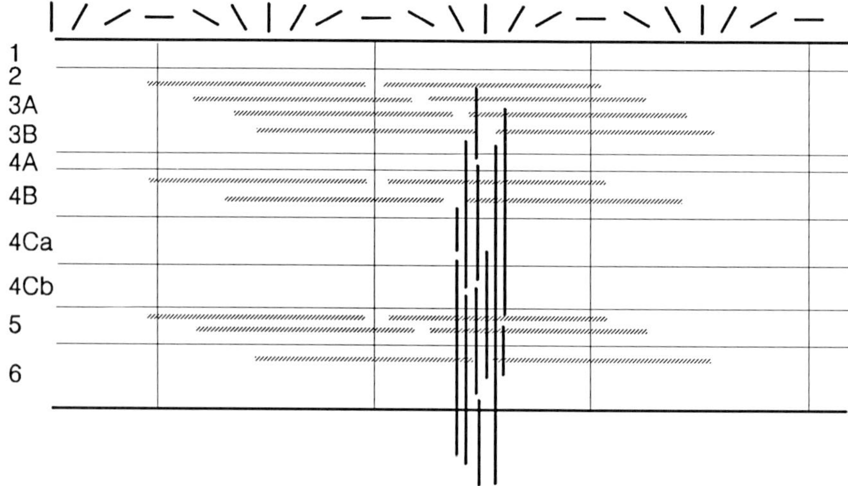

Figure 15.4 Schematic diagram of vertical (*solid lines*) and horizontal (*hatched lines*) connections in visual cortex, compared to the periodicity of orientation columns.

placed within the receptive field. When the local input is removed, however, such as with the laser-induced lesions, the effect of the horizontal connections can be potentiated to suprathreshold levels. There are several possible mechanisms for this, as we have observed in in vitro experiments on conical slices (Hirsch and Gilbert, 1990, 1991). The experiments described here were made in preparations where the connections between layers 3 and 4 were severed by making a cut between the two layers, excluding input from interlaminar connections to the results.

The synaptic potentials elicited by the horizontal input are consistent with the anatomy, which shows that the targets of the horizontal connections are a mixture of excitatory and inhibitory cells (Kisvarday et al., 1986; McGuire et al., 1991). Even if the inhibitory targets are in the minority (approximately 20%), their effect can be large. As shown in figure 15.5, the excitatory postsynaptic potential (EPSP) ordinarily elicited by stimulating the horizontal connections is small and typically unable to drive the cell to fire from its resting potential. Furthermore, as the stimulus strength is raised to recruit greater numbers of horizontal fibers, inhibitory postsynaptic potentials (IPSPs), appear and come to predominate the response at higher stimulus strengths. Even if IPSPs were not an apparent component of the postsynaptic response, removing inhibition pharmacologically by the application of bicuculline led to a dramatic increase in the degree of evoked excitation (figure 15.6). This is due to an unmasking of an underlying polysynaptic network of excitatory connections that can be driven by horizontal input. Thus reducing inhibition would be an effective mechanism for producing the enlarged or shifted receptive fields seen in the laser-induced lesion experiments. Alternatively, the horizontally evoked EPSP could be enhanced directly. We have been able to alter the synaptic efficacy of the horizontal connections by combining direct

     Plasticity of Connectivity in the Visual System

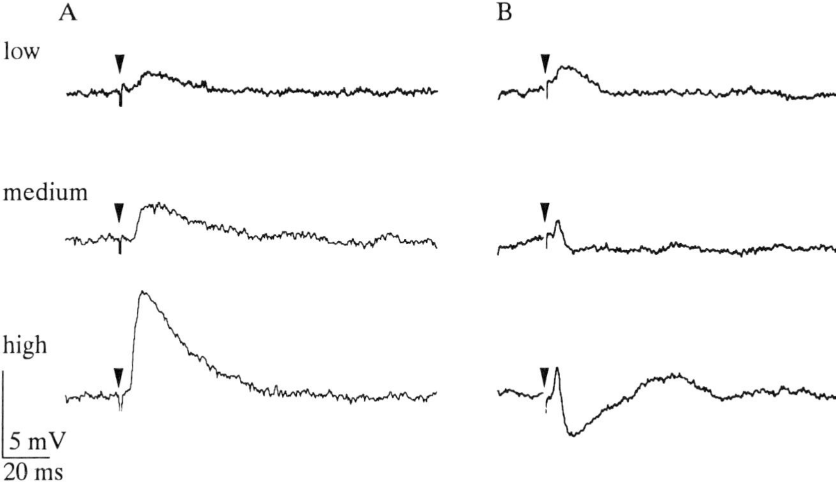

Figure 15.5 Characteristic responses to the activation of horizontal fibers. These records were obtained from two separate pyramidal cells in layers 2 and 3. The stimulating electrode was 1.2 mm away from the recording pipette in both cases. Each trace is the average of three trials. *A,* graded EPSPs recorded from a cell whose response to horizontal inputs was primarily excitatory. *B,* synaptic response of a cell whose response to horizontal input also included a graded fast IPSP at stimulus voltages above threshold. The membrane potential was depolarized from -76 to -58 mV for *A,* and from -77 to -65 mV for *B.* The voltage ranges of the shocks used to stimulate the cells in this figure were: low, 5 to 15 V; medium, 25 to 50 V; and high, 75 to 100 V.

depolarization of the impaled cell with activation of the horizontal inputs. As shown in figure 15.7, this conditioning of the horizontal input leads to a twofold increase in the peak of the EPSP. We currently do not know which, if any, of these possible mechanisms underlie the changes observed in the laser-induced lesion experiments. The mechanism behind the long-term recovery might even involve sprouting of connections, leading to a change in the neuronal circuitry. All told, however, these experiments demonstrate the mutability of the cortical circuit, and suggest ways in which the effects of the inputs to a cell change according to the pattern of their activation.

We have shown that modification of the balance of sensory input can lead to changes in cortical topography and receptive field structure. The mechanism underlying these changes is yet to be established, but experiments in tissue slices show a number of possible sources of dynamic changes in cortical circuitry. Different mechanisms may apply for short-term vs. long-term changes, ranging from reduction in inhibition to potentiation of monosynaptic excitatory potentials to anatomical changes in axonal arbors. We have evidence that the changes are intrinsic to the cortex rather than in subcortical structures. The picture that emerges is that even in the adult, receptive field properties are mutable, influenced by context and modifications of sensory input. These dynamic changes may play a role in normal visual perception as well as in recovery from central nervous system (CNS) lesions, and may also be related to the mechanisms of memory occurring in higher visual areas.

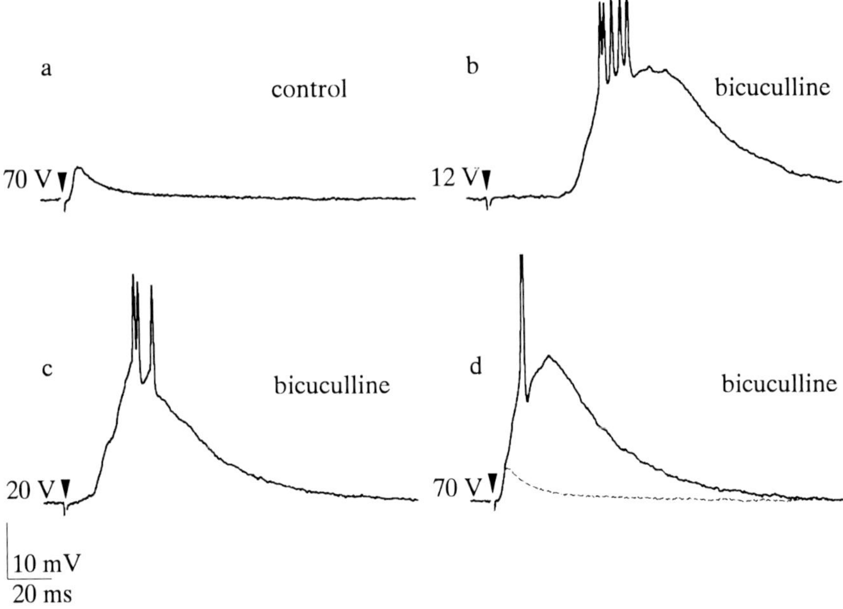

Figure 15.6 Blocking inhibition reveals a polysynaptic network that can be activated by horizontal fibers. Following application of the GABA$_A$ antagonist bicuculline, the threshold stimulus dropped from nearly 70 V (*a*) to 12 V (*b*) and the threshold response changed from a monosynaptic EPSP at short (3.6-ms) latency to a large, suprathreshold potential at long (35-ms) delay. Increasing the shock strength shortened the latency of the burst (*c*) until it overlapped the monosynaptic EPSP at the original threshold voltage (*d*); the trace in *a* is shown there as a *dashed line*. Each trace is the average of three trials recorded from a pyramidal cell while the membrane was at rest, −83 mV.

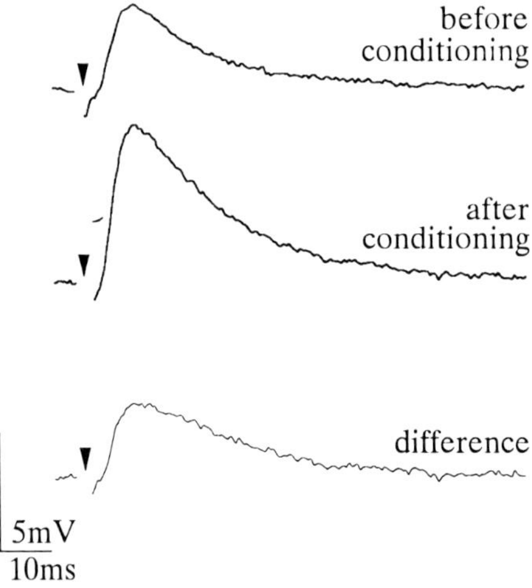

Figure 15.7 The EPSP produced by horizontal fibers can be strengthened by use. The peak of the response was nearly doubled following conditioning. Conditioning was done by pairing the EPSP with a suprathreshold pulse of intracellularly injected current (100 ms, 0.7 nA). The pairs were delivered in volleys of 100 at 1.7 Hz, twice. The top two traces are the average of three trials recorded from a pyramidal cell while the membrane was at rest.

　　Plasticity of Connectivity in the Visual System

REFERENCES

Calford, M.B., and Tweedale, R. (1988). Immediate and chronic changes in responses of somatosensory cortex in adult flying-fox after digit amputation. *Nature* 332:446–448.

Clark, S.A., Allard, T., Jenkins, W.M., and Merzenich, M.M. (1988). Receptive fields in the body-surface map in adult cortex defined by temporally correlated inputs. *Nature* 332:444–445.

Cusick, C.G., Wall, J.T., Whiting, J.H., Jr., and Wiley, R.G. (1990). Temporal progression of cortical reorganization following nerve injury. *Brain Res.* 537:355–358.

Devor, M., and Wall, P.D. (1978). Reorganisation of spinal cord sensory map after peripheral nerve injury. *Nature* 276:75–76.

Eysel, U.T., Gonzalez-Aguilar, F., and Mayer, U. (1981). Time-dependent decrease in the extent of visual deafferentation in the lateral geniculate nucleus of adult cats with small retinal lesions. *Exp. Brain Res.* 41:256–263.

Gilbert, C.D., and Wiesel, T.N. (1979). Morphology and intracortical projections of functionally identified neurons in cat visual cortex. *Nature* 280:120–125.

Gilbert, C.D., and Wiesel, T.N. (1983). Clustered intrinsic connections in cat visual cortex. *J. Neurosci.* 3:1116–1133.

Gilbert, C.D., and Wiesel, T.N. (1989). Columnar specificity of intrinsic connections in cat visual cortex. *J. Neurosci.* 9:2432–2442.

Gilbert, C.D., and Wiesel, T.N. (1990). The influence of contextual stimuli on the orientation selectivity of cells in primary visual cortex of the cat. *Vision Res.* 30:1689–1701.

Gilbert, C.D., and Wiesel, T.N. (1991). Short and long term changes in receptive field size and cortical topography following focal retinal lesions. *Soc. Neurosci. Abstr.* 17:1090.

Gilbert, C.D., Hirsch, J.A., and Wiesel, T.N. (1990). Lateral interactions in visual cortex. *Cold Spring Harbor Symp. Quant. Biol.* 55:663–677.

Heinen, S.J., and Skavenski, A.A. (1991). Recovery of visual responses in foveal V1 neurons following bilateral foveal lesions in adult monkey. *Exp. Brain Res.* 83:670–674.

Hirsch, J.A., and Gilbert, C.D. (1990). Interactions and stimulus-dependent changes of synaptic potentials evoked by activating interlaminar and horizontal pathways in the cat's striate cortex. *Soc. Neurosci. Abstr.* 16:1271.

Hirsch, J.A., and Gilbert, C.D. (1991). Synaptic physiology of horizontal connections in primary visual cortex. *J. Neurosci.* 11:1800–1809.

Kaas, J.H., Krubitzer, L.A., Chino, Y.M., Langston, A.L., Polley, E.H., and Blair, N. (1990). Reorganization of retinotopic cortical maps in adult mammals after lesions of the retina. *Science* 248:229–231.

Kalaska, J., and Pomeranz, B. (1979). Chronic paw deafferentation causes an age-dependent appearance of novel responses from forearm in "paw" cortex of kittens and adult cats. *J. Neurophysiol.* 42:618–633.

Kisvarday, Z.F., Martin, K.A.C., Freund, T.F., Magloczky, Zs., Whitteridge, D., and Somogyi, P. (1986). Synaptic targets of HRP-filled layer III pyramidal cells in the cat striate cortex *Exp. Brain Res.* 64:541–552.

Martin, K.A.C., and Whitteridge, D. (1984). Form, function and intracortical projections of spiny neurones in the striate visual cortex of the cat. *J. Physiol.* 353:463–504.

McGuire, B.A., Gilbert, C.D., Rivlin, P., and Wiesel, T.N. (1991). Targets of horizontal connections in Macaque primary visual cortex. *J. Comp. Neur.* 305:370–392.

Merzenich, M.M., Kaas, J.H., Wall, J.T., Nelson, R.J., Sur, M., and Felleman, D.J. (1983a). Topographic reorganization of somatosensory cortical areas 3b and 1 in adult monkeys following restricted deafferentation. *Neuroscience* 8:33–55.

Merzenich, M.M., Kaas, J.H., Wall, J.T., Nelson, R.J., Sur, M., and Felleman, D.J. (1983b). Progression of change following median nerve section in the cortical representation of the hand in areas 3b and 1 in adult owl and squirrel monkeys. *Neuroscience* 10:639–665.

Merzenich, M.M., Nelson, R.J., Stryker, M.P., Cynader, M.S., Schoppmann, A., and Zook, J.M. (1984). Somatosensory cortical map changes following digit amputation in adult monkeys. *J. Comp. Neurol.* 224:591–605.

Robertson, D., and Irvine, D.R.F. (1989). Plasticity of frequency organization in auditory cortex of guinea pigs with partial unilateral deafness. *J. Comp. Neurol.* 282:456–471.

Rockland, K.S., and Lund, J.S. (1982). Widespread periodic intrinsic connections in the tree shrew visual cortex. *Brain Res.* 169:19–40.

Rockland, K.S., and Lund, J.S. (1983). Intrinsic laminar lattice connections in primate visual cortex. *J. Comp. Neurol.* 216:303–318.

Sanes, J.N., Suner, S., Lando, J.F., and Donoghue, J.P. (1988). Rapid reorganization of adult rat motor cortex somatic representation patterns after motor nerve injury. *Proc. Natl Acad. Sci. U. S. A.* 85:2003–2007.

Sanes, J.N., Suner, S, and Donoghue, J.P. (1990). Dynamic organization of primary motor cortex output to target muscles in adult rats. I. Long-term patterns of reorganization following motor or mixed peripheral nerve lesions. *Exp. Brain Res.*, 79:479–491.

Ts'o, D., and Gilbert, C. (1988). The organization of chromatic and spatial interactions in the primate striate cortex. *J. Neurosci.* 8:1712–1727.

Ts'o, D., Gilbert, C., and Wiesel, T.N. (1986). Relationships between horizontal connections and functional architecture in cat striate cortex as revealed by cross-correlation analysis. *J. Neurosci.* 6:1160–1170.

Plasticity of Connectivity in the Visual System

16 Regrowth and Reconnection of Severed Axons in the Visual System of Adult Mammals

Albert J. Aguayo

The presence in the mature central nervous system (CNS) of a greater number and variety of nerve cells and glia than in the embryo, the intricate course of many normal axonal projections, and the greater separation between neuronal groups that results from the increase in the size of the organism are all potential obstacles to the restoration of neural connectivity in the injured visual system of adult vertebrates. However, the axotomized retinal ganglion cells (RGCs) of large fish and amphibians appear able to recapitulate complex developmental programs for axonal growth and reconnection and to regenerate long retinal projections that retrieve their lost targets in the tectum and restores vision (Grafstein, 1986). An increasingly favored explanation of this paradox is that the lack of axonal regrowth after CNS injury in adult mammals results from complex events that include: the expression by certain glial cells of molecules that inhibit fiber extension (Schwab, 1990), a limited local availability of trophic factors (Lu et al., 1991), changes in the extracellular matrix (Liesi, 1985; Carbonetto, 1990; Reichardt and Tomaselli, 1991), a loss of functional receptors (Cohen et al., 1989), and even the formation of premature aberrant synapses with cells near the site of damage (Bernstein and Bernstein, 1971).

Such a lack of fiber regrowth after CNS injury has also imposed limitations on the study of the end results of axonal regeneration in the brain, particularly as it concerns the reextension of axons along appropriate pathways and the formation of new synapses in correct targets. In this brief review, it is shown that RGCs axotomized in the optic nerve (ON) of adult rodents can respond to experimental manipulations of the milieu of their cut axons and support a long axonal regrowth that leads to the formation of new functional synapses in the superior colliculus (SC).

This in vivo demonstration that injured CNS neurons are capable of regenerating their axons and forming new terminal connections underscores the importance of the non-neuronal environment in the expression of this neuronal capacity. It is anticipated that future advances in the understanding of the molecular events that influence the interactions of axonal growth cones with their non-neuronal substrates and neuronal targets should help develop

This chapter was presented as the 1991 Helmerich Lecture.

better strategies to enhance the regrowth and reconnection of injured nerve cells.

AN EXPERIMENTAL METHOD FOR THE IN VIVO STUDY OF AXONAL REGENERATION

For these studies in adult rodents, nerve grafts that contain the cellular and matrix components of the peripheral nervous system (PNS) have been used as "bridges" between the eye and the dorsal mesencephalon to provide a favorable substrate for the growth of RGC axons to proximity with their post-synaptic targets in the SC. In adult Sprague-Dawley rats or Syrian hamsters, an autologous segment of peripheral nerve (PN) was attached to the ocular stump of the ON transected near the eye. The distal end of the graft was subsequently inserted into the SC (Vidal-Sanz et al., 1987; Carter et al., 1989a) (figure 16.1), the main retinorecipient area of the rodent brain.

At various times after the placement of these grafts, the regeneration of cut RGC axons and their terminals and synapses in the SC was investigated by anterograde labeling of the axonal projections of RGCs with neuroanatomical tracers such as horseradish peroxidase (HRP), tritiated amino acids, or fluorescent dyes. The PN graft and the SC were then surveyed by light and electron microscopy to identify axons or axon terminals containing these markers. In addition electrophysiological responses to visual stimulation of the retina were sought in both the RGC axons and in the SC (Keirstead et al., 1985, 1989) to define functional correlates of the regeneration of RGC axons and the formation of RGC synapses in the SC.

RETINAL GANGLION CELL AXONS REGENERATE ALONG NEVER GRAFTS

After the ON is sectioned near the eye of adult rats, regenerating axons of RGC neurons have been shown to extend within the PN grafts for 3 to 4 cm, distances that are approximately twice the length of the normal retinocollicular projection of these animals (Vidal-Sanz et al., 1987). The growth cones

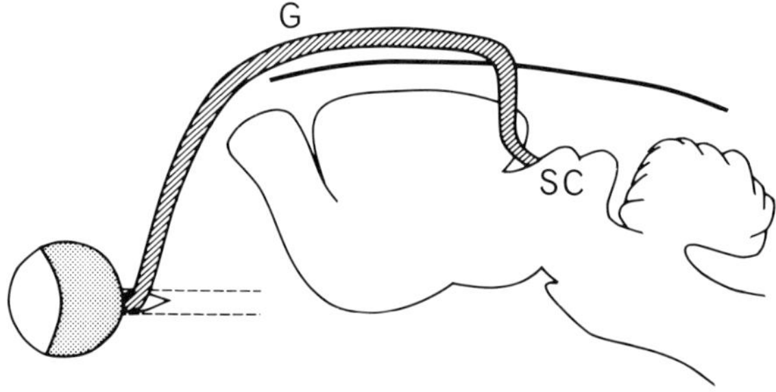

Figure 16.1 Diagram of method used in adult rodents to guide the regrowth of cut retinal ganglion cell axons from the eye to the superior colliculus (*SC*) via a peripheral nerve graft (*G*).

    Plasticity of Connectivity in the Visual System

of these axons extend in close apposition to the plasma membrane of Schwann cells and their basal lamina, an anatomical relationship that suggests these contacts mediate critical neuronal-substrate interactions. Along the PN grafts, RGC axons extend at rates of 1 to 2 mm/day (Cho and So, 1987), a phenomenon that correlates well with the speed at which the main cytoskeletal proteins are transported in these regenerating axons (McKerracher et al., 1990).

It is of interest that RGC axons regenerate when the PN grafts are inserted into the retina (So and Aguayo, 1985) or are apposed to the ocular stump of ONs cut near the eye (Vidal-Sanz et al., 1987); no regrowth is observed, however, when the PN segments are attached to the ON at distances of 8 to 10 mm from the retina (Richardson et al., 1982). While the mechanisms that influence these peculiar responses to axotomy and PN grafting remain unknown, it has also been observed that only lesions near the RGC somata lead to an enhanced immunoreactivity for the growth-associated protein GAP-43 in RGCs (Lozano et al., 1987; Doster et al., 1991) and to a marked increase in the transport of this protein along the proximal stump of the ON (Doster et al., 1991). The apparent relationship between successful axonal regrowth into PN grafts and the enhanced expression of GAP-43 suggests that this molecule may be involved in cellular mechanisms that modulate the responsiveness of injured neurons to the substrate components that influence axonal regrowth. The more recent observation of similar increases in GAP-43 messenger RNAs (mRNAs) after intraorbital or intracranial ON section (Jones and Aguayo, 1991) may indicate that axonal lesions at various distances from the cell body can trigger and increase in GAP-43 mRNA levels while the expression of the protein requires additional conditions that are optimized when RGC axons are damaged near the perikaryon (P.S. Jones, personal communication, 1991).

The components of the PN grafts that permit or promote the elongation of RGC and other CNS axons may include: longitudinally aligned Schwann cells within basal lamina tubes that express growth factors and critical receptors (Richardson and Ebendal, 1982; Heumann et al., 1987; Taniuchi et al., 1986), macrophages that influence the synthesis of neurotrophins and partake in the removal of neuronal and non-neuronal debris (Lindholm et al., 1987; Brown et al., 1991), and extracellular matrix molecules (Reichardt et al., 1989). Moreover, there is no indication that PNS myelin or other Schwann cell components express molecules that inhibit growth cone extension (Schwab, 1990).

Interactions between the regrowing axons and some of the PNS cellular and substrate constituents have been investigated in tissue culture. In vitro, two major classes of molecules appear to influence nerve cell growth and survival: growth factors and adhesive molecules. Although there are major overlaps in structure and function, and adhesive molecules can be differentiated functionally into cell adhesion molecules (e.g., N-CAM, N-cadherin) and extracellular matrix (ECM) proteins (e.g., laminin) (see chapter 15). The availability of antibodies and peptides known to disrupt the function of integrins has stimulated studies on the role of these molecules in regeneration and development. For example, laminin, which is expressed transiently in the ECM of the developing vertebrate CNS (Liesi, 1985), facilitates the regeneration of axons in PNS injury (Sandrock and Matthew, 1987). Furthermore, integrins on developing neurons undergo a functional down-regulation (Reichhardt and Tomaselli, 1991) that involves posttranslational modification of these receptors influenced by the connection or neurons with their targets (Cohen et al., 1989). After axotomy in adult animals, integrins function in the PNS is also restored (Toyota et al., 1990). Thus, integrin and their ECM proteins are involved in aspects of neural development that appear to be recapitulated during regeneration.

Changing the adult mammalian CNS non-neuronal environment of injured axons to that of the PNS also appears to influence neuronal mechanisms that regulate the transport of cytoskeletal proteins essential for the maintenance and regrowth of axons. In the ocular stumps of intracranially transected ONs not exposed to PN grafts, there is a ten-fold decrease in the transport of tubulin and neurofilaments (McKerracher et al., 1990). This decrease in rates of slow transport is not accompanied by comparable changes in fast axonal transport. In contrast, when the ON was cut near the eye and replaced by a PN graft, the rates of tubulin and neurofilament transport doubled and the rate of actin transport decreased (McKerracher et al., 1990), a pattern that resembles slow transport in the developing ON (Willard and Simon, 1983).

FORMATION OF NEW SYNAPTIC CONNECTIONS IN THE INJURED CNS

In animals with PN grafts bridging the retina and the superior colliculus, the RGCs were labeled intravitreously with tracer substances and the region of the SC near the end of the PN graft was surveyed by light or electron microscopy to identify axon terminals containing the orthograde transported markers. It was shown that the RGC axons that emerged from the caudal end of these long PN grafts penetrated into the superficial layers of the SC for up to 500 μm at 2 months (Carter et al., 1989a) and 1,000 μm at 8 to 10 months (Carter et al., 1989b). Such limited extension into the SC contrasts sharply with the lengthy elongation of the RGC axons in the PN bridges.

Upon penetration into the SC, the regenerating RGC axons extended toward the laminae that normally receive most retinal projections: the stratum griseum superficialis (SGS) and the stratum opticum (SO) (Carter et al., 1989a). The patterns of RGC arborization in the SC were studied by filling the regenerating RGC axons with HRP, applied near the insertion of the PN graft into the dorsal mesencephalon. The branches formed by the regenerated RGC arbors in the SC tended to be shorter than in controls and their boutons were more densely packed than normal. However, many of the re-formed arbors exhibited normal numbers of boutons (Carter et al., 1991). Moreover, the regenerating RGC axons formed normally appearing terminals and synapses that were confined to the SGS and the SO of the tectum (figure 16.2). These synapses persisted for the entire period spanned by this study: up to 10

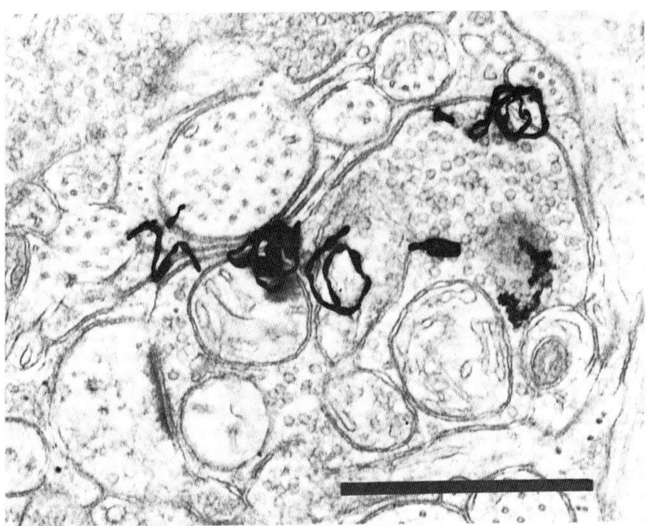

Figure 16.2 Electron micrograph of a radiolabeled regenerated retinal ganglion cell terminal in the SC of a 21-month-old rat 16 months after the eye and the SC were linked by a nerve graft. The animal received [^{3}H]-labeled amino acids intraocularly 2 days before perfusion fixation. As in age-matched controls the regenerated terminals contained round vesicles and pale mitochondria, and contact postsynaptic profiles. Scale bar: 1 μm. (Reproduced with permission from Vidal-Sanz et al., 1991.)

months in hamsters and 18 months in rats (Vidal-Sanz et al., 1991; Carter et al., 1989b). In addition, the proportion of contacts made by the RGC terminals on the dendritic shafts and on the spines of SC neurons closely resembled the normal (Carter et al., 1989a). It has not been determined if the regenerated projections are deployed retinotopically.

While the predilection of the regenerating RGC axons in the SC for certain neuronal domains and laminae could reflect the high density of dendritic processes that exists in such layers or be dictated by the extensive tectal denervation caused by ON interruption, additional studies of the synaptic distribution of RGC axons guided to nondenervated targets (Zwimpfer et al., 1992) suggest that affinities between pre- and postsynaptic neuronal components play a role in determining such synaptic preferences.

In addition to the anatomical evidence of capacities for axonal regrowth and synaptic differentiation exhibited by the injured RGC neurons, the newly established retinotectal projections have been shown to display two important functional attributes: (1) in the retina, the RGCs remain responsive to the illumination of the eye (Keirstead et al., 1985); and (2) in the tectum, the regenerated synapses can transmit impulses to SC neurons (Keirstead et al., 1989). The functional responsiveness of these nerve cells was established by demonstrating that, 2 to 3 months after placement of the PN graft, some of the RGCs with regenerated axons fired in characteristic on and off patterns after light was directed onto discrete receptive fields of the retina (Keirstead et al., 1985). This finding suggests that following axotomy near their somata and the regrowth of their axons into a PNS environment, the RGCs had retained or regained inputs that mediate these responses to light.

Transynaptic activity in the vicinity of regenerated terminals was subsequently demonstrated in the region neighboring the insertion site of the PN grafts where differentiated RGC terminals had been observed by electron microscopy in the anatomical studies described above. In the superficial 450 μm of the SC, microelectrode recordings revealed both excitatory and inhibitory responses to light flashed into the PN-grafted eye (Keirstead et al., 1989). Some of these responses were shown to reflect activity in postsynaptic neurons rather than in RGC-regenerated axons that penetrated the SC (Keirstead et al. 1989).

It is unclear to what extent the efficacy of the retinotectal transynaptic activation thus far observed in these animals resembles that of normal retinotectal connections. Furthermore, the possible behavioral effects of the reinervation of the SC by these axons have not been determined.

CONCLUSIONS

As in most regions of the vertebrate brain, the retina, the visual cortex, and the tectum are mainly composed of interneurons whose activity is conveyed by a smaller population of projection neurons with lengthy axons. The demonstration that functional synapses can be made by the long-range growth of axons from the retina to the SC when the ON is replaced by a PN graft raises the possibility that connections may also be restored in the CNS between neighboring nerve cells, such as interneurons, whose somata and cellular appendages are so close to each other. If this assumption were to be proved correct, it can be anticipated that further progress in the understanding of the molecular determinants of neuronal responses to injury may provide new means to foster the restoration of lost connections in circumstances where the long-range growth and guidance of axons within the injured CNS are not required.

While it is becoming clear that certain capacities for axonal growth and synaptogenesis may be retained in the adult CNS, it is still difficult to envisage how the developmental conditions that guide a multitude of axonal projections to more distant fields of innervation can be replicated in the injured CNS. The precision with which RGCs in amphibian and fish restore lost connections in the tectum provides an encouraging argument for studying regeneration in the CNS of adult mammals.

Acknowledgments

The Medical Research Council of Canada and the Multiple Sclerosis Society of Canada supported these studies. A.J.A. is a member of the Canadian Network for the Study of Neural Regeneration of Functional Recovery.

REFERENCES

Bernstein, J.J., and Bernstein, M.E. (1971). Axonal regeneration and formation of synapses proximal to the site of lesion following hemisection of the rat spinal cord. *Exp. Neurol.* 30: 336–351.

Brown, M.C., Perry, V.H., Lunn, E.R., Gordon, S., and Heumann, R. (1991). Macrophage dependence of peripheral sensory nerve regeneration: Possible involvement of nerve growth factor. *Neuron* 6:359–370.

Carbonetto, S. (1990). Laminin receptors: From PC12 cells to PNS. In *Brain Repair*, ed. A. Björklund, A.J. Aguayo, and D. Ottoson, 185–197. New York: Stockton Press.

Carter, D.A., Bray, G.M., and Aguayo, A.J. (1989a). Regenerated retinal ganglion cell axons can form well-differentiated retinal ganglion cell axons in the superior colliculus of adult hamsters. *J. Neurosci.* 9:4042–4050.

Carter, D.A., Bray, G.M., Aguayo, A.J. (1989b). Extension and persistence of regenerated retinal ganglion cell axons in the superior colliculus of adult hamsters. *Soc. Neurosci. Abstr.* 15:872.

Carter, D.A., Bray, G.M., and Aguayo, A.J. (1991). Patterns of the arborizations made by retinal ganglion cell axons regenerating into the superior colliculus of adult hamsters. *Soc. Neurosci. Abstr.* 17:568.

Cho, E.Y.P., and So K.-F. (1987). Retinal ganglion cell axons regenerating in a peripheral nerve graft in adult hamsters. *Brain Res.* 419:369–374.

Cohen, J., Nurcombe, V., Jeffrey, P., and Edgar, D. (1989). Developmental loss of functional laminin receptors on retinal ganglion cells is regulated by their target tissue, the optic tectum. *Development* 107:381–387.

Doster, S.K., Lozano, A.M., Aguayo, A.J., and Willard, M.B. (1991). Expression of the growth-associated protein GAP-43 in adult rat retinal ganglion cells following axon injury. *Neuron* 6:635–647.

Grafstein, B. (1986). Regeneration in ganglion cells. In *The Retina*, ed. R. Adler and D, Farber, 275–335. Orlando, Fla: Academic Press.

Heumann, R., Korsching, S., Bandtlow, C., and Thoenen, H. (1987). Changes in nerve growth factor synthesis in non-neuronal cells in response to sciatic nerve transection. *J. Cell Biol.* 104:1623–1631.

Jones, P.S., and Aguayo, A.J. (1991). Axotomy enhances GAP-43 mRNA levels in adult rat retinal ganglion cells. *Soc. Neurosci. Abstr.* 17:555.

Keirstead, S.A., Vidal-Sanz, M., Rasminsky, M., Aguayo, A.J., Levesque, M., and So, K.F. (1985). Responses to light of retinal neurons regenerating axons into peripheral nerve grafts in the rat. *Brain. Res.* 359:402–406.

Keirstead, S.A., Rasminsky, M., Fukuda, Y., Carter, D.A., Aguayo, A.J., and Vidal-Sanz, M. (1989). Electrophysiologic responses in hamster superior colliculus evoked by regenerating retinal axons. *Science* 246:255–258.

Liesi, P. (1985). Laminin immunoreactive glia distinguish regenerative adult CNS systems from non-regenerative ones. *EMBO J.* 4:2505–2511.

Lindholm, D., Heumann, R., Meyer, M., and Thoenen, H. (1987). Interleukin-1 regulates synthesis of nerve growth factor in non-neuronal cells of rat sciatic nerve. *Nature* 330:658–659.

Lozano, A.M., Doster, S.J., Aguayo, A.J., and Willard, M.B. (1987). Immunoreactivity to GAP-43 in axotomized and regenerating retinal ganglion cells of adult rats. *Soc. Neurosci. Abstr.* 13:1389.

Lu, B., Yokoyama, M., Dreyfus, C.F., and Black, I.B. (1991). NGF gene expression in actively growing brain glia. *J. Neurosci.* 11:318–326.

McKerracher, L.J., Vidal-Sanz, M., and Aguayo, A.J. (1990a). Slow transport rates of cytoskeletal proteins change during regeneration of axotomized retinal neurons in adult rats. *J. Neurosci.* 10:641–648.

McKerracher L.J., Vidal-Sanz, M., and Essagian, C., and Aguayo, A.J. (1990b). Selective impairment of slow axonal transport after optic nerve injury in adult rats. *J. Neurosci.* 10:2834–2841.

Reichardt, L.F., and Tomaselli, K.J. (1991). Extracellular matrix molecules and their receptors: Functions in neural development. *Annu. Rev. Neurosci.* 14:531–370.

Reichardt, L.F., Bixby, J.L., Hall, J.L., Ignatius, M.J., Neugebauer, K.M., and Tomaselli, K.J. (1989). Integrins and cell adhesion molecules: Neuronal receptors that regulate axon growth on extracellular matrices amd cell surfaces. *Dev. Neurosci.* 11:332–347.

Richardson, P.M., and Ebendal, T. (1982). Nerve growth activities in the rat peripheral nerve. *Brain Res.* 246:57–64.

Richardson, P.M., Issa, V.K.M., and Shemie, S. (1982). Regeneration and retrograde degeneration of axons in the rat optic nerve. *J. Neurocytol.* 11:949–966.

Sandrock, A.W., and Matthew W.D. (1987). Identification of a peripheral nerve neurite growth-promoting activity by development and use of an in vitro bioassay. *Proc. Natl. Acad. Sci. U. S. A.* 84:6934–6938.

Schwab, M.E. (1990). Myelin-associated inhibitors of neurite growth. *Exp. Neurol.* 109:2–5.

So, K.-F., and Aguayo, A.J. (1985). Lengthy regrowth of cut axons from ganglion cells after peripheral nerve transplantation into the retina of adult rats. *Brain Res.* 328:349–354.

Taniuchi, M., Clark, H.B., and Johnson, E.M. (1986). Induction of nerve growth factor receptor in Schwann cells after axotomy. *Proc. Natl. Acad. Sci. U. S. A.* 83:4094–4098.

Toyota, B., Carbonetto, S., and David, S. (1990). A dual laminin-collagen receptor acts in peripheral nerve regeneration. *Proc. Natl. Acad. Sci. U. S. A.* 87:1319–1322.

Vidal-Sanz, M., Bray, G.M., Villegas-Pérez, M.P., Thanos, S., and Aguayo, A.J. (1987). Axonal regeneration and synapse formation in the superior colliculus by retinal ganglion cells in the adult rate. *J. Neurosci.* 7:2984–2909.

Vidal-Sanz, M., Bray, G.M., and Aguayo, A.J. (1991). Regenerated synapses persist in the superior colliculus after the regrowth of retinal ganglion cell axons. *J. Neurocytol.* 20:940–952.

Willard, M.B., and Simon, C. (1983). Modulations of neurofilament axonal transport during the development of rabbit retinal ganglion cells. *Cell* 35:551–559.

Zwimpfer, T.Z., Aguayo, A.J., and Bray, G.M. (1992). Synapse formation and preferential distribution in the granule cell layer by regenerating retinal ganglion cell axons guided to the cerebellum of adult hamsters. *J. Neurosci.* 12:1144–1159.

Plasticity of Connectivity in the Visual System

Retina Research Foundation

The Retina Research Foundation is a publicly supported, tax-exempt charitable organization headquartered in Houston, Texas. Since 1973 the Foundation has sustained a multifaceted basic science and clinical research program to find the causes of and cures for the many retinal diseases that annually threaten millions of citizens worldwide with the prospect of blindness or serious visual impairment. It is dedicated to the prospect that blindness is a foe that can be fought successfully through research.

Officers

Emmett A. Humble, Chairman of the Board
Alice R. McPherson, M.D., President and Scientific Director
Robert W. Phillips, Vice Chairman of the Board
Carl G. Mueller, Jr., Secretary
James M. Barr, Treasurer

Board of Directors

Laura Lee Blanton	Nancy Japhet	Carl G. Mueller, Jr.
Harry G. Austin	Saunders Gregg	Robert W. Phillips
James M. Barr	August C. Bering, III	Cecil C. Rix, Ph.D.
L. Henry Gissel, Jr.	Baine P. Kerr	Henry O. Weaver
Emmett A. Humble	Alice R. McPherson, M.D.	James N. Winfrey

Board of Advisory Directors

Thomas D. Anderson
John T. Cater
Bertha Miller
E. J. Hagstette, Jr.,
E. C. Japhet
Fred E. Wallace
R. Bruce LaBoon

The Retina Research Foundation offices are located at 6560 Fannin, Suite 2200, Houston, Texas 77030

Index

Axotomy (cont.)
  responses of retinal ganglion cells after,
    111*f*
  of retinal ganglion cells, death and survival
    of, 29–38
  retrograde effects of, 29
  strategies to enhance survival of, 37–38

Behavioral testing, following retinal
  transplantation, 168, 170–172
BDNF. *See* Brain-derived neurotrophic factor
  (BDNF)
bFGF injection, effect of on dystrophic
  retinas, 158
Binocularity, vulnerability of, 45
Brain-derived neurotrophic factor (BDNF)
  activity of, 17
  neuron dependence on during development,
    30
  trkB response to, 26
  trophic influence of on retinal ganglion
    cells, 36

C6 glioma cells, migration of into white
  matter, 84–86
CaM II kinase
  associated with synaptic function, 177
  changes in affecting cortical neuron
    function, 178, 179
  changes in following monocular deprivation,
    180
  in forebrain, 188
  immunoreactivity associated with, 187
  in situ hybridization of in monkey visual
    cortex, 181–186
  long-lasting effects of changes in levels of,
    189
  mRNA levels of in normal vs. monocularly
    deprived monkey, 184*f*
  oligonucleotides for, 178
  regulation of by neural activity, 188–189
Carbocyanine dye, retinal ganglion cell
  labeling by, 33–34
Casein kinase II, in GAP–43 phosphorylation,
  101
CDF. *See* Cholinergic differentiation factor
Cell adhesion molecules
  differentiation of, 235
  importance of differences in, 66–67
  interaction of in extracellular matrix, 59
Cell death
  during development, 29–30
  mechanisms of, death of, 29–33. *See also*
    Neurons

physiological, 31
Central nervous system
  ability of injured neurons of to regenerate
    in adult mammals, 233–238
  brain-derived neurotrophic factor in, 17
  formation of new synaptic connections in
    following injury, 236–238
  neural activity in maturation of, 177
  number and variety of nerve cells and glia
    in, 233
  refractoriness of axons to regeneration, 197
  response of to injury, 3–4
  terminals of axons in, 199
ChAT, nerve growth factor effects on
  activity of, 55
Chick embryo, regeneration of retina in, 5
Cholinergic differentiation factor, 59
Chondroitin sulfate proteoglycans, inhibition
  of regeneration by, 86
Chromatolysis, 3
CNS. *See* Central nervous system
Collagens
  extracellular, 61–62
  interaction of embryonic chick retinal
    neurons with, 62–64
Colliculus, superior
  ablation of, 197, 198–199*f*
  grafts bridging retina and, 236–237
  projections to from transplanted retinas,
    131*f*
  reinervation of, 238
  relay circuitry of, 139
Contour orientation, 211
Cortical cells
  binocular, visual inputs on, 45
  contextual sensitivity of, 221–223
Cross-correlation analysis, 223
Cyclic adenosine monophosphate (cAMP),
  regulation of SCIP gene in cultured
  Schwann cells, 72–73
Cycloheximide, 73
Cysteine proteases, 81
Cytoskeletal proteins, role of in axonal
  regeneration, 4

Dendrites
  branching pattern analysis of, 121*f*
  morphology of in retinal RGCs
    regenerating axon along peripheral nerve
    graft, 119–121
  variations in complexity of in regenerating
    RGCs, 120
2-Deoxyglucose autoradiography technique,
  223

     Index